T
a

1

2

# Epidemiology

*Principles and Methods*

Brian MacMahon, M.D., Ph.D., D.P.H.
Thomas F. Pugh, M.D., M.P.H.

Department of Epidemiology
Harvard University School of Public Health

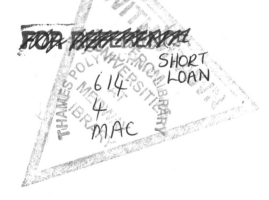

*Little, Brown and Company*
*Boston*

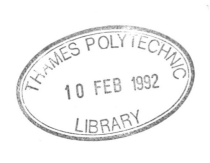
First Edition

*Thirteenth Printing*

Library of Congress catalog card No. 73-127122

ISBN 0-316-54259-8

Printed in the United States of America

*HAL*

# *Preface*

The objective of this book is to introduce the principles and methods of epidemiology, particularly as they are applied in the study of those chronic diseases for which preventive measures are now unknown or inadequate. The book began as a new edition of *Epidemiologic Methods,* published ten years ago, but, as we contemplated a revision, it seemed to us preferable to write a new book emphasizing principles as well as methods, giving more consideration to the historical roots of epidemiology and dealing somewhat more broadly with the interaction of genetic and environmental factors in the etiology of disease. Methodologic approaches that have seen important developments in the last decade—notably studies of migrant populations and the detection of low-intensity disease clustering—have been included.

There is, at the present time, considerable concern over the possible effects on human health of environmental contaminants. It is evident that much more knowledge of the long-range effects of these substances must be obtained. In that this book's major emphasis is on the elucidation of cause-effect relationships, it has relevance to this problem.

The study of chronic disease epidemiology is inconceivable without knowledge of biostatistics. Elementary statistical techniques are essential to our subject. However, because accounts of these techniques appear in many textbooks of biostatistics, we have avoided the repetition of such material. It is also evident that biostatistics is providing some of the most important methodologic advances in epidemiology. Detailed accounts of these more advanced statistical methods are also not included, since we have attempted to produce a book that is intelligible to a person with medical or biologic, but not necessarily statistical, training. For this reason, the book should be considered an introduction to chronic disease epidemiology rather than a comprehensive account of the subject.

B. M.
T. F. P.

*Boston*

# *Acknowledgments*

The difficulty of defining accurately the sources of one's ideas, points of view, and information is well known. This book has been influenced by the thoughts and efforts of so many colleagues and students that to most of them we can offer only this general acknowledgment of our indebtedness.

To Dr. Jane Worcester, however, who has been an unfailing source of constructive advice throughout the years when this book was taking shape, we express our gratitude specifically. For much immediate help and many suggestions in the preparation of the text, we thank Dr. Philip Cole, Dr. Olli Miettinen, and Dr. Dimitrios Trichopoulos.

Finally, we are deeply grateful to Miss Kathleen Shreeve, administrative assistant to the Department. We thank her for the patience, tact, and efficiency with which she has helped sustain the operation of the Department and for the many hours she has devoted to this manuscript over and above her other responsibilities.

B. M.
T. F. P.

# Contents

# Epidemiology

*Principles and Methods*

# 1

## Epidemiology

### DEFINITION

Epidemiology is the study of the distribution and determinants of disease frequency in man.

Two main areas of investigation are indicated in this definition—the study of the *distribution* of disease and the search for the *determinants* of the observed distribution. The first area, describing the distribution of health status in terms of age, sex, race, geography, etc., might be considered an extension of the discipline of demography to health and disease. The second area involves explanation of the patterns of distribution of a disease in terms of causal factors. Many disciplines seek to learn about the determinants of disease; the special contribution of epidemiology is its use of knowledge of the frequency and distribution of disease in populations.

Like many sciences epidemiology has developed from the study of the exotic and the unusual into the elucidation of general principles. Epidemiology is now no more restricted to the study of striking outbreaks of disease than meteorology is to the study of hurricanes or astronomy to eclipses of the sun. Yet an epidemiologist might today still consider his concern to be primarily the study of epidemics, if a broad view is taken as to what constitutes an epidemic and if it is recognized that research designed to explain epidemics cannot be restricted to periods during which the epidemics prevail.

## Concept of an Epidemic

In the past the term *epidemic* was used almost exclusively to describe an acute outbreak of infectious disease. More current definitions stress the concept of *excessive prevalence* as its basic implication in both lay [132] and professional [13] usage. This characteristic is exemplified by many noninfectious diseases as well as by diseases known to be associated with microorganisms. The United States, for example, is at the present time in the grip of epidemics of at least two seemingly noninfectious diseases—coronary atherosclerosis and lung cancer—which easily satisfy the criterion of excessive frequency. Lung cancer is now over 30 times more common in this country than it was 50 years ago; coronary heart disease accounts for nearly one-third of all deaths in the United States, although there are areas of the world where it is relatively infrequent. In noninfectious, as in infectious, diseases the idea that the frequency of a particular disease is excessive may be gained by following its frequency over time, by comparing its frequency in different places, or by comparing one subgroup of the population with another. That the excessive frequency must come about within a period as short as a few days or weeks is no longer considered an essential part of the meaning of epidemic.

## Epidemic and Nonepidemic Frequency

Even when the predominant concern is the explanation of epidemics, knowledge of disease frequency and distribution during nonepidemic times may be crucial. There are several bases for this.

1. Without knowledge of nonepidemic frequency, how can the existence of an epidemic be demonstrated? How can it be determined that the frequency of a disease in a particular population at a particular time is in excess? Clearly it is necessary to know the frequency of the disease in other populations and in the same population at other times.

Sometimes the existence of an epidemic is obvious. This is so when the epidemic involves a large number of persons, produces a distinctive illness, and occurs over a short period of time. Thus there is little difficulty in detecting epidemics of cholera, plague, smallpox, or the common infections of childhood. In all these the disease is familiar, the difference between epidemic and nonepidemic prevalence is large, and the transition is rapid. In contrast, the risk to an American male of dying of coronary heart disease is currently quite as large as the risk of death experienced during some of the major historical epidemics of infectious disease, yet the general population remains almost unaware of the existence of an epidemic of coronary heart disease. The slow growth of this epidemic has concealed its size.

Even acute epidemics may pass unnoticed if they appear in unfamiliar form. For example, during the intense London fog of 1952 there was very limited realization of the effects of the fog on the population's health. The full effect was appreciated only when deaths for the period were counted (Fig. 1) and compared with deaths during the preceding and subsequent periods of the same year and during similar periods of previous years. It then became apparent that the fog had been responsible for over 4000 deaths.

2. An unusually low disease frequency in a population may be just as significant in understanding the causes of epidemics as a high frequency. For example, the very low attack rates from cholera observed by John Snow [376] among two groups of people (workers in a brewery and denizens of a workhouse) in the center of an otherwise epidemic area led to a strengthening of the belief that the water supply was responsible for the epidemic since these two groups did not share the general water supply of the neighborhood. Similarly, the virtual absence of cancer of the uterine cervix in nuns is an important consideration in the formation of hypotheses regarding the etiology of this disease.

3. In the chronic diseases, which have prolonged upswings and downswings of the epidemic wave, it may be difficult to decide whether or not a given frequency qualifies as epidemic (or excessively prevalent) even if all the necessary comparative information is available. It is common to find a gradient in the frequencies of a disease in different populations. While the dis-

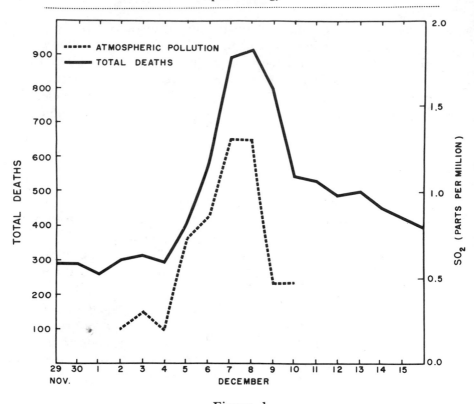

Figure 1

Atmospheric pollution (parts per million of sulfur dioxide) and numbers of deaths per day in London, Nov. 29 to Dec. 16, 1952. (Data from a report of the Ministry of Health [257].)

ease may be considered definitely epidemic when populations with the highest frequencies are compared with those with the lowest rates, the applicability of the term to populations with intermediate frequencies will depend largely on the observer's point of view. Under such circumstances attempts to correlate quantitative statements of disease frequency with quantitative statements of the frequency of the suspected factors are more revealing than attempts to correlate the dichotomy of epidemicity and nonepidemicity with the dichotomy of presence or absence of specific factors.

## HISTORICAL BACKGROUND

Some of the basic concepts underlying the practice of epidemiology can be illustrated by reference to historical episodes and personalities. A few episodes which seem particularly relevant to the development of current concepts and methods—as distinct from substantive knowledge of the epidemiology of particular diseases—are outlined in this section. While in one sense epidemiology is almost as old as medicine itself, in another sense it is a very new discipline. Although Hippocrates spoke in terms that have meaning to epidemiologists today, it is only in the last few decades that epidemiology has become recognizable as a named discipline with which investigators, research groups, and academic departments are identified.

The history of epidemiologic methodology is largely the history of the development of four ideas: (1) human disease is related to man's environment; (2) the counting of natural phenomena may be instructive; (3) "natural experiments" can be utilized to investigate disease etiology; and (4) under certain conditions, experiments on man can also be utilized for this purpose.

## Disease and Environment

The idea that disease may be connected with a person's environment was expressed by Hippocrates almost 2400 years ago. Today the concept seems self-evident, but the clarity of his statement, and its relevance to the objectives of epidemiology today, deserve recognition. In *On Airs, Waters and Places* [163] Hippocrates states:

Whoever wishes to investigate medicine properly should proceed thus: in the first place to consider the seasons of the year, and what effects each of them produces. Then the winds, the hot and the cold, especially such as are common to all countries, and then such as are peculiar to each locality. In the same manner, when one comes into a city to which he is a stranger, he should consider its situation, how it lies as to the winds and the rising of the sun; for its influence is not the same whether it lies to the north or the south, to the rising or to the setting sun. One should consider most attentively the waters which the inhabitants use, whether they be marshy and soft, or hard and running from elevated and rocky situations, and then if saltish and unfit for cooking; and the ground, whether it be naked and deficient in water, or wooded and well watered, and whether it lies in a hollow, confined situation, or is elevated and cold; and the mode in which the inhabitants live, and what are their pursuits, whether they are fond of drinking and eating to excess, and given to indolence, or are fond of exercise and labor.

In light of this clear and firm admonition from such an influential teacher, it is remarkable that virtually nothing was discovered about the specific characteristics of unhealthy environments during the subsequent 2000 years. Greenwood [135] attributes this to the fact that the operative word in Hippocrates' statement was *consider*—not *count*. However full of insight an investigator's considerings may be, they are unlikely, if not supported by observations objectively recorded in quantitative terms, to form a basis for the considerings of successive generations of investigators.

## Counting and Measurement

The introduction of quantitative methods to epidemiology—indeed, to biology and medicine in general—is credited to John Graunt, who in 1662 published his *Natural and Political Observations . . . on the Bills of Mortality* [134]. Graunt analyzed the weekly Bills of Mortality and the parish registers of christenings in London during the previous decades, noting the excess of males over females among births and deaths, the high rate of mortality among infants, seasonal variation in mortality, and many other features of birth and death data. He provided a numerical account of the impact of the plague on the population of the city and examined the meteorologic and other ecologic characteristics of the years in which plague struck. He made pioneering attempts at two basic biostatistical procedures—the estimation of population and the construction of a life table. More significantly, however, he demonstrated "the uniformity and predictability of . . . biological phenomena taken in the mass" [418] and thus is widely regarded as the founder of the science of biostatistics. Since these new techniques saw no further epidemiologic application for almost 200 years, Graunt might more appropriately be regarded as a forerunner than a founder of epidemiology.

## "Natural Experiments"

The roots of today's epidemiology are more clearly detectable in the work of William Farr, a physician given responsibility for medical statistics in the Office of the Registrar General for England and Wales in 1839. The Annual Reports of the Registrar

General during the subsequent 40 years established a tradition of careful application of vital data to problems of public health and to other broad public concerns. Some of the matters to receive Farr's attention included mortality in the Cornish metal mines and other occupational settings, in prisons and other institutions, and among married and single persons, fluctuations in the marriage rate as an index of the economic health of the country, the distribution of cholera, trends in the literacy rate, the value of a person in terms of money, and the consequences to England and Wales of the 19th century emigration. The thoroughness of Farr's analyses can be illustrated by his attempt to ascertain the effect of imprisonment on mortality [172]. He determined the population at risk as well as the number of deaths, compared the prison death rate with that in the general population, took into account the age of the prisoners and the duration of their stay in prison, and considered the fact that "prisoners rarely labour under any serious disease at the time of their committal." Finally, he computed what we shall later refer to as an attributable risk and concluded, "Only 8 criminals were executed (in) 1837, while . . . the average annual number of deaths due to imprisonment was 51." In considering the population at risk, the need to take into account differences in the characteristics of compared groups, the biases involved in the selection of persons exposed to a suspected cause, and ways of measuring excess risk, Farr identified some of the major concerns of epidemiologists today.

One of Farr's contemporaries was a physician most widely known for his administration of chloroform to Queen Victoria during childbirth, but remembered among epidemiologists for his demonstration of the spread of cholera by fecal contamination of drinking water. We shall refer to the work of John Snow in several contexts but, from the methodologic point of view, his most interesting investigation was the demonstration that cholera risk was related to the drinking water supplied by a particular commercial company in London and, by inference, to the source from which the company obtained its water [376].

Snow noted that in 1849 cholera rates were particularly high in areas of London supplied with water by the Lambeth Company and by the Southwark and Vauxhall Company, both of which drew their water from the Thames River at a point heavily polluted with sewage. Subsequent to the relocation between 1849 and 1854 of the Lambeth Company's source to a less polluted area of the river, the incidence of cholera declined in the areas of the city supplied by that company. During the same time period there was no change in the incidence of the disease in areas supplied by the Southwark and Vauxhall Company which continued to draw its water from the most polluted area of the river. The situation in 1854 is illustrated in Table 1. The

## Table 1

Mortality from cholera in the districts of London supplied by the Southwark and Vauxhall Company and by the Lambeth Company, July 8 to August 26, 1854*

| Districts with water supplied by | Population, 1851 | Deaths from cholera | Cholera death rate per 1000 population |
|---|---|---|---|
| Southwark and Vauxhall Company only | 167,654 | 844 | 5.0 |
| Lambeth Company only | 19,133 | 18 | 0.9 |
| Both companies | 300,149 | 652 | 2.2 |

* From Snow [376].

areas of London supplied entirely by the Southwark and Vauxhall Company experienced a rate of 5.0 deaths from cholera per 1000 population, whereas the death rate in the areas supplied entirely by the Lambeth Company was only 0.9 per 1000. A large area supplied by both companies experienced 2.2 deaths per 1000, a rate midway between those for the areas supplied by either company alone.

Snow saw that these observations were consistent with the hypothesis that persons drinking water supplied by the Southwark and Vauxhall Company had greater risks of cholera than those drinking Lambeth Company water. However, he also realized that many factors other than water supply could differ between these geographic areas and parallel the observed variations in cholera rates. Snow's genius lay in his recognition of a circumstance by which the hypothesis implicating the water supply could be put to a crucial test. In his own words [376]:

. . . the intermixing of the water supply of the Southwark and Vauxhall Company with that of the Lambeth Company, over an extensive part of London, admitted of the subject being sifted in such a way as to yield the most incontrovertible proof on one side or the other. In the sub-districts enumerated in the above table as being supplied by both Companies, the mixing of the supply is of the most intimate kind. The pipes of each Company go down all the streets, and into nearly all the courts and alleys. A few houses are supplied by one Company and a few by the other, according to the decision of the owner or occupier at that time when the Water Companies were in active competition. In many cases a single house has a supply different from that on either side. Each company supplies both rich and poor, both large houses and small; there is no difference either in the condition or occupation of the persons receiving the water of the different Companies. Now it must be evident that, if the diminution of cholera, in the districts partly supplied with the improved water, depended on this supply, the houses receiving it would be the houses enjoying the whole benefit of the diminution of the malady, whilst the houses supplied with the water from Battersea Fields would suffer the same mortality as they would if the improved supply did not exist at all. As there is no difference whatever, either in the houses or the people receiving the supply of the two Water Companies, or in any of the physical conditions with which they are surrounded, it is obvious that no experiment could have been devised which would more thoroughly test the effect of water supply on the progress of cholera than this, which circumstances placed ready made before the observer.

The experiment, too, was on the grandest scale. No fewer than three hundred thousand people of both sexes, of every age and occupation, and of every rank and station, from gentlefolks down to the very poor, were divided into two groups without their choice, and, in most cases, without their knowledge; one group being supplied with water containing the sewage of London, and, amongst it, whatever might have come from the cholera patients, the other group having water quite free from such impurity.

To turn this grand experiment to account, all that was required was to learn the supply of water to each individual house where a fatal attack of cholera might occur.

Within the districts supplied by both companies, Snow inquired of relatives and others as to which company supplied water to every house in which a death from cholera had occurred between July 8 and August 26, 1854. The results are shown in Table 2. The cholera death rates for customers of each company

Table 2

Mortality from cholera in London, July 8 to August 26, 1854, related to the water supply of individual houses in districts served by both the Southwark and Vauxhall Company and the Lambeth Company*

| Water supply of individual houses | Population, 1851 | Deaths from cholera | Cholera death rate per 1000 population |
|---|---|---|---|
| Southwark and Vauxhall Company | 98,862 | 419 | 4.2 |
| Lambeth Company | 154,615 | 80 | 0.5 |

* From Snow [376].

were similar to those (seen in Table 1) of the same company's customers in the districts supplied exclusively by that company. Moreover, the death rate for customers of the Lambeth Company was no higher than that for the rest of London, even though the majority of the Lambeth Company's customers were located in the area supplied also by the Southwark and Vauxhall Company—an area in which the epidemic raged severely. The hypothesis that the drinking of water supplied by the Southwark and Vauxhall Company was associated with death from cholera was therefore supported.

Snow's utilization of this "natural experiment" focuses attention on the value of searching out unusual circumstances that can be used to test hypotheses. In his determined exploitation of the circumstance when found, Snow demonstrated the force of the arguments that can be developed from nonexperimental kinds of hypothesis testing. Sometimes, the test provided by such natural circumstances approaches the rigor of that of actual experimentation. In recent years, a series of studies remarkably comparable to those of Snow has resulted in the linking of "Blackfoot Disease" (peripheral vascular disease and gangrene)

in certain areas of Taiwan to the drinking of water from artesian, rather than shallow, wells [52]. The provision of piped
water to the affected areas has resulted in a dramatic reduction
in frequency of the disease [53], even though the suspected etiologic agent—arsenic in the artesian well water—has been in-
criminated only inferentially.

*Intervention Studies*

While epidemiologic knowledge will no doubt continue to be
based predominantly on nonexperimental observations, experiments on man have played decisive roles in some instances.
Well-known among these are Lind's trial of fresh fruit in the
treatment of scurvy in 1747 [203], Jenner's experiments with
cowpox vaccination in 1796 [183], the demonstration of the mosquito-borne nature of yellow fever by Finlay in 1881 [115] and
by Reed et al. in 1900 [338], and Goldberger's induction of pellagra by deficient diet in 1915 [131]. In these instances the interest of the experiments lies in the advances they produced in
understanding the etiology of the specific diseases, rather than in
their contribution to the development of new methodology.
The feature that makes *epidemiologic methodology* particularly
relevant to an experiment on man is the use of a large experimental population. In such experiments, as in the laboratory,
the use of randomization in the assignment of individuals to
groups receiving different experimental treatments is an important component of the design.

In this context the experiment of Fletcher [116] assessing the
protective effect of cured* rice against beriberi was ahead of its
time. In 1905 there was a severe epidemic of the disease in the
Kuala Lumpur Lunatic Asylum. Fletcher described his experiment as follows:

The lunatics are housed in two exactly similar buildings on opposite sides of a quadrangle surrounded by a high wall. On Dec. 5th
[1905] all the lunatics at that time in the hospital were drawn up in

* Cured rice is rice that is parboiled in its husk prior to milling. In the
process of parboiling, the thiamine diffuses from the husk and germ and becomes fixed in the starchy kernel. Subsequent milling does not, therefore, remove
the thiamine. "Indian" rice was prepared in this way. "Siamese" rice was milled
without parboiling.

the dining shed and numbered off from the left. The odd numbers were subsequently domiciled in the ward on the east side of the courtyard and no alteration was made in their diet, they were still supplied with the same uncured rice (Siamese) as in 1905. The even numbers were quartered in the ward on the west of the quadrangle and received the same rations as the occupants of the other ward, with the exception that they were supplied with cured (Indian) rice. . . . On Dec. 5th there were 59 lunatics in the asylum; of these 29 were put on cured rice and 30 on Siamese rice. The next patient admitted to the asylum was admitted to the Bengal rice ward, and the one admitted after him to the uncured rice ward, the next to cured, and so on alternately to the end of the year.

In the middle of the year the patients in the east ward were moved to the west and those in the west ward to the east, but they continued to receive the same diets. By the end of 1906, among 120 patients eating uncured rice there had been 34 cases of beriberi and 18 deaths. Among the 123 patients assigned to cured rice there had been only 2 cases and no deaths and both cases had been manifested at the time the patients were admitted to the asylum.

The recognition of the need for safeguards against damage to persons participating in experiments has increased substantially since the beginning of the century, and attempts at formalization of such safeguards have recently been made [72]. In addition, the methodology of large-scale experimental studies has been extensively developed, largely in connection with trials of vaccines against specific infectious diseases conducted since the Second World War [327]. Experiments of the U.S. Public Health Service in evaluating the addition of fluoride to drinking water for the prevention of dental caries [17, 19, 31] will also figure prominently in future historical accounts of the development of epidemiologic methodology.

AIMS

Knowledge of the distribution of disease may be utilized to elucidate causal mechanisms, explain local disease occurrence, describe the natural history of a disease, or provide guidance in the administration of health services.

## Understanding the Causation of Disease

The most significant purpose of epidemiology is to acquire knowledge of causal mechanisms that can form a basis for preventive measures against diseases not currently preventable. This aim encompasses a number of subsidiary objectives:

1. Developing hypotheses that explain patterns of disease distribution in terms of specific human characteristics or experiences.
2. Testing such hypotheses through specially designed studies.
3. Testing the validity of the concepts on which disease control programs are based, through the use of epidemiologic data collected in conjunction with the programs.
4. Aiding in the classification of ill persons into groups that appear to have etiologic factors in common. Even if the etiologic factors are not fully identified, similarity of epidemiologic behavior may point to etiologic similarity even of clinically distinct entities. Conversely, differences in the epidemiologic distributions of subgroups of a clinical entity may suggest that such subgroups should be regarded as separate disease entities for purposes of etiologic investigation.

Most frequently epidemiologists are concerned with elucidating the causes of *disease*. However, other biologic processes, including growth, multiple pregnancy, sex determination, intelligence, and fertility, may be studied by similar methods.

It is sometimes suggested that epidemiology should also be concerned with the positive components of health implicit in the definition used by the World Health Organization. According to this definition, "Health is a state of complete physical, mental and social well-being and not merely the absence of disease or infirmity" [422]. However, the number of widespread and serious diseases of which the etiology is unknown is more than sufficient to occupy epidemiologists for some years to come. Concentration of effort on these diseases appears to be indicated by the urgent need for knowledge leading to their prevention, as well as by the practical difficulties in quantitative investigation of concepts that have not been defined in clinical, pathologic, or other operational terms.

### Explaining Local Disease Patterns

Frequently the epidemiologist is concerned not so much with the acquisition of new knowledge about the origin of a disease as with understanding the causes of specific epidemics of a disease whose nature is generally well understood. For example, he may utilize what is already known about the etiology of typhoid fever to explain and deal with a particular outbreak and to formulate preventive measures suitable to a particular community.

A fine distinction cannot be drawn between these two types of investigation since new knowledge may be derived during the course of any routine study. Nevertheless, in a great deal of epidemiologic work new knowledge of disease causation is not purposefully sought. Typical are the large numbers of investigations of localized outbreaks of food poisoning and salmonellosis undertaken to find the local source of infection, halt the epidemic, and prevent its recurrence. At the present time, because of inadequacies of knowledge concerning other illnesses, such practical uses of epidemiology are largely confined to infectious diseases and certain industrial intoxications.

### Describing the Natural History of Disease

While most epidemiologic work is directed towards elucidating causal factors, the same methods are used in studies that seek to identify factors related to the course of a disease once established. Thus it is useful to know how the duration of a disease and the probability of the various possible outcomes (recovery, death, specific complications, etc.) vary by age, sex, geography, and so on. Such information is useful not only for prognostic purposes but also in stimulating hypotheses as to what specific factors may be more directly involved in determining the course of a disease in an individual.

In addition, the relations between various measures of disease frequency (to be discussed in Chap. 5) sometimes allow inferences about the course and duration of a disease when such measures cannot be derived by direct follow-up of patients. For example, data on incidence and prevalence of carcinoma of the cervix have been used to estimate the average duration of the several stages of this disease [96, 97, 99, 186]. Such estimates cannot be made by following patients, since once the disease is diagnosed its natural course is interrupted by therapy.

The amount of epidemiologic work in this field is still quite small.

*Administrative Uses*

Knowledge of the frequency of disease in a population serves a number of administrative purposes. It is essential to the logical planning of facilities for medical care. For example, estimation of the number of hospital beds required for patients with specific diseases (chronic nephritis, mental illness) or for given segments of the population (prematurely born infants, the elderly) requires knowledge of the frequency and natural history of the specific diseases, or of all diseases in the given segments of the population. The planning of efficient research, whether clinical, therapeutic, or preventive, also requires knowledge of how many cases of a particular disease are likely to be found in a given population during a given period.

Knowledge of the relative frequencies of a disease in subgroups of the population is also useful if it enables programs and studies to be directed toward the population group manifesting the greatest concentration of the disease. For example, if facilities are limited, epidemiologic information should assist in deciding which age, occupational, sex, geographic, or ethnic group should be the target for a tuberculosis, diabetes, or cancer screening program. Similar considerations apply to the choice of a subgroup of the population for any study that requires the maximum yield of cases for a given size of population studied.

## RELATED DISCIPLINES

Epidemiology is an applied discipline—that is, one concerned with the solution of practical problems. The epidemiologist needs the contributions of many other disciplines in order to pursue his own. Two such disciplines—clinical medicine and pathology—provide the means for describing and defining disease. Without such definition no determination of disease frequency can be made. The reference already made to the importance of quantitative methods in the historical development of epidemiology marks biostatistics as a third discipline on which epidemiologic investigation depends. While epidemiologic information is at times derived from a much wider spectrum of biologic and medical disciplines, these three—clinical medicine, pathology, and biostatistics—have almost universal application in epidemiology. Indeed, epidemiology may be thought of as the joint application of the three in the search for further understanding of disease etiology.

# 2

Concepts of Cause

## DEFINITION

Certain events or circumstances tend to follow others in time. Some of these temporal associations have qualities that lead the observer to speak of them as associations between cause and effect—the earlier event or characteristic being denoted the cause of the later. The repeated observation of a sequence of events or circumstances gives confidence that a particular effect is likely to succeed a particular cause. However, as Hume [171] noted: "We are never able, in a single instance, to discover any power or necessary connection, any quality which binds the effect to the cause, and renders the one an infallible consequence of the other. We only find that one does actually, in fact, follow the other."

What, then, leads one to think of certain relationships as causal? The word *cause* is an abstract noun and, like *beauty*, will have different meanings in different contexts. No definition will be equally appropriate in all branches of science. Epidemiology has the practical purpose of discovering relations which offer possibilities of disease prevention and for this purpose a causal association may usefully be defined as an association between categories of events or characteristics in which an alteration in the frequency or quality of one category is followed by a change in the other. In many instances the possibility of alteration must be presumed; human genetics, for example, is a science based almost entirely on associations that can only presumptively be classified as causal. Nevertheless, the idea of changeability is a basic component of epidemiologic concepts of causation.

## TYPES OF ASSOCIATION

To understand the implications of the use of the term *causal association,* it is necessary to describe some of the ways in which categories of events or circumstances may be related. By a category of things is meant all those having specific characteristics that permit their classification together; for example, diabetics, as distinct from a person with diabetes, or deaths, as distinct from the death of an individual. With respect to each other, two categories may be:

A. Not statistically associated (independent)
B. Statistically associated
   1. Noncausally (secondarily) associated
   2. Causally associated
      a. Indirectly associated
      b. Directly causal

This classification illustrates a common progression in the investigation of a relationship—from demonstration of statistical association to demonstration that the association is causal, and ultimately to ascertainment of its directness.

### Statistical Association

If one category of events occurs in a certain proportion, $x$, of a group of persons and another category in a proportion, $y$, the two types of events will occur together among some members of the group—in a proportion, in fact, equal to the product of the separate proportions, $xy$.

When one of these categories is a disease and the other is an attribute or experience of man there will be a certain number of individuals who exhibit both the experience and the disease. While the disease and the experience are in a nontechnical sense associated in these individuals, this is not evidence of statistical association. Statistical association, or simply *association* in the scientific sense, means that the proportion of persons exhibiting both events is either significantly higher or significantly lower than the proportion predicted on the basis of simultaneous consideration of the separate frequencies of the two categories of events.

While the content of the last paragraph is obvious enough, its main implication should not be overlooked. Statistical associations are determined for *categories,* and not for individual instances. For example, suppose that 100 persons are inoculated with a vaccine against a certain infectious disease and that 100 persons indistinguishable from the first group receive a placebo. During a subsequent epidemic the two groups have similar exposure; 20 of the vaccinated persons and 50 of the unvaccinated contract the disease. Since this difference is unlikely to be due to chance, we would say that a statistical association exists between vaccination and remaining free of the disease and, in view of criteria discussed later (p. 21), that this association is probably a causal one. However, it is not possible to say that vaccination caused any individual person in the vaccinated group to remain disease-free, since there were instances of vaccinated persons who contracted the disease and of unvaccinated who remained free. Within the framework of these results, it is even possible that there were persons who contracted the disease *because* of vaccination, even though the over-all tendency was in the opposite direction.

This is not to deny, however, that information from a group experience may suggest the likelihood of causal association in an individual instance. The stronger the association between the two categories of events revealed by the group experience, the more likely is the assumption of causal association in a specific instance to be correct. Thus, if the disease frequency in the unvaccinated series had been 99 percent and that in the vaccinated series 1 percent, there would be a very high probability that the absence of disease in any one vaccinated individual was related to the vaccination, and the statement that the vaccination of any one individual was causally related to his freedom from disease would probably be correct. The validity of the statement would depend, however, on the total experience and not on any observations made on this one individual (other than that he was one of those who were vaccinated and remained free of disease).

## Causal and Noncausal Association

Only a minority of statistical associations are causal within the sense of the definition, which requires that change in one party to the association alters the other. The large number of statistical associations which do not satisfy this requirement are sometimes referred to as secondary associations. Noncausal statistical associations usually result from association of both categories of events with a third category. For example, if category A is causally associated with both category B and category C (i.e., A precedes and influences both B and C), B and C will also be associated statistically. However, the association between B and C is noncausal, since there is no prospect of altering C by manipulating B, or of altering B by manipulating C. This type of association is common. For example, injection of neoarsphenamine (B) in outpatient clinics for venereal disease has been noted to be associated with jaundice—salvarsan icterus (C). For a long time, as the name indicated, the drug was regarded as the cause of the icterus, until it was discovered that the association was the result of causal association of both icterus and injection of neoarsphenamine with a third factor—treatment for syphilis (A).

Once a statistical association has been demonstrated, how can it be determined whether or not it is causal—that is, is B affected if A is altered? The most satisfactory procedure is direct experiment. While freely available to the laboratory worker, this procedure is infrequently available to the epidemiologist. Further, in certain associations, the presumed cause may not be susceptible to manipulation; while knowledge of whether the relationship is or is not causal may in such an instance be of little immediate value, it may nevertheless be important from the standpoint of the development of knowledge about the disease.

In the absence of experimental data, three types of consideration are useful in distinguishing between epidemiologic associations that are causal and those that are secondary:

1. Time sequence. For a relationship to be considered causal, the events that are considered causative must precede those thought to be effects. When the sequence of events cannot be determined precisely (a frequent situation in chronic disease), at least the possibility of such a sequence must exist.

2. Strength of the association. The stronger the association between two categories of events (for example, the higher the ratio of the incidence of B following A to the incidence of B without A), the more likely it is that the association is causal. If the suspected cause is a quantitative variable, the existence of a dose-response relationship—that is, an association in which the frequency of the effect increases as the exposure to the cause increases—is usually considered to favor a causal relationship, although even in a causal relationship, such an association may not exist over the entire range of exposures to the cause.

3. Consonance with existing knowledge. Here several considerations come into play:

a. A causal hypothesis based on epidemiologic evidence is supported by knowledge of a cellular or subcellular mechanism that makes it reasonable in the light of existing knowledge in relevant sciences. In the absence of this support, there should at least be the belief that such mechanisms are possible.

b. Evidence that the distribution of the disease in populations follows the distribution of the supposed causal factor supports a causal hypothesis. Major discrepancies between the two patterns, not reconcilable in terms of other causal factors or explanations, tend to weaken a causal hypothesis.

c. Evidence obtained through exclusion may be pertinent. The more extensive the efforts have been to identify non-causal explanations of an association, the more one is likely to believe, if these efforts have been unsuccessful, that the association is causal.

The evaluation of the causal nature of a relationship, in the absence of direct experiment, is neither easy nor objective. Differences of opinion resulting from subjective assembly and interpretation of evidence are common. Caution in judging relationships to be causal is laudable. On occasion, however, such caution appears to be carried to an unrealistic extreme. As Thoreau noted [367]: "Some circumstantial evidence is very strong, as when you find a trout in the milk." When the derivation of experimental evidence is either impracticable or unethical, there comes a point in the accumulation of evidence when it is more prudent to act on the basis that the association is causal rather than to await further evidence. If there is controversy or argument, it should center around the decision as to where this point lies, and not on the unanswerable question of whether the causal hypothesis is or is not "proven."

### Direct and Indirect Causal Association

At the beginning of the preceding section (p. 20), we discussed a noncausal statistical association between two categories of events that was explicable in terms of the association of both with a third category. This type of secondary association must be distinguished from causal associations in which a third variable occupies an intermediate stage between cause and effect. Thus, if A is causally related to D (A being the cause and D the effect) and D is causally related to B (D the cause, B the effect), there will be a causal relationship between A and B, but the association is indirect. For example, treatment for syphilis is not of itself productive of icterus, but it is one of the factors associated with the use of unclean syringes. Further investigation of salvarsan icterus indicated that the unclean syringe component rather than the treatment of the syphilis was responsible for the icterus. However, since a certain number of cases of icterus would presumably be prevented by failure to treat syphilis, the association of syphilis treatment with icterus is, in terms of our definition, a causal one, even though indirectly so.

The distinction between direct and indirect causal relationships is a relative one. Apparent directness depends on the limitations of current knowledge. In the example, the association of icterus with syphilis treatment was indirect, and that with the use of unclean syringes direct. Further investigation, however, revealed that the icterus was associated not with unclean syringes per se, but with the injection of minute amounts of human serum that remained in unclean syringes after their previous use. This discovery resulted in a change of the name of the condition to serum hepatitis. Still later, the icterus was found to be associated directly, not with serum, but with the presence in the serum of a specific virus. Thus the association with the virus is currently considered the direct one and that with serum indirect. Further studies might in due course reveal what specific attributes or molecular components of the virus might be considered more direct causal factors. Knowledge of causal mechanisms is not refined to the degree that makes it possible to state that *this* is the ultimate direct association and that no other associations intervene.

The practical significance of causal associations in the development of preventive programs does not necessarily depend on the degree of directness. First, more direct associations may not yet have been identified and so there may be no choice but to make use of obviously indirect associations in preventive programs. For example, knowledge of the association of freedom from scurvy with diets containing fresh fruits and vegetables was put to practical use hundreds of years before the identification of vitamin C, and prevention of smallpox antedates modern virology by almost 200 years. Second, more direct causes, although known, may not be susceptible to economical alteration, whereas the indirect ones may be. For example, preventive measures against serum hepatitis are directed against poor syringe hygiene and not specifically toward removal of the hepatitis virus. And decades after the discovery of the microorganisms associated with enteric disease, preventive measures are still directed, at least in the United States and Europe, primarily toward the provision of clean water and food, rather than against specific microorganisms.

## THE WEB OF CAUSATION

We have discussed the types of association that may exist between two categories of events. In fact, effects are not dependent on single causes. The concept of chains of causation, although useful has the defect of oversimplification. In Figure 2 are shown some of the components that enter into the causal association between treatment for syphilis and serum hepatitis. When it is considered that only a few of the major components are shown, that these are indicated as broad classes of events rather than as the multiple minor events which make up each class,

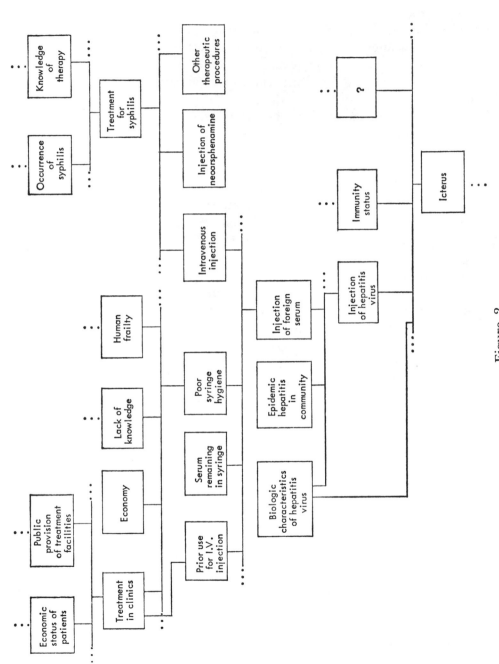

Figure 2

Some components of the association between treatment for syphilis and icterus.

that each component shown is itself the result of a complex genealogy of antecedents, and that the myriad effects of these components other than those contributing to the development of icterus are not shown, then it becomes evident that the chains of causation represent only a fraction of the reality, and the whole genealogy may be thought of more appropriately as a web, which in its complexity and origins lies quite beyond our understanding.

Fortunately it is not necessary to understand causal mechanisms in their entirety to effect preventive measures. Knowledge of even one small component may allow significant degrees of prevention.

The concept of the chain mechanism is that many variables may be related to a single effect through a direct-indirect mechanism in which C is causally related to D, D to E, E to F, and so on, until finally maybe Q plays an important part in the development of the disease. We may note that many variables other than those directly in the selected chain enter the genealogy at each link. Consequently, the longer the chain, the weaker the association. Successful prevention of the disease depends on finding an element in the chain which can be eliminated and which is sufficiently close to Q in the mechanism for its elimination to have a substantial effect on Q. Thus the injection of hepatitis virus in venereal disease clinics can be prevented at a number of different points in the chain, and wherever the chain is broken the disease will be prevented, even though no attempt has been made to alter, for example, the immunologic status of the patients receiving treatment.

The effect that the elimination of Q will have on the total incidence of the disease will depend on the importance of Q relative to other factors that, descended independently of the selected chain, are causally related to the disease. The effect of these independent variables may be thought of as additive: the elimination of any one of them may have an appreciable effect on the disease frequency, but nevertheless the effect of the other factors remains. For example, the elimination of serum hepatitis associated with the use of unclean syringes in the treatment of syphilis will have only very indirect effects on the disease arising from other sources such as blood transfusion.

## CAUSATION AND PREVENTION

The etiology of a disease may be thought of as having a sequence consisting of two parts: (1) causal events occurring prior to some initial bodily response, and (2) mechanisms within the body leading from the initial response to the characteristic manifestations of the disease. For example, it may be that penetration of a marrow cell by ionizing rays will lead to a specific mutation in a very high proportion of instances, and, if circumstances are appropriate for the reproduction of the altered cell, to the patient's becoming leukemic. Thus we may describe the etiologic sequence as (1) the series of prior events which brought the ionizing rays in contact with a susceptible marrow cell, followed by (2) the series of events initiated by the mutation and terminating in the death of the patient.

This simplification enables the recognition that prevention, and therefore epidemiology, is concerned predominantly with those successions of events which result in the exposure of specific types of individuals to specific types of environments, whereas therapy is concerned with the bodily mechanism which finally results in the manifest signs and symptoms of the disease. This distinction may lead to differences between practitioners of prevention and of therapy in their concepts of what constitutes an important causal association. For example, the therapist may be satisfied to know that deficiency of a pancreatic secretion is an important cause of diabetes mellitus, since if this deficiency is remedied the symptoms of the disease are significantly modified. For purposes of prevention, however, it is more pertinent to know what caused the pancreatic deficiency.

If knowledge of causal associations is sought predominantly for its practical application, there is one other aspect that it is desirable to determine—the side-effects of alteration of the cause. For, just as any effect has multiple causes, the alteration of any cause may be expected to have multiple effects besides the one intended, and in any prevention program the side-effects of alteration of the cause must be acceptable. On the one hand, a certain loss of character in the taste of public water supplies is apparently an acceptable price to pay for a typhoid-free existence, but, on the other, the citizens of many communities have expressed their view that a predictable reduction of dental decay is not worth the conjectured risks that fluoridation of water supplies might entail.

Knowledge of causal associations that do not offer preventive possibilities, either because the cause is unalterable or because the side-effects are unacceptable, is nevertheless important. Such knowledge allows more effective studies directed toward the identification of causal associations that do offer preventive possibilities. For example, knowledge of the association of disease rates with age is a basic requirement for epidemiologic studies of chronic disease, although this association is not one with preventive application.

# 3

*Strategies of Epidemiology*

As stated in Chapter 1, the predominant purpose of epidemiology is the search for causal associations between diseases and environmental exposures. In epidemiology, as in other sciences, progress in this search results from a series of cycles in which investigators (1) examine existing facts and hypotheses, (2) formulate a new or more specific hypothesis, and (3) obtain additional facts to test the acceptability of the new hypothesis. A fresh cycle then commences, the new facts, and possibly the new hypothesis, being added to the available knowledge.

Before the various strategies commonly applied in this process are described, the elements of an epidemiologic hypothesis should be considered. Ideally an epidemiologic hypothesis should specify:

1. The population—the characteristics of the persons to whom the hypothesis applies
2. The cause being considered—the environmental exposure
3. The expected effect—the disease
4. The dose-response relationship—the amount of the cause needed to lead to a stated incidence of the effect
5. The time-response relationship—the time period that will elapse between exposure to the cause and observation of the effect

A well-developed hypothesis describes each of these elements with a high degree of specificity. For example, current knowledge might allow us to formulate the hypothesis that among adults without previous exposure to typhoid fever the ingestion of ten million viable typhoid bacilli will result in an attack rate of typhoid fever of 50 percent within a period of 30 days.

In practice, the components of an epidemiologic hypothesis are often less well-specified and may indeed be no more than implied. The hypothesis that dirty water causes diarrhea lacks specificity in the two components which are stated (cause and effect), and leaves implied the concepts that the population involved is man (or at least animal), that the amounts of cause and effect are finite, and that the time relationship is such as to be within the attention span of man. Even though unstated, these last components must be implied if the hypothesis is to be testable and therefore useful.

Although a relatively unspecific hypothesis may have practical significance—as does that linking dirty water with diarrhea—its potential usefulness is enhanced by increasing the specificity of any one of its five components. The added specificity may not lead immediately to a more practical preventive program, but it may provide the basis for further investigation which does.

## ASSEMBLING THE FACTS

Whatever the existing level of knowledge, the formation and testing of hypotheses is the basis of scientific progress. In epidemiology the procedure may involve simply the further specification of the population to which an already highly specific causal hypothesis has relevance. Let us suppose, however, that we are dealing with a disease whose causes are quite unknown. At this level the data needed for developing a hypothesis include facts about the clinical nature and pathology of the disease and the pathophysiology of affected and related organ systems—indeed, the entire accumulation of medical knowledge—together with information on the types of people affected with the disease and the various circumstances in which it occurs. While an epidemiologist must consider information from all these areas in developing hypotheses, it is the collection of information on the distribution of disease in the population which is his particular responsibility.

An inquiry into the nature of an unknown quantity opens logically with general questions. For example, in a well-known parlor game an unseen object must be identified on the basis of the answers to 20 questions. Since the object is frequently of great rarity, such as the mummified left great toe of Ramses II, the chance of success through unguided guesses is small. The devotees of this game have developed opening questions aimed at rapidly reducing the number of possibilities. For example, the inquiry usually opens with the question, "Is it animal, vegetable, or mineral?" If a helpful answer is received to this question (and in the present example it may not be), the inquiry proceeds with further general questions as to the object's age, color, consistency, and so on. Eventually the number of possibilities compatible with the answers resulting from these general questions may be sufficiently reduced to enable specific guesses.

Similarly, epidemiologists have developed their own set of general limiting questions. Since the epidemiologist's questions are not so readily answered as those in the parlor game, he must weigh the value of an answer to a general question against the expense and time involved in deriving it. The collection of data being expensive, the exploratory phase of epidemiologic investigation is heavily influenced by what information is available, and the questions most frequently asked are those on which information is already assembled and published in reports of census bureaus, vital statistics centers, and other agencies dealing with health statistics.

The variables most commonly examined can be classified as descriptive of time, place, and person. They include:

1. Characteristics describing the *time* in which persons were found affected. For example, is there any unusual feature of the distribution of cases by year, month, or day of occurrence?

2. Characteristics describing the *place* in which persons were found affected. For example, are cases equally distributed with respect to country, state or district within countries, urban-rural residence, or within the affected local communities?

3. Characteristics describing the *persons* affected. For exam-

ple, what is their age, sex, ethnic group, occupation, education, socioeconomic class, and marital status?

It is evident that the variables listed are not necessarily those which have causal association with the disease being examined, but are simply the things that have been measured. Thus an association of a disease with a particular place might well be due to the type of person that inhabits that place, and an association with a variable that is descriptive of a person, such as his race, might be the result of factors peculiar to the place of residence of that race. The grouping of variables into categories of time, place, and person should be thought of as an initial separation helpful to the investigator (like the grouping into animal, vegetable, or mineral in the parlor game) rather than as a classification of causal factors.

## FORMING HYPOTHESES

In epidemiology, as in science in general, a new and convincing hypothesis can be one of the most powerful forces influencing the direction of future research, and the success or failure of that research frequently depends on the soundness of the hypothesis. Yet the thought processes involved in forming hypotheses are not clearly formalized and classified.

In the early cycles of epidemiologic investigation of a disease, hypotheses are formed that seek to identify causes that explain the patterns of its distribution in populations. Four methods of reaching these hypotheses will be discussed. The first three are patterned after three of Mill's five canons of inductive reasoning [255], which dealt with the definition and proof of causation.

### Method of Difference

If the frequency of a disease is markedly different under two different circumstances and some factor can be identified in one circumstance that is absent in the other, this factor, or its absence, may be a cause of the disease.

The difficulty with this method of forming epidemiologic hypotheses is usually not one of being unable to identify a factor that is present in one circumstance and not in the other (or relatively so), but rather of the multiplicity of hypotheses which are often suggested on the basis of the difference. For example, literally dozens of possibilities may be suggested to explain differences in disease frequency between males and females, or between the United States and India, or between certain age groups. For this reason any one descriptive observation, even though revealing a marked characteristic of the disease under study, usually is not sufficient for the establishment of a sound hypothesis. Occasionally, however, a single descriptive feature of a disease is sufficiently striking to favor it as a likely basis for a hypothesis. For example, although carcinoma of the cervix is one of the commonest forms of cancer in females, it is extremely rare in nuns. The differences between nuns and other females are few enough to make attractive the hypothesis that some aspect of the reproductive process predisposes to carcinoma of the cervix.

## Method of Agreement

If a factor is common to a number of different circumstances that have been found to be associated with presence of a disease, this factor may be a cause of the disease. For example, cholera is associated with patient contact, with overcrowding, and with sewage-contaminated water supply. A common factor is the opportunity to ingest fecal discharges from cholera patients. This may be a cause of cholera. Again, cancer of the cervix is associated with sexual intercourse at an early age, multiple sexual partners, and low socioeconomic status. A common factor may be a venereally transmitted virus.

## Method of Concomitant Variation

The method of concomitant variation involves the search for some factor whose frequency or strength varies with the frequency of the disease. It is a quantitative rather than a dichotomous way of looking at the same ideas that are involved in the methods of agreement and difference. A well-known example is the attempt to relate the relative frequencies of various dietary constituents to the incidence of coronary artery disease in different areas of the world [187]. Another is the comparison of the fluoride concentration in drinking water in various areas with the frequency of dental caries in the inhabitants [77].

*Method of Analogy*

The distribution of a disease may be sufficiently similar to that of some other disease that has been more completely and successfully investigated to suggest that certain causes may be common to the two. This method of arriving at hypotheses is related to the process of deductive reasoning, whereby epidemiologic principles already established are applied to specific situations. Thus we tend to associate diseases occurring in certain places during the summer months with vector transmission, and, until the identification of the slow viruses, we were reluctant to accept as infectious those diseases that did not spread rapidly.

Even in the absence of general laws or principles, however, this method may be of service. For example, the observation that the age and sex pattern for pulmonary tuberculosis in adults had features similar to those of pulmonary cancer and the knowledge that lung cancer is related to smoking led Lowe [208] to formulate and test the hypothesis that smoking may also be a factor in progressive pulmonary tuberculosis in later life. Likewise, the similarity of the geographic distribution of Burkitt's lymphoma in Africa to that of yellow fever led to the hypothesis that a mosquito vector may be involved in the former as well as in the latter disease [141]. The similarity of the shape of the age incidence curve in Burkitt's lymphoma to the increase with age in prevalence of antibodies to yellow fever virus strengthened the hypothesis [142]. The similarity of the geographic distribution and certain other epidemiologic features of multiple sclerosis to those of paralytic poliomyelitis led Poskanzer et al. [328] to suggest that the clinical illness of multiple sclerosis might also be an occasional manifestation of a widespread infection usually acquired at an early age.

The method of analogy, while useful, can also be treacherous; major errors have been made as the result of false analogies. Thus, because genetically determined diseases tend to run in families, there is a temptation to assume that all familial concentration of a disease is evidence of genetic determination. This view is, of course, false. In a different connection, John Snow, having demonstrated the sewage-water transmission of cholera and having observed that plague and yellow fever shared the association of cholera with crowding, lack of personal cleanliness, and a tendency to attack towns located on freshwater rivers, was led to the mistaken idea that plague and yellow fever were transmitted in the same way as cholera [376].

## Some Considerations in the Formation of Hypotheses

While any one or any combination of the methods and variables described may lead to a useful hypothesis, it is helpful to consider situations that have been particularly productive in the past.

1. New hypotheses are commonly formed by relating observations from several different fields. In the area of disease causation, epidemiologic findings are most profitably viewed in the light of clinical, pathologic, and laboratory observations. Thus Snow interpreted the epidemiologic characteristics of cholera in the light of clinical and pathologic observations that the intestine was the apparent focus of the disease. In Vienna in 1847 an obstetrician, Ignaz Semmelweis, was attempting to explain the high incidence of puerperal fever in women delivered by medical students compared to those delivered by midwives. The clinical observation that certain features of the disease were evidenced by a colleague who died following a cut received in the autopsy room led Semmelweis to suspect that their attendance at autopsies might be the characteristic that made medical students more dangerous than midwives to puerperal women [361]. More recently, the observation of radiation dermatitis in a patient with carcinoma of the breast led MacKenzie [218] to explore the possible role of multiple fluoroscopy in the etiology of breast cancer.

2. The stronger a statistical association, the more likely it is to suggest a causal hypothesis. Strength here does not mean the degree of statistical significance, but the degree to which the situation of a disease being entirely absent in one circumstance and invariably present in another is approached. The fact that this situation is more nearly approached for the association between

smoking and lung cancer than for that between smoking and cardiovascular disease, makes the former association a firmer basis for considering etiologic possibilities. Associations of low strength, however significant statistically, are rarely immediately productive of strong hypotheses.

3. Observations of change in frequency of a disease over time have been very productive of hypotheses. This is particularly true of changes that occur over a relatively short period. For example, the rapidity of the rise of an epidemic of unusual congenital malformations in the period 1959 to 1961 called immediate attention to the fact that some new factor must be operative and led to the rapid identification of thalidomide as the cause [199, 210]. However, even changes taking place over several decades can be productive of hypotheses if the changes are striking, as was the case with lung cancer [79], or if they follow unusual patterns, as did an epidemic of chronic nephritis in Queensland, Australia [157] and Parkinson's disease in the United States [329.]

4. An isolated or unusual case should receive particular attention in the formation of hypotheses. Such cases—for example, in persons living in communities otherwise free of the disease—have been of great value in the study of infectious diseases and figure prominently in the investigations of Snow on cholera [376], Budd on typhoid fever [35], and Panum on measles [309]. The occurrence of typhus in areas of the United States where the disease was not known to exist, and where opportunities for infection seemed remote, led to recognition of the possibility of recrudescence of this disease many years after infection [434].

5. Observations that appear in conflict or to create a paradox are particularly worthy of consideration. For example, the fact that nurses and attendants in asylums did not develop pellagra, in spite of their close contact with the inmates who did, led Goldberger [130] to favor hypotheses relating the disease to diet rather than to infectious agents. The fact that high levels of estrogens increase breast cancer risk, but that childbearing—which is associated with high estrogen levels—appears to decrease the risk, supports a hypothesis regarding the specific types of estrogen which may be productive of breast cancer [428].

*Selection and Evaluation of Hypotheses*

Almost any set of observations will be compatible with more than one hypothesis. From all the possibilities it is necessary to select some few that seem particularly worthy of test. This process of evaluating one hypothesis against another usually proceeds concurrently with the formation of the hypotheses. The following considerations must be kept in mind.

First, the value of a hypothesis is inversely related to the number of acceptable alternatives. The number of these alternatives in turn depends on a variety of circumstances:

a. The greater the number of separate associations that could be explained by association between the suspected factor and the disease, the fewer the number of acceptable alternatives. While an association involving only one variable occasionally leads to the development of a productive hypothesis, an association with two independent variables may narrow the field considerably. For example, several hypotheses could explain the high incidence of leukemia observed in radiologists [201]. Relatively few would explain both this observation and the high leukemia rate in patients given x-ray therapy for ankylosing spondylitis [69]. When yet a third observation is added—the increased rate of leukemia in survivors of the atomic bombs in Nagasaki and Hiroshima [30]—the possibilities are reduced even further.

b. The more closely two variables both found to be associated with a disease are themselves associated, the less is their independent value in the formation of a hypothesis. For example, many factors may be conceived that are common to one of the Census Bureau's professional occupations and to residence in a favored residential district. Any disease associated with one of these variables will almost always be associated with the other. Much more limited in number are factors common to holding a professional occupation and, say, being single, since the correlation between most occupations and marital status is weak.

c. Associations with certain variables—for example, occupation and religion—may be of greater value than those with others, such as age and sex, since the unique environmental circumstances associated with the former may be fewer than those associated with the latter.

Second, in evaluating a hypothesis that is in process of development, it is useful to make a deliberate search for specific demographic information that may be relevant to it. For example, if a genetic predisposition to cancer of the stomach is hypothesized on the basis of the high frequency of the disease in Japan, one would predict that stomach cancer would be common in all persons of Japanese ancestry, regardless of current residence. In fact, Americans of Japanese ancestry have stomach cancer rates quite similar to those of Americans of European origin, and the genetic explanation of the high rates in Japan must be discarded [145]. Similarly, the low rate of cervix cancer in Jewish women has for many years suggested that circumcision of the sexual partner might be protective against this disease. Abou-Daoud [1] therefore compared cervix cancer rates among religious groups in Lebanon, where the Moslem men are circumcised and the Christians not. The fact that there was no apparent difference in cervical cancer rates in the two groups weakens the circumcision hypothesis. To evaluate the hypothesis that benign gastric ulcer predisposes to gastric malignancy, Hirohata and Kuratsune compared the distributions of mortality rates from the two diseases in Japan [165]. They found that the two conditions had entirely different distributions—a finding that weakens the hypothesis that they are causally associated. Although this kind of hypothesis evaluation can be very valuable, it should be noted that the population groups used have special characteristics other than the exposure which is the subject of the hypothesis, and the inferences regarding the specific exposure (e.g., circumcision) are indirect.

Third, a hypothesis need not be consistent with all existing observations. Inconsistencies may be due to several factors:

a. Multiple causes of a single disease. As was discussed in Chapter 2, concern in epidemiology is with *a* cause of a disease, not *the* cause. Causes other than the one suspected may be responsible for observations that do not fit into the hypothesis. For example, differences between ethnic groups in frequency of tuberculosis may be contributed to by genetic differences in susceptibility to the organism as well as by differences in the frequency or intensity of exposure. Conceivably, Lebanese Moslems have high rates of cervix cancer for reasons quite different from those which explain a difference between circumcised and uncircumcised groups in other countries.

b. Crudity of the disease classification. The disease entity under investigation—for example, anemia—may in fact comprise several different entities that have not yet been distinguished, and the particular hypothesis may account for the features of only one of these subentities. Epidemiologic variations in the other subentities may appear inconsistent with the hypothesis. The hypothesis, if otherwise supported, may in fact provide the basis for separating the subentity to which it relates from the other components of the crude entity (see Chap. 4).

Furthermore, observations that appear to be inconsistent with a hypothesis may be particularly worthy of investigation in that valuable information may turn up in attempts to explain the inconsistency. For example, in evaluating the evidence that water from deep artesian wells was causally related to the occurrence of "blackfoot disease" in Taiwan, Chen and Wu [52] observed five cases of the disease in persons drinking water from shallow wells. These cases appeared to be inconsistent with the hypothesis. Investigation revealed, however, that all five persons had changed their source of drinking water from artesian to shallow wells a few years prior to onset of the disease.

## TESTING EPIDEMIOLOGIC HYPOTHESES

An epidemiologic hypothesis generally specifies a cause-effect relationship between two categories of things. As outlined in Chapter 2, several considerations enter into the determination of whether or not such a relationship exists. First is the question whether a statistical association exists between the two categories, and second is whether the association is causal in nature. If the relationship can be studied experimentally, its causal aspect may be evaluated readily. If experimental evidence is not available, the assessment of causation is more difficult and must take into account a wide variety of information about the supposed cause, the postulated effect, and their observed relationship. The particular contributions of epidemiology to the assessment are provision of information on whether an association exists between the cause and the effect in man, and, if an association does exist, a description of its characteristics—particularly, its strength and constancy.

## Experimental Studies

The experimental method of testing a cause-effect hypothesis is the deliberate application or withholding of the supposed cause and observation for the subsequent appearance or lack of appearance of the effect. Although there are examples of the experimental testing of epidemiologic hypotheses in man (see Chap. 1), opportunities for such tests are uncommon. Ethical considerations usually restrict such experiments to those that involve the addition of things presumed to be beneficial or the removal of things presumed to be noxious. At the same time, if benefit from the procedure appears very likely, the withholding of it in order to obtain additional evidence may be unethical. Further limiting factors in epidemiologic experiments are the practical considerations of gaining the cooperation of a sufficiently large number of subjects and of maintaining this cooperation long enough to complete the experiment.

However, it may be possible to test an epidemiologic hypothesis by evaluating the efficacy of a preventive measure suggested by the hypothesis. If properly designed and carried out—as were the trials of fluoridation of drinking water for the prevention of dental caries and the several trials of vaccines referred to in Chapter 1—tests of preventive measures can offer powerful support of epidemiologic hypotheses.

## Nonexperimental Studies

In assembling evidence to test a hypothesis without recourse to experiment, epidemiologists seek to identify natural circumstances that mimic an experiment. For example, a human experiment to test the hypothesis that cigarette smoking causes lung cancer is impracticable, but advantage can be taken of the fact that, without any encouragement from epidemiologists, people have separated themselves into groups of smokers and nonsmokers. This at least allows determination of whether the two categories of things (smoking and lung cancer) are statistically associated and investigation of the characteristics of the association.

Since the information needed to test for the existence of most associations of interest in epidemiologic hypotheses is rarely available in routine sources of data, special studies are usually necessary. To illustrate the methods used, suppose that a study is planned to test the hypothesis that a particular drug taken during pregnancy causes congenital malformation in the offspring. With respect to the two events—exposure to drug and occurrence of malformation—each individual belongs to one of the cells in Table 3, the numbers of individuals in each cell being indicated by the letters $a, b, c,$ and $d$.

### Table 3

Distribution of individuals with respect to presence
or absence of two characteristics

| Drug during pregnancy | Malformation in offspring | | |
|---|---|---|---|
| | Present | Absent | Total |
| Exposed | $a$ | $b$ | $a + b$ |
| Not exposed | $c$ | $d$ | $c + d$ |
| Total | $a + c$ | $b + d$ | $a + b + c + d$ |

The question at issue is whether the proportion malformed is higher in the offspring of mothers who took the drug than in the offspring of those who did not. In other words, is the number of individuals in cell $a$ (infants who were exposed *and* exhibited the effect) higher than would be expected if the two events were unrelated? The method by which the expected number of individuals in cell $a$ is obtained distinguishes two basic types of study —cohort studies and case-control studies.

COHORT STUDIES. In this type of study the investigator may select a study population consisting of some pregnant women who took the drug and some who did not. He then observes the groups over time to determine how many exposed and nonexposed infants developed malformation. He can then compare the proportion of malformed infants in the nonexposed group, $c/(c + d)$, with the proportion of malformed in the exposed group, $a/(a + b)$. Note that this approach permits direct comparison of the rates of malformation in exposed and nonexposed infants.

CASE-CONTROL STUDIES.* An alternative approach is to select a study population consisting of some infants who were malformed (cases) and some who were not (controls). The investigator must then determine the frequency with which the mothers of the two groups took the drug. The frequency of exposure in the cases, $a/(a + c)$, is compared with that in the unaffected controls, $b/(b + d)$. Although in a study of this type the study groups are selected from the affected $(a + c)$ and unaffected $(b + d)$ populations, they represent unknown proportions of those populations, since the number of controls included is usually determined by the available number of cases; for example, it may be decided to include two controls for each case. Consequently, the cells $a$ and $b$ as represented in the study group do not represent the relative frequencies of such individuals in the population, and in this kind of study a *rate* of malformation is not obtained in either exposed or nonexposed individuals. There are methods by which such rates can be estimated (see p. 273), but they are rarely obtained directly from the study population.

CHOICE OF STUDY DESIGN. More detailed descriptions and examples of cohort and case-control studies and of their many variations and special features are given in Chapters 11 and 12. However, it may be useful here to note the special features that influence the choice of one or another type for study of a particular relationship. Cohort studies, while providing the most complete picture of the association between the disease and the exposure, are economical only when the disease under investigation is relatively frequent. For infrequent diseases very large cohorts are required to obtain firm estimates of disease rates, and the case-control approach is usually preferable.

---

* In our previous text [229], we referred to these studies as "case-history" studies, to emphasize the focus of obtaining historical information on the antecedents of affected individuals. However, to avoid confusion with clinical and other studies in which such historical information is collected for a series of cases but no comparison group is used, we now prefer the term "case-control" study.

A considerable limitation of the case-control study, however, is that information on the supposed cause must be retained—either in memories of persons or in written documents—until after the person can be identified as having the disease. Written documentation is lacking for many variables of epidemiologic interest, and information drawn from memory must be carefully evaluated for possible biases relating to the development of the disease in one group (the cases) and not in the other (the controls).

A case-control study is usually less costly than a cohort study—in terms of both time and resources—and is therefore frequently undertaken as a first step to determine whether or not an association exists between the suspected cause and effect, or to select between several hypotheses that may explain the observed characteristics of the disease. Cohort studies may then be undertaken to gain added confidence in the existence of a relationship and to measure more accurately its strength. For example, some 15 case-control studies of the relationship between smoking and lung cancer had been published before the appearance of the first cohort study in 1954 [82].

RETROSPECTIVE AND PROSPECTIVE COHORT STUDIES. An important element of the cost of a cohort study is the waiting time that elapses between the selection of exposed and nonexposed cohorts and the development of the disease. In a typical *prospective* cohort study—such as the Framingham Heart Study of the U.S. Public Health Service [75]—even when a relatively common disease, such as coronary artery disease, is under investigation, many years must elapse between the selection of the study groups and the appearance of sufficient cases for the computation of reliable disease rates among the exposed and nonexposed subgroups.

The cost of such a study can be substantially reduced if the cause and effect under investigation are such that they can both be ascertained *retrospectively* from existing records. For example, in 1960 Beebe [23] assembled from U.S. Army records a cohort of men who were hospitalized for mustard gas poisoning in 1918. Two comparison cohorts were also assembled from military records of the same vintage. Mortality of the cohorts between 1919 and 1955 was ascertained from Veterans Administration records, a significant excess of deaths due to lung cancer being found in the cohort exposed to mustard gas. Since both the exposure and the effects had occurred prior to the time the investigation began, the waiting period required in a prospective study was eliminated. Such retrospective studies combine the economy of the case-control study with the advantages of the cohort study in providing direct estimates of risk.

Note that the words *retrospective* and *prospective,* in this terminology, are used to describe the time of occurrence of the events being studied relative to the investigator's place in time. In contrast to this usage, the terms *retrospective* and *prospective* have been used by some workers to refer to what we have called case-control studies and cohort studies [118, 162, 202, 393]. The rationale for this latter special use of the words lies in the idea that retrospective studies involve looking backward from effects to preceding causes, and the prospective approach involves looking forward from causes to effects. This terminology does not specify any necessary relation in calendar time of the observer and the events. White and Bailar [415] have pointed out that such terminology gives rise to considerable confusion, since the terms have everyday meanings closely connected with calendar time. In the everyday sense, a retrospective study is one based on past data or past events, whereas a prospective study is one planned to observe events that have not yet occurred. In addition, White and Bailar pointed out that there is lack of agreement as to the precise meanings of the terms prospective and retrospective, even when used in a special sense. For these reasons we prefer to use these terms only in a context in keeping with their everyday meanings.

CROSS-SECTIONAL AND LONGITUDINAL STUDIES. Epidemiologic studies can also be characterized by whether the ascertainment of cause and effect relate to two different points in time or to a single point. In a *longitudinal* study the observations relate to two different points in time—even if both items of information are collected simultaneously. Most cohort and case-control studies are longitudinal in nature. In a *cross-sectional* study, on the other hand, measurements of cause and effect are made at the same point in time. Although the cross-sectional study is easier and more economical than the longitudinal, it is limited to studies of causes that are permanent, or reasonably permanent, characteristics of the individual, so that his status with respect to the cause measured at the time he has the disease has a high probability of reflecting his status at the time the disease was induced. For example, a cross-sectional study would be a reasonable way of investigating the relationship between blood group and disease. A longitudinal study, however, would be required to study the effect of neonatal jaundice on mental development. In practice, the distinction between cross-sectional and longitudinal studies often is not clear-cut. Cigarette consumption, for example, is a variable that may or may not be a long-term characteristic of the individual, and a great variety of degrees of permanency of individual characteristics can be visualized.

Cross-sectional studies are frequently made on total population samples. For example, the U.S. National Health Survey [117, 305, 347] has reported a number of studies in which correlations between possible causal factors (current occupation, parity, blood glucose) and diseases (hearing deficiency, diabetes, high blood pressure) have been based on observations made at a single examination of a random sample of the United States population. It should be borne in mind that such studies describe the patterns of disease prevalence, rather than incidence, and that these will be affected by factors determining duration as well as incidence. Studies of blood group and disease [7], however, exemplify cross-sectional studies that may use the case-control method of subject selection, and in these instances may be based on incident rather than prevalent cases of disease. A study of the prevalence of respiratory disease in workers in a flax mill [114] would be an instance of the cross-sectional approach in a study using the cohort method of study group selection.

The categorizations and terminology just given are presented solely for the purpose of describing some of the techniques and problems associated with particular aspects of study design. While many studies may be described as "typical" examples of, say, a case-control study or a retrospective cohort study, there are also studies that defy such classification. For example, there are studies that have been designed as cohort studies but analyzed as case-control studies [306, 307], and there are case-control studies that permit rather direct estimates of disease rates in exposed and nonexposed groups [351]. It would be unfortunate if epidemiologic methodology were to lose flexibility and become constrained within these or any other definitions of "typical" kinds of study.

## SEARCH FOR A MECHANISM

The over-all evaluation of an epidemiologic hypothesis, in addition to including an assessment of whether the hypothesis seems reasonable when viewed against the results of epidemiologic tests and general biologic and medical knowledge, may include attempts to reproduce the circumstances of the association in an experimental animal and efforts to find cellular or biochemical mechanisms that explain the association. The mechanism sought would substitute for the direct jump from cause to effect a series of smaller steps involving associations at the level of organs, cells, or their components that conform to knowledge based on a broader foundation than that supporting this particular hypothesis.

Success, either in demonstrating the association in animals other than man or in identifying a plausible micromechanism for the association, will usually profoundly increase the acceptability of a hypothesis. Failure to reproduce in another animal a cause-effect relationship that is suspected in man, however, may simply be a reflection of the uniqueness of man in regard to this particular association. Similarly, failure to identify a biologic mechanism for such a relation may be a reflection of the limitations of existing techniques. The macromechanisms of contagion, of transmission of cholera and typhoid by the fecal-oral route, of disease due to specific nutritional deficiency, and of the deleterious effects of cigarette smoke on health were all identified with sufficient certainty to provide effective means of disease prevention before the micromechanisms were clearly delineated.

# 4

## Classification of Disease

As noted in Chapter 2, inferences that an association is more than a random phenomenon can be made only when the elements of the association are considered in groups or *classes*. Such inferences cannot be made from isolated observations of individual events or circumstances. The grouping of events or things into classes is therefore an essential scientific procedure. The basic objective is to form classes that allow generalizations regarding the behavior or features of the members of a class in some dimension other than that used in its formation [156]. For example, a disease entity based on similarity of symptoms and signs would be useful if it allowed generalizations regarding its causes or its prognosis. Likewise, an entity based on similarity of cause might allow prediction of the symptoms and signs that occur in exposed persons or of the course of their illness.

The process of disease classification may be thought of as having two components. The first is the grouping of ill persons into categories such that the characteristics of the members of one category permit them to be distinguished from the members of another. These categories are then viewed as being disease entities, and the members of a category are thought of as suffering from *a* disease. The second component is the arrangement of the disease entities themselves into groups having common characteristics. In this chapter the concern is primarily with the first aspect of the process.

47

CLASSIFICATION OF ILL PERSONS

*Manifestational and Causal Entities*

Two distinct types of criteria are used to categorize ill persons into groups (disease entities):

1. Manifestational criteria. The ill persons are grouped according to their similarity with respect to symptoms, signs, changes in body fluids or tissues, physiologic function, behavior, prognosis, or some combination of these features. Examples of diseases defined by manifestational criteria are fracture of the femur, diabetes mellitus, mental retardation, the common cold, schizophrenia, and cervical cancer.

2. Causal criteria. Here the grouping depends on similarity of individuals with respect to a specified experience believed to be a cause of their illness. Examples of diseases defined by causal criteria are birth trauma, silicosis, syphilis, and lead poisoning.

There is no logical reason to suppose that the ill persons classified together by the one kind of criterion will remain as a group if the other kind of criterion is used. For example, the identification of the tubercle bacillus by Koch [191], and the consequent decision to group ill persons in terms of having a disease causally associated with this bacillus, led to a classification which removed individuals from several of the manifestational entities in the nosologies of preceding times. In 1785 Cullen's classification of ill persons [71] consisted of the four manifestational categories indicated in Figure 3. Each of the four categories no doubt included persons who today are said to be suffering from tuberculosis.

It is true that examples may be found of close correspondence between the two types of grouping. Thus the gross manifestations of rubeola are so distinctive that a group of persons classified together on the basis of similarity of manifestations corresponds closely to the group of persons having an illness caused by the rubeola virus. Even when the gross manifestations of a causal entity seem heterogeneous, a more refined manifestation may be identified that gives unity to the seemingly heterogeneous

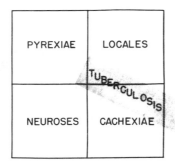

Figure 3

Classification of a group of ill persons according to manifestational (unshaded) and causal (shaded) criteria.

group. For example, the tubercle of tuberculosis is a histologic manifestation common to most persons with illness causally associated with tubercle bacillus. Therefore the correspondence between the group of persons with illness supposedly caused by the tubercle bacillus (causal criterion) and the group characterized by the histologic presence of tubercles (manifestational criterion) would be quite close. Such unifying manifestations are by no means common, however, and it is important to recognize that considerable violence to existing disease entities may result from a decision to change the axis of classification from manifestational to causal criteria.

Appreciation of the lack of necessary congruence between the two ways of classification is important to epidemiologists from several points of view:

1. Polymorphous effects (manifestations) of newly isolated causal agents may be understood, indeed expected. For example, the fact that cigarette smoking is associated with several other diseases besides lung cancer was for several years used as an argument against the acceptance of the associations as causal, since it was felt that truly causal agents would have more specific effects [27, 28]. In fact, even if cigarette smoke contained only a single disease-causing agent, past experience would lead to the expectation of a diversity of effects.

2. It can be understood that an agent causally associated with a certain manifestational disease entity may not be causally in-

volved with *all* the ill persons manifesting "the" disease. Following the identification of a causal association, the examination of subcategories of the manifestational entity may reveal groups that are not involved. For example, it has been determined that epidermoid, but not oat cell, carcinomas of the lung are associated with cigarette smoking. On the other hand, because of lack of appropriate techniques, such subcategories may not be identifiable even though they exist. For example, no particular manifestational category of coronary heart disease has been found to be associated with cigarette smoking, although the high frequency of the disease in nonsmokers indicates clearly that this factor is not involved in all cases of the disease.

3. The arbitrariness of the frequent distinction between necessary causes—those without which the disease does not occur—and contributing causes may be realized. Thus *Mycobacterium tuberculosis* is often spoken of as the necessary cause of tuberculosis, and other factors such as age, nutritional status, and genetic constitution as contributing factors. Most commonly the chosen factor is the necessary cause only by definition, in the sense that automobiles are the necessary cause of automobile accidents. Thus *M. tuberculosis* may be the necessary cause of tuberculosis as it is presently defined, but had medical knowledge developed differently this pathologic state might have been included in the definition of a specific nutritional defect. In that case the nutritional defect would have been the necessary cause and the bacillus a contributory factor. In this connection it may be pointed out that the first of the postulates attributed to Koch [398]—a set of conditions commonly thought of as criteria to be satisfied in establishing causal association between microorganisms and disease—is in fact an example of circular reasoning related to the concept of necessary cause. The postulate states that for a microorganism to be considered a cause of a disease it should be found "in all cases of the disease in question." The postulate implies that the microorganism necessarily be the cause of an already-defined manifestational entity. In actuality, however, the "disease in question" cannot be defined until a particular causal criterion has been arbitrarily selected as the "necessary" cause.

4. The fact can be recognized that not all persons experienc-

ing the cause must become diseased as a result of the experience. For example, while there is a definite statistical association between the tubercle bacillus and tuberculosis, evidence of interaction with the bacillus is found in many persons who have no evidence of illness, just as many persons who smoke cigarettes fail to develop cancer of the lung.

## Selection of Criteria for Classification

Classifications themselves are traditionally designated as artificial or natural. Linnaeus's system of dividing plants into 24 classes according to the stamens is often cited as an example of an artificial system, while classifications which fit in with current evidence on plant evolution are said to be natural.

The distinction between these two types of classification does not seem particularly clear. The level of existing knowledge largely determines what criteria are used to arrange things into groups. In a time not yet influenced by Darwinian theory it seems not at all unnatural that differences between plants in the characteristics of the stamens were considered important. Today the usefulness of the Darwinian concept of species as a natural classification is being questioned [106].

Further, the particular interest of the observer to a large extent determines the kind of criteria selected; for example, a landscape gardener may find it useful for his purposes to classify bushes as large or small. Similarly, usefulness for particular purposes is a major determinant of the type of criterion used for disease classification in medical practice.

In the absence of knowledge of causal factors, manifestational criteria provide the only basis for such classification. Here the setting of the limits of disease entities appears to be a highly intuitive process, having as a governing principle the assumption that the greater the similarity of the manifestations of illness the more properly the illness of the persons exhibiting the manifestations may be considered an entity.

As causal factors are identified, some are used to define new disease entities. Predominant among these have been the microbial agents. The acceptance of these agents as the basis for creation of new disease entities seems to stem from the usefulness, for preventive as well as therapeutic purposes, of the categories so created. Other causal factors, however, have not been used to develop new classifications. For example, "cigarette-smoker's disease"—which could incorporate most cases of emphysema, epidermoid carcinoma of the lung, and peripheral vascular disease, and some cases of coronary heart disease and bladder cancer—might be a very useful disease entity if looked at solely from a preventive point of view. But therapy remains the predominant purpose of medicine, and from that point of view it is much more useful to group a case of epidermoid carcinoma of the lung with a case of oat cell cancer than with a case of peripheral vascular disease. Since the objective of prevention is not seriously jeopardized in this instance by retention of the existing classification, it is unlikely that the concept of cigarette-smoker's disease will replace the current manifestational entities used to classify ill persons.

Use of one classificatory scheme does not exclude concurrent use of another. Thus the emergency department of a hospital may categorize injured persons into manifestational groups such as fractures, sprains, concussions, and cases of suspected internal hemorrhage, while an accident prevention program would be more likely to use causal criteria such as automobile accidents, fires, falls, and industrial accidents. This duality of needs is given recognition in the International Classification of Diseases [426] which has two distinct classifications for accidents, poisonings, and violence—one based on the nature of the injury (the N code) and one based on the external cause (the E code). Such dual classificatory systems arise, obviously, in situations where classifications useful for one purpose are not useful for another. Neither is more correct or more "natural" than the other.

## Role of Epidemiologic Observations

The epidemiologist frequently has no alternative but to undertake studies based on manifestational entities and to hope that the manifestations have a strong enough tie to etiologic factors to allow the identification of these factors. The results of a successful study may reveal causal criteria around which revised groupings of ill persons could be made. Thus, disease classification is not only a prerequisite of epidemiologic study but also one of its goals.

Even in the absence of identification of direct causal factors, epidemiologic criteria may be used to classify, or subclassify, groups of persons with particular manifestational diseases. In some instances epidemiologic observations assist in identifying a subcategory of patients who also are found to be distinguishable on the basis of more refined manifestational criteria. For example, Caverly [48], describing an outbreak of paralytic disease in Vermont in the summer of 1894, included in his arguments for its being a separate disease (poliomyelitis) the season of the year during which the illness occurred. The classic distinction between typhus and typhoid fever by Lombard [207] was based on differences he observed between the disease he saw in Ireland and the one he saw in France and Switzerland. In addition to differences in postmortem findings, Lombard noted that the Irish disease (typhus) occasionally attacked breast-feeding infants and the elderly and frequently attacked nurses and those in attendance on the sick, whereas on the Continent infants on the breast and the elderly were never, and hospital attendants only rarely, attacked by the illness (typhoid). These differences attracted his attention to the existence of differences in the clinical manifestations of the two diseases which up to that point had not been noted.

Epidemiologic characteristics may be sufficient to justify separation of disease entities even in the absence of observed manifestational differences. For example, the 1909 edition of Osler's *Principles and Practice of Medicine* [304] describes an entity known as infectious jaundice, and notes that Weil had recently categorized a group of these cases (Weil's disease) because "the cases occurred in groups, and a very large proportion in butchers." This subgroup was subsequently shown to be caused by a specific spirochete. Other subgroups of the entity "infectious jaundice" that were identified on epidemiologic grounds, and prior to the isolation of specific causal agents, include infectious hepatitis and serum hepatitis.

Occasionally epidemiologic evidence suggests that two categories may usefully be merged—at least for the purpose of further investigation of etiology. For example, the similarity of behavior of anencephaly and spina bifida with respect to association with sex, socioeconomic status, ethnic group, and maternal age and parity, together with similarity in trends of frequency over time and the occurrence of both anomalies in the same sibships, provide a reasonable basis for considering them as one causal entity rather than two [228]. However, epidemiologic evidence has been less commonly brought forward to suggest that categories may usefully be merged than to suggest the separation of categories into subgroups. Furthermore, since as in the present example categories that might usefully be merged for the purpose of studying etiology may for the purposes of therapy be more usefully considered separately, such evidence does not ordinarily lead to revision of existing classifications.

## CLASSIFICATION OF DISEASE ENTITIES

Classification of ill persons into groups, whatever the criteria for their classification, and agreement as to the boundaries of the groups, are followed by the assignment of names to the groups. This results in a *nomenclature* of disease entities, or *nosology*. However arbitrary the processes leading to the nosology, agreement on some standard nomenclature is essential for communication between workers in a field.

Beyond this, there is also convenience in arranging the entities themselves into categories sharing similar features. Such an arrangement is referred to as a *classification* of disease. Unlike the creation of entities of disease, the process of disease classification has little immediate relevance to the practitioner of medicine. Its usefulness lies primarily in efforts to achieve standardization, and therefore comparability, in the methods of presentation of mortality and morbidity data from different sources.

An internationally accepted classification, now published by the World Health Organization, has been in use since 1900, and is presently in its eighth (1968) revision [426]. Originally designed for the purpose of classifying causes of death, its scope was expanded in the sixth (1948) revision to cover morbidity from illness and injury. An adaptation of the International Classification has been prepared by the U.S. National Center for Health Statistics [276]; it retains the structure of the International Classification but incorporates illnesses and syndromes not listed in the parent classification and is an attempt to satisfy both clinical and statistical needs. The classification of mental disorders recently published by the American Psychiatric Association [12] is compatible with the relevant section of the World Health Organization classification and in addition contains rough indications of the boundaries of the entities which it classifies.

# 5

## Measures of Disease Frequency

Statements of disease frequency in terms which permit comparisons between populations, or between subgroups within a population, are essential to epidemiology. In this chapter the most commonly used measures of frequency are described.

### RATES

In simplest terms a statement of frequency might be, "There were 500 cases of tuberculosis." Such a statement has little utility, however, until it is further qualified with respect to two features: (1) in what population were these cases observed, and (2) when were they observed. Thus the statement would gain needed specificity if it read, "On Jan. 1, 1970, in the population of this town there were 500 cases of tuberculosis." For administrative purposes such a measure of frequency might be entirely satisfactory. For example, information in this form would facilitate the planning of medical facilities for the tuberculous patients of the town, since basically such planning requires only knowledge of the number of cases.

If, however, the purpose of the frequency statement is to determine whether the inhabitants of one town have a greater or lesser probability of having tuberculosis than those of another, such a statement has obvious shortcomings. The second town may have more or fewer cases than the first simply because its population is larger or smaller. To allow for differences in population size, the frequencies must be expressed in the form of *rates*.

In epidemiologic usage, a rate is the frequency of a disease or characteristic expressed per unit of size of the population or group in which it is observed. The time at or during which the cases are observed is a further specification needed for epidemiologic purposes. Thus the tuberculosis frequency rate in a city on Jan. 1, 1970, might be expressed as 500 cases per 2,000,000 persons (the actual population of the city). In practice, to enable ready comparison, rates are expressed in terms of certain conventional units of population size—usually some multiple of ten. The tuberculosis rate in the city with 500 cases per 2,000,-000 might then be expressed as 0.025 per hundred, 0.25 per thousand, or 250 per million.

It is evident, therefore, that three items of information are necessary for a rate to have epidemiologic usefulness—the numerator of the fraction (the number of persons affected), the denominator (the population among whom the affected persons are observed), and a specification of time. The denominator is commonly called the *related* or *reference* population.

The numerator and denominator of a rate should be similarly restricted; if the numerator is confined to a certain age, sex, or racial group, the denominator should be similarly limited. For example, if the denominator population is the number of residents of a town, cases appearing in the numerator should also be limited to residents of that town. Similarly, if the numerator consists of the number of cases of a disease limited to females, the denominator would preferably be the related female population. When the denominator is restricted solely to those persons who are capable of having or contracting the disease, it is sometimes referred to as a population *at risk*.

The denominator of a rate may not be a population in the ordinary demographic sense. For example, a hospital may express its maternal mortality rate as the number of maternal deaths per thousand deliveries. The women delivered do not form a geographic population, but they do make up the group within which the deaths were observed, and it is customary to refer to such a group as a population. Similarly, the *case fatality rate* is the number of deaths due to a disease per so many patients with the disease; here the individuals with the disease constitute the observed population.

### Ratios

Certain measures, although sometimes loosely called rates, are more correctly called ratios. A common form of ratio expresses the number of affected persons relative to the number of unaffected persons and not relative to the total population (affected plus unaffected persons). For example, in the United States it is common to express the number of fetal deaths relative to the number of livebirths. This is called the *fetal death ratio* and should be distinguished from the *fetal death rate,* which is the number of fetal deaths expressed as a proportion of the related total births (livebirths plus fetal deaths). Ratios have the disadvantage of being less amenable than rates to treatment as probability statistics.

### Proportional Rates

Numbers of cases of a disease are sometimes expressed relative to the total number of cases of all diseases, rather than to the population. For example, the number of deaths ascribed to a particular disease may be expressed as a proportion of all deaths. This value is known as the *proportional mortality rate.* Similarly, in clinical studies the incidence of a disease is sometimes reported as the number of patients with that disease as a proportion of all patients seen at the same institution.

Such proportional rates do not, of course, express the risk of members of the population contracting or dying from the disease. Comparison of such rates between areas or between population subgroups may suggest that a difference exists that is worth investigating. But until rates can be computed against a population base, it will not be known whether the difference relates to differences in the sizes of the numerators or the denominators of the compared rates.

For example, Berman [29] noted that 91 percent of cancers seen in Bantu laborers in Witwatersrand gold mines were primary cancers of the liver. In this instance all cancers, rather than all diseases, were used as the denominator of the rate. Since the liver generally contributes only about 1 percent of cancers, it was inferred that the Bantus suffered an extraordinarily high rate of primary liver cancer. However, Gilliam [125] estimated population rates on the basis of the data given by Berman. The results, shown in Table 4, indicated that the Bantus do indeed

### Table 4
Mortality rates from cancer in Bantu mine workers and American Negroes*

|  | Mortality rate† | |
| --- | --- | --- |
| Site | Bantu | American Negro |
| Liver cancer | 12.7 | 3.0 |
| Other cancer | 1.3 | 61.5 |
| All cancer | 14.0 | 64.5 |

* From Gilliam [125].
† Rates are annual mortality rates per 100,000 population, and are not age-standardized.

have higher rates of liver cancer than American Negroes, but an even greater discrepancy existed with respect to the other cancers that, with the liver cancers, made up the denominators of the proportional percentages. Thus the proportional rates greatly overstated the difference in frequency of liver cancer and did not reveal the marked difference in the other sites.

A similar situation exists when the frequency of a disease is expressed in relation to the frequency of some other disease. For example, one sees many comparisons of the ratio of cases of cancer of the body of the uterus to cases of cancer of the cervix. Such comparisons may suggest that a difference exists between two populations, but they do not reveal which of the two diseases is unusually common or uncommon.

## DEFINITIONS OF MEASURES

### Incidence

The incidence of a disease is the number of cases of the disease which come into being during a specified period of time. The incidence *rate* is this number per specified unit of population.

In practice it is usually not possible to measure incidence directly, since the exact time of onset of an illness is uncertain. Instead, such occurrences as onset of symptoms, time of diagnosis, or date of notification or of hospitalization are used. It should be noted that incidence is the frequency of *events* during a period of time.

ATTACK RATE. Under certain circumstances, a population may be at risk of a disease for a limited period of time only. The limitation of the period of risk may be due to the fact that etiologic factors operate for only a short period of time, such as the duration of an epidemic, or to the fact that risk is restricted to certain age groups. In such circumstances it may be possible to express a total incidence that would remain the same even if the length of observation were increased. For example, many diseases are limited to infancy. Thus in a study of 194,000 liveborn infants, 578 developed hypertrophic pyloric stenosis [230]. Since this condition occurs predominantly in the first 3 months of life and is practically unknown over 6 months of age, a short observation period ensures the derivation of total incidence. The incidence of pyloric stenosis may therefore be expressed as $578 \times 1000/194,000$, or 3.0 per 1000 livebirths, without any specification of the duration of observation since it is understood that it exceeded the period during which the infants were at risk. Similarly if, during an outbreak of measles in a school of 400 boys, 60 developed the disease, the total incidence during the epidemic would be 15 percent.

This special form of incidence rate, in which there is a limited period of risk, is frequently called an attack rate.

A *secondary attack rate* is a measure in which the numerator consists of the number of cases of a disease which occur within the same household following the occurrence of a first, or primary, case. It is usually used in studies of infectious disease, and there is a stated or implied time limitation that, on the basis of the incubation period of the particular disease, indicates that the secondary cases probably derived from the primary case. For diseases conferring prolonged immunity, the denominator in a secondary attack rate usually excludes persons who have previously had the disease.

## Prevalence

*Point prevalence* of a disease is a census type of measure. It is the frequency of the disease at a designated point in time. Expressed for a specified population at a specified time, point prevalence *rate* is the proportion of that population which exhibits the disease at that particular time. The numerator includes all persons having the disease at the given moment, irrespective of the length of time which has elapsed from the beginning of the illness to the time when the point prevalence is measured. The denominator is the total population (affected and unaffected) within which the disease is ascertained. In contrast to incidence rates, which measure events, point prevalence rates are measures of what prevails or exists.

*Period prevalence* is a measure that expresses the total number of cases of a disease known to have existed at some time during a specified period. It is the sum of point prevalence (the number of cases existent at the beginning of the period) and incidence (the number of cases coming into existence during the period).

Period prevalence is of limited usefulness, since both the epidemiologist and the administrator will generally require knowledge of whether the cases being counted are new or old. Period prevalence data are therefore more useful when separated into their two components—point prevalence and incidence. For this reason period prevalence is not considered further in this text, and the word prevalence in subsequent sections refers to point prevalence.

### Death

Since rates of death measure the frequency of events, they resemble incidence rates in requiring specification of a period of time during which the deaths have been counted.

It is necessary to distinguish between two rates which deal with the frequency of death: (1) the disease-specific *death* or *mortality rate,* and (2) the disease-specific *case fatality rate.* Both have the same numerator—the number of persons dying of the disease during a stated period—but the denominators are different. In a mortality rate the denominator is the total population within which the deaths occurred, while in a case fatality rate it is restricted to persons with the disease. Thus the mortality rate expresses the frequency with which members of a general population die of the disease, while the case fatality rate expresses the frequency with which affected individuals die of the disease.

## EXAMPLES OF MEASURES

To illustrate some of the measures of disease frequency, use will be made of the data shown in Tables 5 and 6 on cases of leukemia in Brooklyn, New York, between 1948 and 1952 [223]. We shall assume that these represent all the cases of leukemia in the white population, which in 1950 numbered 2,525,000.

### Table 5

Data on patients with acute leukemia, Brooklyn, New York, whites, 1948–1952

| Year | (1) Patients alive at beginning of year | (2) New cases diagnosed in year | (3) Deaths in year | (4) Patients lost to trace |
|------|------|------|------|------|
| 1948 | 7 | 69 | 54 | 7 |
| 1949 | 15 | 91 | 86 | 3 |
| 1950 | 17 | 83 | 73 | 3 |
| 1951 | 24 | 99 | 101 | 1 |
| 1952 | 21 | 68 | 81 | 1 |
| *Total* | 84 | 410 | 395 | 15 |

### Table 6

Data on patients with chronic leukemia, Brooklyn, New York, whites, 1948–1952

| Year | (1) Patients alive at beginning of year | (2) New cases diagnosed in year | (3) Deaths in year | (4) Patients lost to trace |
|------|------|------|------|------|
| 1948 | 129 | 79 | 50 | 8 |
| 1949 | 150 | 83 | 71 | 5 |
| 1950 | 157 | 90 | 90 | 6 |
| 1951 | 151 | 61 | 84 | 7 |
| 1952 | 121 | 53 | 89 | 4 |
| *Total* | 708 | 366 | 384 | 30 |

PREVALENCE. Patients alive at the beginning of the year whose disease was diagnosed in a previous year (column 1) are in fact the cases of leukemia existent on Jan. 1 of each year. They form, therefore, estimates of prevalence. Prevalence rates can be derived by relating these numbers to the population. For acute leukemia (Table 5) the average prevalence for these five points in time is:

$$\frac{84}{5} \times \frac{10^6}{2,525,000} = 6.7 \text{ per million}$$

INCIDENCE. Time of diagnosis is used here as the basis for determining incidence. Incidence rates are derived from column 2. The 5-year incidence rate for acute leukemia is:

$$\frac{410 \times 10^6}{2,525,000} = 162.4 \text{ per million per 5 years}$$

Since incidence rates are usually expressed per annum, the 5-year rate is divided by 5 to derive an average annual incidence rate of 32.5 per million per year.

MORTALITY RATE. The mortality rate is derived from column 3. For acute leukemia the average annual death rate is:

$$\frac{395}{2,525,000} \times \frac{10^6}{5} = 31.3 \text{ per million per year}$$

These rates are shown in Table 7 for the two forms of leukemia.

Table 7

Measures of frequency of acute and chronic leukemia
derived from data in Tables 5 and 6

|  | Rates per million population | |
|---|---|---|
| Measure | Acute leukemia | Chronic leukemia |
| Prevalence | 6.7 | 56.1 |
| Incidence per annum | 32.5 | 29.0 |
| Death (mortality) per annum | 31.3 | 30.4 |

## INTERRELATION OF MEASURES

An important relation exists between prevalence and incidence. It may be expressed as follows:

*P varies as* the product of *I* and *D*

where *P* is prevalence, *I* is incidence, and *D* is the average duration of the disease from onset to termination, measured in the same time units used to specify the incidence. Duration of the disease is measured from the same point as that used to approximate its time of incidence (e.g., date of diagnosis) and prevalence likewise includes only cases existent at or subsequent to that point.

A change in prevalence from one period to another may be the result of changes in (1) incidence, (2) duration, or (3) both incidence and duration. For example, improvements in therapy, by preventing death but at the same time not producing recovery, may give rise to the apparently paradoxical effect of an increase in prevalence of the disease. And decrease in prevalence may result not only from decrease in incidence but also from a shortening of the duration of illness—through either more rapid recovery or more rapid death. Further, if duration decreased sufficiently, a decrease in prevalence could take place despite an increase in incidence. The recent decline in prevalence of in-patients in mental hospitals seems to be an example of the last phenomenon.

Note that prevalence was said to *vary with* the product of incidence and duration. In the theoretical circumstance that incidence and duration remained constant over time, the disease is said to be stable and the relation between prevalence, incidence, and duration would be such that

*P equals* the product of *I* and *D*

Given two of the values in this equation, it is possible to compute the third. For example, from the estimates of prevalence and incidence of leukemia in Table 7 the average duration of the disease can be calculated from the relationship $D = P/I$.

$$\text{For acute leukemia: } D = \frac{6.7}{32.5} = 0.21 \text{ years} = 2.5 \text{ months}$$

$$\text{For chronic leukemia: } D = \frac{56.1}{29.0} = 1.93 \text{ years} = 23 \text{ months}$$

These are close to the values of 2.4 months for acute leukemia and 20 months for chronic leukemia derived independently from special follow-up studies of the same patients. These durations represent the interval between diagnosis and death, since incidence here was based on date of diagnosis. Note that these data relate to a time preceding the widespread use of antileukemic drugs.

The requirements of "stability" for a disease include constancy of incidence for a period corresponding to the longest duration of the disease in an individual, and constancy of the distribution of cases by duration of illness. Calculation of one component of the equation from observed values for the other two should be made with the knowledge that the result will be an approximation, since the conditions for stability are never fully met. If the formula is applied to a disease which is not stable but has increasing or decreasing incidence, the estimates of duration will be lower or higher, respectively, than the true values.

Another relation that exists if the disease is stable—or nearly so—is between incidence ($I$) and mortality ($M$), from which the case fatality rate ($F$) may be estimated:

$$F = \frac{M}{I}$$

Thus, for acute leukemia (see Table 7), $F = 31.3/32.5 = 0.96$, or 96 percent; for chronic leukemia, $F = 30.4/29.0 = 1.05$, or 105 percent. The findings are consistent with the knowledge that both forms of leukemia are invariably fatal. An additional requirement for stability in this situation is that the proportion of patients with various possible outcomes—e.g., death or recovery—must also be constant.

## SPECIFICATION OF TIME

We have shown that specification of time is essential for both prevalence and incidence rates. In the former it is a point in time *at* which the observations are made; in the latter it is a period *during* which events are counted. So far we have spoken of time as if calendar time were necessarily implied. Actually there are several ways of specifying time.

### Calendar Time

If one wished to estimate the incidence of coronary occlusion, one could count all cases of coronary occlusion occurring between Jan. 1 and Dec. 31 of a particular year, and relate this number to the population at the middle of the year, to derive an annual incidence rate. This is the most common way of specifying the beginning and end of a period of observation.

Similarly, it is common practice to measure prevalence at a point in calendar time. National censuses, for example, which measure the prevalence of people, refer to a specified date.

### Age

A second way to specify time is by using chronologic age of the population. Chronologic age is commonly used in situations in which there is interest in a disease occurring shortly after birth. For example, suppose that in a maternity hospital over a certain period of time there were 2000 deliveries of liveborn children, 22 of whom died in the first week after birth. The death rate in the first week of life may then be expressed as 11 per 1000 livebirths. Not all these children were observed during the same period in calendar time, and it does not matter for this purpose whether the 2000 births occurred over a period of 1 year or 10 years. The period of observation is specified as beginning at a certain age (birth) and continuing for 7 days thereafter.

In the case of prevalence data, an example of the use of chronologic age in specifying time would be a statement that, by age 10 years, 20 percent of a certain population are tuberculin positive.

A rate may be expressed as if it were defined in terms of chronologic age, while in truth this is not entirely the case. In the neonatal mortality example just given, the hospital might have been able actually to observe each of the infants born for a period of 7 days and to include in the numerator of the rate only those deaths occurring in the denominator population. However, this is commonly not possible. For example, in an infant mortality rate (death rate of infants less than 1 year of age), this would necessitate observation of the denominator population for a full year. Thus it is usual to express the infant mortality rate as:

$$\frac{\text{Number of deaths of infants aged less than 1 year}}{\text{Number of livebirths during the same year}} \times 1000$$

The assumption is that the number of livebirths that occurred during the period in which the deaths were observed is the same as the number of livebirths that was the source of the infant deaths.

Again with the proviso that the disease is stable, the theoretical relation, $P = ID$, holds whether time is specified in the form of age or calendar time. In the situation where age is the point of reference, this means that neither incidence nor duration changes with age. Since changes in incidence with age are usually marked, calculations from the formula would be of little value. However, the general principle that prevalence is a function of incidence and duration remains the same, prevalence at a specified age depending on incidence at younger ages and the duration of incident cases. For example, although rates of congenital malformations expressed per thousand births are frequently thought of as incidence rates, they are in fact prevalence rates, since they depend on the frequency of existence of certain states at a specified age (birth). The events which might be used to determine incidence rates occurred at least 6 months before birth. What such a rate is called is of less concern than the realization that it has the characteristics of a prevalence rate in being influenced by both incidence and duration. In the case of congenital malformation, an important determinant of duration is survival of the fetus. Differences in the frequency with which congenitally malformed fetuses die and are aborted without being counted will produce differences in the prevalence of congenital malformations at birth, even though the incidence of malformation remains constant.

## Other Ways of Specifying Time

Without direct reference to either age or calendar time, the occurrence of some circumstance may be used to time the point at which an observation is made or a period of observation is begun. For example, one can measure the prevalence of certain serologic findings at the time of premarital examination, or the incidence of psychotic reactions occurring within a specified period after childbirth. The time of the premarital test or the delivery are the points which define the observations in time, and these need not occur at any specified point in age or calendar time.

Case fatality rates and disease complication rates are also of this nature, the time of observation beginning when the disease is diagnosed, regardless of the calendar time or age of the affected individual. There may, of course, be specification of age or calendar time in addition, if these are relevant variables, but they are not the characteristics which define the onset of the observation period.

Similarly, we can speak of the prevalence of impairments among military inductees or among school entrants, or the incidence of certain disabilities within a specified period following retirement. Although age is highly related to these circumstances, it is not the defining element.

## OTHER SPECIFICATIONS

The general type of event which goes into the numerator of incidence rates—onset of illness—deserves further consideration.

When expressed as a rate, incidence (unlike prevalence) is not necessarily a fraction of the population. The numerator may be made up of cases or attacks rather than individuals, since in some illnesses, such as acute alcoholic delirium or the common cold, some individuals may experience more than one attack during the period of observation. In such a circumstance the rate describes the risk of episodes of the illness occurring among the population rather than the risk of individuals becoming ill. It would seem preferable, for epidemiologic purposes, to reduce the numerator to individuals, so that a probability of individuals having one or more attacks during the interval might be expressed. Further subdivision into risks of having one, two, three, . . . attacks during the period are useful in identifying and describing groups of individuals who have an abnormal frequency of attack.

In addition, although attacked only once during the period of observation, some individuals may be experiencing a recurrence of an illness such as reactive depression, their initial attack having occurred several years before the period. Under this condition an incidence rate expresses the risk of individuals having an attack during the period of interest, whereas it would usually be more helpful to an understanding of basic causal mechanisms to identify those individuals having their initial episode of illness during the period.

The denominators of incidence rates may also be limited to specific components of a population under observation. For example, if the denominators of incidence rates contain people who are not at risk of contracting the disease, important epidemiologic differences between rates may be obscured. Thus, in those infectious diseases in which an attack confers permanent immunity, the majority of a specified population may not be at risk because of past encounter with the disease. As already noted, for this reason the denominator in a secondary attack rate excludes previously affected persons when the disease is one for which immunity follows a first attack. An analogous situation may exist in common chronic or relapsing diseases of long duration where the denominator may contain an appreciable proportion of persons who are either currently ill with the disease or have had it in the past and are therefore not at risk of having an initial attack. Ideally an incidence rate would have its population base confined to those persons who have not in the past had and do not presently have the disease under study, but this is a refinement which has not been commonly practiced, and which in fact may be ignored without serious error unless the proportion of such persons in the population is large.

## SELECTION OF MEASURES

A variety of rates have been described which are related to the frequency of a disease in a population. The utility of one rather than another is dependent on the problem under study.

### Incidence

Attempts at elucidation of causal factors focus on explaining the occurrence of illness, and the measure most descriptive of this occurrence is the incidence rate. Causal factors necessarily operate prior to the onset of disease, and the closer in time that the stage of disease at which incidence is measured comes to the time of actual onset, the more directly will the measure be influenced by the operation of causal factors. For these reasons, incidence measured as early in the disease as practicable is the measure of frequency most useful to studies of causal factors.

Because of their ready availability, death rates are sometimes used as indices of incidence. Routine registration of deaths together with specification of cause of death enables death rates to be derived for many diseases and among many populations for which more direct measures of incidence are not available. Death rates are most reliable as indices of incidence rates when the interval between incidence and death is short and when the disease has a high case fatality rate.

### Prevalence

For epidemiologic purposes prevalence measurements are inferior to incidence, since two sets of factors determine them: those connected with the occurrence of cases, and those connected with course and duration of the cases once established. There would appear to be a better chance of identifying causal factors by separate investigation of incidence rates and prognosis. When incidence data are unobtainable, patterns in prevalence rates may give clues to variations in incidence rates, but the contribution of duration to prevalence must constantly be borne in mind.

The main value of prevalence rates is in administrative situations requiring knowledge of how many patients with a given disease exist in the community. Incidence rates are of uncertain value in these situations, since for a given incidence rate diseases of long duration often impose a greater burden on the community than those of short duration. Here too, however, knowledge of incidence rates is important when facilities for new cases differ from those for patients who do not recover within a short period of time.

# 6

## Sources of Data

During the course of an individual's life, many records are created which contain information relevant to his health status. These include documents required for legal purposes, as well as records designed primarily for medical reasons. Some of the documents are used by governmental and other agencies as the source of information on the frequency of disease in the population. The published tabulations allow the health of the population to be monitored, and also provide the descriptive information used in the formation and evaluation of epidemiologic hypotheses. In addition, information from the primary documents is frequently used in hypothesis-testing epidemiologic studies [260].

In this chapter we will describe the principal sources of epidemiologic data and the kinds of analyses for which they are used. Both the sources and the analyses vary considerably from one country to another. While this discussion will deal primarily with the situation in the United States, the description of the strengths and weaknesses of particular sources of data is widely applicable to similar sources in other countries.

In introducing *Natural and Political Observations . . . on the Bills of Mortality* in 1662 (see p. 6), Graunt [134] described some of the uses to which the Bills were put by the families that subscribed to them. These included looking to see whether the burials had increased or decreased over the previous week, searching for unusual or interesting events that might form a topic of conversation at the next social gathering, and watching for the rise or decline of the plague—"so the Rich might judge of the necessity of their removal, and Trades-men might conjecture what doings they were like to have in their . . . dealings." Greenwood [135] suggests also that the published figures provided a resource for a 17th century numbers game.

By making epidemiologic use of documents produced for other purposes, Graunt established a lasting tradition. Indeed, until 20 or 30 years ago, all the regular sources of epidemiologic data were produced for other purposes. Certificates of birth and death and census data served legal purposes primarily. Systems of disease notification and registration were introduced for control, rather than investigation. In recent decades, with the recognition of the usefulness of information on the health of populations, existing sources of data have been modified and new data sources established to serve epidemiologic purposes primarily.


## VITAL RECORDS

Vital records are the certificates of birth, death, marriage, and divorce required for legal and demographic purposes in most industrialized countries. In the United States the content of these records is determined by the individual states and certain independent registration cities, although most areas follow closely the Standard Certificates developed by the National Center for Health Statistics of the U.S. Public Health Service after consultation with registration authorities. For an account of the content of the present certificates of birth, death, and fetal death in the U.S., and of how this has varied over the years, the reader is referred to a recent publication of the National Center for Health Statistics [137].

The registration states and cities in the United States are responsible for registration procedures and maintenance of records. On the other hand, while most states prepare tabulations for their own purposes, the detailed tabulation and analysis of data from vital records is predominantly a function of the federal National Center for Health Statistics.

## Death Certificates

The introduction of death registration was the foundation of modern epidemiology; it changed the subject from a narrative discipline into a quantitative science. The roles of Graunt and Farr in this change were referred to in Chapter 1. Even today, changes in the death rate may give the first indication of epidemic conditions (see Fig. 1, p. 4), and cause-specific death rates are the single most useful source of information on the distribution of many diseases. The mortality rate from a particular disease is, of course, a result of the case fatality rate of the disease as well as its incidence. The fact that death rates are most reliable as indices of disease occurrence when the interval between incidence and death is short and the case fatality rate of the disease is high (see Chap. 5) applies whether one is estimating the total disease frequency or attempting to interpret a change over time in the distribution of a disease in the population.

COMPLETENESS OF DEATH REGISTRATION. Insofar as recording the fact of death is concerned, death registration is virtually complete in North American and European countries. This is not the case, however, in most areas of the world, and differences in completeness of registration must be considered when evaluating statistics based on death certificates. Even in countries in which levels of registration are generally high, it may be deficient in small, ethnically or culturally isolated groups.

In considering United States data it may also be necessary to consider that satisfactory levels of registration were achieved by the different states at different times. Admission to the National Death Registration Area—the geographic area for which mortality data are published by the federal government—has been dependent upon satisfactory levels of registration, and consequently the area for which statistics have been published has varied from time to time. At its formation in 1880 the Death Registration Area included only two states, Massachusetts and New Jersey. The Area became complete, that is, comprised all the then-existent states, only in 1933, with the inclusion of

Texas. Since death rates vary from state to state, as well as from time to time, these changes in the Registration Area must be considered in the interpretation of time trends. Trends for the years between 1900 and 1933 are most accurately determined by restriction of data to the 10 states which provided acceptable data throughout that period.

CAUSE OF DEATH.    Unlike *fact* of death, *cause* of death as recorded on death certificates cannot be accepted without question. Ascertainment of cause of death is a problem enmeshed in concepts of what constitutes a cause, adequacy of diagnostic acumen, classification of disease, and other questions that have much broader implications than the interpretation of death certificates. In addition, in the present context, is the question of how much of what the certifying physician knows is recorded on the certificate. Autopsy findings, for example, usually do not enter into the cause as recorded on the certificate—at least in the United States—since the certificate is usually completed prior to the autopsy and not amended in the light of the later findings. The certifying physician may in some instances not be the attending physician, and there may be lack of communication between the two [262].

A number of ad hoc studies [8, 154, 178, 182, 217, 261, 262, 264] have been undertaken in several countries in order to evaluate the diagnostic basis of the certified cause and the correspondence between the certified cause and the opinion of the medical informant. These studies indicate that blanket evaluations cannot be made. Some diseases—for example, most cancers —are recorded on a very high proportion of certificates if they are present at death. Others—for example, diabetes, hypertension, and pneumonia—are not, even if there is a reasonable basis for believing that they contributed to the death. The accuracy of diagnosis appearing on the death certificate may vary not only with the specific diagnosis, but with the age and sex of the decedent, the area of the body affected by the disease, and the specific wording on the certificate [217]. With respect to cardiovascular disease, in which significant diagnostic problems might be expected to exist, Moriyama et al., on the basis of questionnaires to certifying physicians and others with knowledge of the case, estimated [262] that the classification of deaths as due to cardiovascular disease was a "reasonable inference" in 70 to 75 percent of the deaths so classified.

MULTIPLE CAUSES OF DEATH. The 1968 U.S. Standard Certificate of Death is shown in Figure 4. It is apparent that more than one diagnosis may be entered in the section dealing with cause of death. The physician may, for example, specify pneumonia as the immediate cause on line 18(a), listing cerebral hemorrhage and hypertension on lines 18(b) and (c), and diabetes in Part II (other significant conditions). Two or more diagnoses appear on 58 percent of United States certificates [262]. However, practically all published statistics deal with deaths as if each person died of but one disease. Clearly this detracts from the value of the tabulations prepared from the certificates. Moreover, since changes have occurred in the manner of selecting the single cause to be tabulated, comparability of statistics over time and between countries is impaired.

For many years it was customary to select diagnoses for tabulations on the basis of arbitrary rules [286]; thus a certificate mentioning both heart disease and diabetes mellitus was automatically assigned to diabetes, even though the certifying physician might have considered heart disease the underlying cause of death and diabetes only a coincident condition. Following the recommendations of various international bodies, Great Britain in 1940 and the United States in 1949 began assigning certificates bearing multiple causes on the basis of the certifying physician's opinion as to the underlying cause of death. This change had a marked effect on the statistics of some diseases. For example, diabetes mellitus showed an abrupt decline of between 30 and 50 percent in the number of assigned deaths. Studies have been undertaken of the effect of these changes in trends for various causes of death [110, 288, 340].

Dorn [88, 89] and Guralnick [140] have discussed the issues in tabulating multiple causes of death, and an evaluation of the content of U.S. certificates—particularly with respect to deaths from cardiovascular disease, in which the problem is especially serious—has been undertaken by Krueger [193]. Other recent ad hoc studies are those of Markush [240] and Cohen and Steinitz [60]. Computers would now appear to make practicable the preparation of multiple-cause tabulations on a regular basis,

FORM APPROVED
BUDGET BUREAU NO. .68—R1901

U.S. GOVERNMENT PRINTING OFFICE : 1967 OF—241-661

(PHYSICIAN)
U.S. STANDARD
CERTIFICATE OF DEATH

TYPE, OR PRINT IN
**PERMANENT INK**
SEE HANDBOOK FOR
INSTRUCTIONS

LOCAL FILE NUMBER

STATE FILE NUMBER

**DECEASED**

1. DECEASED—NAME — FIRST | MIDDLE | LAST

2. SEX
3. DATE OF DEATH ( MONTH, DAY, YEAR )

4. RACE WHITE, NEGRO, AMERICAN INDIAN, ETC. ( SPECIFY )
5a. AGE—LAST BIRTHDAY (YEARS)
5b. UNDER 1 YEAR — MOS. | DAYS
5c. UNDER 1 DAY — HOURS | MIN.
6. DATE OF BIRTH (MONTH, DAY, YEAR )

7a. CITY, TOWN, OR LOCATION OF DEATH
7b. INSIDE CITY LIMITS ( SPECIFY YES OR NO )
7c. COUNTY OF DEATH
7d. HOSPITAL OR OTHER INSTITUTION—NAME (IF NOT IN EITHER, GIVE STREET AND NUMBER )

8. STATE OF BIRTH ( IF NOT IN U.S.A., NAME COUNTRY )
9. CITIZEN OF WHAT COUNTRY
10. MARRIED, NEVER MARRIED, WIDOWED, DIVORCED ( SPECIFY )
11. SURVIVING SPOUSE (IF WIFE, GIVE MAIDEN NAME )

USUAL RESIDENCE
WHERE DECEASED LIVED. IF DEATH OCCURRED IN INSTITUTION, GIVE RESIDENCE BEFORE ADMISSION.

12. SOCIAL SECURITY NUMBER
13a. USUAL OCCUPATION ( GIVE KIND OF WORK DONE DURING MOST OF WORKING LIFE, EVEN IF RETIRED )
13b. KIND OF BUSINESS OR INDUSTRY

14a. RESIDENCE—STATE
14b. COUNTY
14c. CITY, TOWN, OR LOCATION
14d. INSIDE CITY LIMITS ( SPECIFY YES OR NO )
14e. STREET AND NUMBER

**PARENTS**

15. FATHER—NAME — FIRST | MIDDLE | LAST

16. MOTHER—MAIDEN NAME — FIRST | MIDDLE | LAST

17a. INFORMANT—NAME
17b. MAILING ADDRESS (STREET OR R.F.D. NO., CITY OR TOWN, STATE, ZIP)

**CAUSE**

PART I. DEATH WAS CAUSED BY: [ENTER ONLY ONE CAUSE PER LINE FOR (a), (b), AND (c)]

APPROXIMATE INTERVAL BETWEEN ONSET AND DEATH

IMMEDIATE CAUSE (a)
DUE TO, OR AS A CONSEQUENCE OF:

CONDITIONS, IF ANY, WHICH GAVE RISE TO IMMEDIATE CAUSE (a), STATING THE UNDER-LYING CAUSE LAST
(b)
DUE TO, OR AS A CONSEQUENCE OF:
(c)

PART II. OTHER SIGNIFICANT CONDITIONS: CONDITIONS CONTRIBUTING TO DEATH BUT NOT RELATED TO CAUSE GIVEN IN PART I (a)

AUTOPSY ( YES OR NO)
IF YES WERE FINDINGS CONSIDERED IN DETERMINING CAUSE OF DEATH

AND WELFARE—PUBLIC HEALTH SERVICE—NATIONAL CENTER FOR HEALTH STATISTICS
1968 REVISION

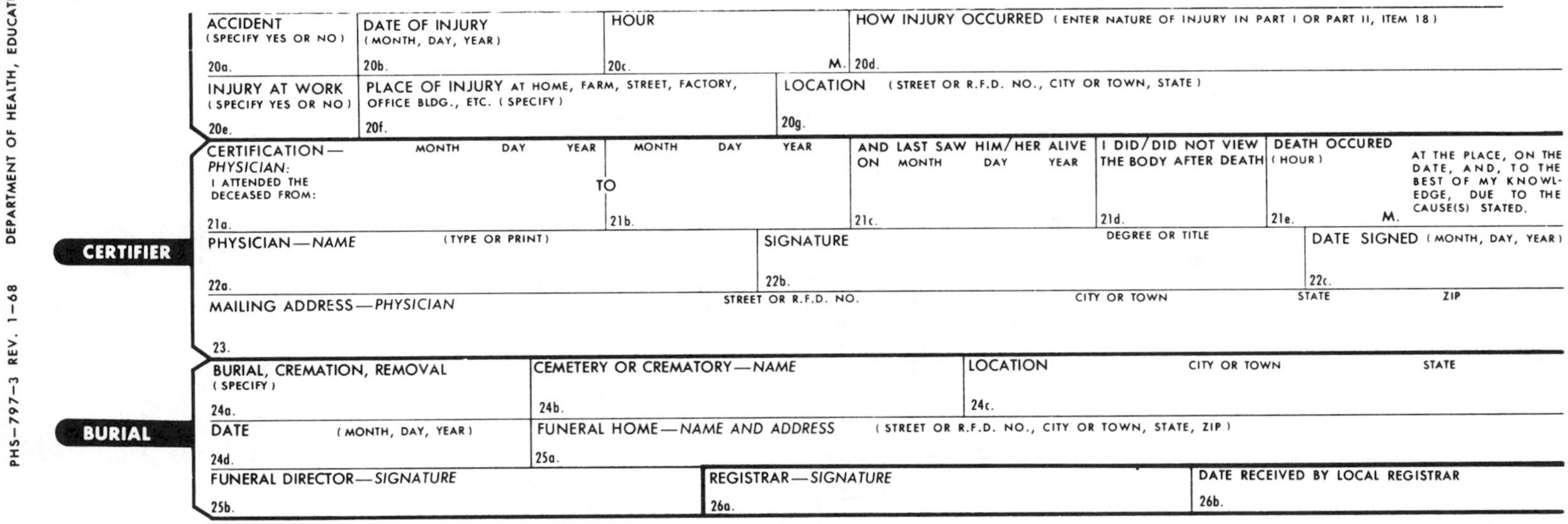

PHS–797–3 REV. 1–68 DEPARTMENT OF HEALTH, EDUCATION

ACCIDENT (SPECIFY YES OR NO) 20a. | DATE OF INJURY (MONTH, DAY, YEAR) 20b. | HOUR 20c. M. | HOW INJURY OCCURRED (ENTER NATURE OF INJURY IN PART I OR PART II, ITEM 18) 20d.

INJURY AT WORK (SPECIFY YES OR NO) 20e. | PLACE OF INJURY AT HOME, FARM, STREET, FACTORY, OFFICE BLDG., ETC. (SPECIFY) 20f. | LOCATION (STREET OR R.F.D. NO., CITY OR TOWN, STATE) 20g.

CERTIFIER

CERTIFICATION—*PHYSICIAN:* I ATTENDED THE DECEASED FROM: MONTH DAY YEAR 21a. TO MONTH DAY YEAR 21b. | AND LAST SAW HIM/HER ALIVE ON MONTH DAY YEAR 21c. | I DID/DID NOT VIEW THE BODY AFTER DEATH 21d. | DEATH OCCURED (HOUR) 21e. M. AT THE PLACE, ON THE DATE, AND, TO THE BEST OF MY KNOWLEDGE, DUE TO THE CAUSE(S) STATED.

PHYSICIAN—*NAME* (TYPE OR PRINT) 22a. | SIGNATURE DEGREE OR TITLE 22b. | DATE SIGNED (MONTH, DAY, YEAR) 22c.

MAILING ADDRESS—*PHYSICIAN* STREET OR R.F.D. NO. CITY OR TOWN STATE ZIP 23.

BURIAL

BURIAL, CREMATION, REMOVAL (SPECIFY) 24a. | CEMETERY OR CREMATORY—*NAME* 24b. | LOCATION CITY OR TOWN STATE 24c.

DATE (MONTH, DAY, YEAR) 24d. | FUNERAL HOME—*NAME AND ADDRESS* (STREET OR R.F.D. NO., CITY OR TOWN, STATE, ZIP) 25a.

FUNERAL DIRECTOR—*SIGNATURE* 25b. | REGISTRAR—*SIGNATURE* 26a. | DATE RECEIVED BY LOCAL REGISTRAR 26b.

Figure 4

The U.S. Standard Certificate of Death, as recommended by the National Center for Health Statistics, 1968.

but this has not yet been attempted. If it is achieved, a major effort will be required to interpret the data.

CHANGES IN THE INTERNATIONAL CLASSIFICATION. The successive revisions of the International Classification of Diseases (see p. 54), an internationally accepted guide for classification and coding of causes of death, may profoundly influence the apparent trends of mortality of certain diseases as reported in published material. This is particularly true with respect to the Sixth Revision in 1948 [421]. Changes attributable to such revisions are usually easily identified by noting the abruptness of the changes and their coincidence with institution of the revisions. Ascertaining the amount of change due to the revisions is less easy, although there have been special studies of their effects on various causes of death [95, 270, 273, 288, 406, 423].

USE OF TOTAL DEATH RATE. In investigating disease etiology, epidemiologists are usually concerned with specific diseases, and the above discussion has focused on the use of cause-specific death rates to draw inferences about the frequency of individual diseases. Sometimes, however, trends in the total numbers of deaths, or in death rates without respect to cause, may be more revealing than cause-specific rates. For example, the total impact of a noxious agent may be underestimated if attention is restricted to deaths ascribed to specified pathologic conditions. During the London fog of 1952, referred to in Chapter 1, all major causes of death, except automobile accidents, showed an increase in frequency (Table 8). This episode focused attention on the value of observing excess total deaths—the number of deaths over and above those which would have been expected on the basis of the usual level of the death rate in the population under observation. This index has on several occasions shown the consequences of influenza epidemics whose total impact would otherwise have been underestimated. For example, Figure 5 shows the number of deaths per week in 122 cities in the United States during the epidemic of "Hong Kong" influenza of 1968-1969. At the peak of this epidemic (in the week ending Jan. 11, 1969) the number of deaths attributed to influenza and pneumonia in these cities was approximately 1200 greater than that reported during nonepidemic times. Yet Figure 5 suggests

## Table 8

Numbers of deaths assigned to various causes, London
Administrative County: Weeks ended November 29
to December 27, 1952*

| | Week ended | | | | |
|---|---|---|---|---|---|
| Cause of death | 29 Nov. | 6 Dec. | 13 Dec.† | 20 Dec. | 27 Dec. |
| Respiratory tuberculosis | 19 | 14 | 77 | 37 | 21 |
| Cancer of lung | 27 | 45 | 69 | 32 | 36 |
| Vascular lesions of central nervous system | 98 | 102 | 128 | 119 | 91 |
| Coronary disease | 131 | 118 | 281 | 152 | 109 |
| Myocardial degeneration | 79 | 88 | 244 | 131 | 108 |
| Influenza | 7 | 2 | 24 | 9 | 6 |
| Pneumonia‡ | 28 | 45 | 168 | 125 | 91 |
| Bronchitis | 73 | 74 | 704 | 396 | 184 |
| Other respiratory diseases | 8 | 9 | 52 | 21 | 13 |
| Motor vehicle accidents | 1 | 8 | 4 | 10 | 4 |
| Suicide | 5 | 10 | 10 | 7 | 5 |
| Other causes | 377 | 430 | 723 | 484 | 361 |
| *Total* (all causes) | 853 | 945 | 2484 | 1523 | 1029 |

* From a Report of the Ministry of Health [257].
† The fog covered the period Dec. 5–8, and the week ending Dec. 13 was the week of heaviest mortality.
‡ Excluding deaths at ages under 4 weeks.

that the total number of deaths in this week was more than 4000 greater than that in weeks preceding and succeeding the epidemic.

A further reason for monitoring total deaths is that reports can often be made without the delays involved in coding and tabulating cause-specific data. Noting an increase in the over-all death rate may thus provide the first warning of the existence of a situation requiring control measures.

### Birth Certificates

Until recently the predominant epidemiologic purpose served by birth certificates was to provide denominators (number of livebirths) for the computation of rates of diseases of infancy. The great variation that may occur from year to year in the number of births (Fig. 6) points to the importance of such denominator information, not only with respect to diseases of in-

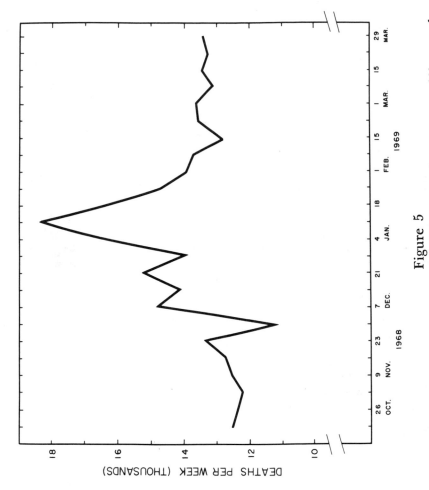

Figure 5

Total deaths in 122 U.S. cities by week, from week ending Oct. 19, 1968, to week ending Mar. 29, 1969. (From *Morbidity and Mortality Weekly Reports* [284].)

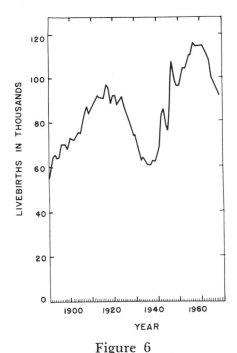

Figure 6

Annual number of livebirths in Massachusetts, 1890 to 1968. (Provisional figures for recent years.) (From *Annual Reports* [67].)

fancy but for use in predicting changes in the size of various age groups in the population as the birth-cohorts age.

Recent requirements that birth certificates include information on complications of the pregnancy and abnormalities of the infant, as well as highly pertinent characteristics such as birth weight of the child, duration of the pregnancy, and duration of education and blood group of the mother, make birth certificates an increasingly valuable source of information on diseases of pregnancy and childhood.

Many studies of the distribution of congenital malformations have utilized information from birth certificates [109, 128]. In the United States, birth certificates in certain states provide reasonably good information on severe malformations of unequivocal diagnosis, but they are still inadequate for surveillance of congenital malformations as a whole, even those obvious at birth. Maternal complications of pregnancy are even less well

*83*

reported. On the other hand, population variations in the distribution of infant weight and of multiple births are problems on which a great deal of knowledge has been gained from studies utilizing birth certificate information.

### Certificates of Fetal Death

In most countries with well-developed registration procedures, fetal deaths are legally required to be certified. In Great Britain certification is required for all deaths after the 28th week of gestation and probably has presented a reasonably complete picture of fetal mortality in the later months of pregnancy for several decades. In the United States, certificates are required in most jurisdictions for deaths after the 20th week, and in some areas for all fetal deaths regardless of the length of gestation. Completeness of reporting falls off markedly for deaths in the early months of pregnancy, and varies considerably by time, geographic area, and population group. Statistics based on such certificates are therefore notoriously unreliable. Further, the general difficulties of determining cause of death in instances of fetal death are reflected in the unsatisfactory nature of the diagnostic information recorded on fetal death certificates. Nevertheless, where certification is reasonably complete, as in Britain, analyses of fetal death reports have enabled useful studies of anomalies, such as anencephaly, for which information based only on livebirths would not be adequate [103].

The United Nations has published a review [405] of the definitions and reporting of fetal deaths in many countries, with information as to completeness and accuracy of reporting.

### Reporting of Vital Statistics

Analyses of vital records are published annually by most countries. The most widely used are probably *The Registrar General's Statistical Review of England and Wales* [343] and *Vital Statistics of the United States* [278]. Valuable summaries of U.S. data for the periods 1900 to 1940 and 1940 to 1960 have been published separately [138, 205]. The United Nations Demographic Yearbook, in addition to regular tabulations of data from many countries, selects a special topic for detailed presentation each year. Special presentations were given on mortality in 1967 [403] and on natality in 1965 [402].

Since there is usually a delay of one or more years between the events that are being reported and the appearance of the published annual report, attempts have been made to provide more rapid publication of preliminary data. In its *Monthly Vital Statistics Report* [279] the National Center for Health Statistics publishes provisional statistics on births and deaths current to within two or three months of the publication. The National Communicable Disease Center's *Morbidity and Mortality Weekly Report* [284] includes, in addition to reports of notifiable diseases and comments on infectious diseases currently epidemic, preliminary data on deaths in 122 selected cities during the previous week. Local communities may also attempt to monitor deaths closely, especially when episodes of atmospheric pollution or epidemics of influenza or other infectious diseases are anticipated [211].

In its *World Health Statistics Report* [427] the World Health Organization publishes, for selected countries with satisfactory levels of registration, periodic data on mortality and on births, as well as reports of notifiable diseases and periodic analyses of special problems.


## MORBIDITY SURVEYS

### U.S. National Health Survey

The National Health Survey was established in 1956, and has provided data on the health of the U.S. population continuously from 1957. A Subcommittee of the U.S. National Committee on Vital and Health Statistics, in recommending the creation of a National Morbidity Survey in 1953 [281], envisioned the following uses for such data:


1. To guide administrative planning and evaluation of public and voluntary health programs
2. To facilitate estimations of needs for medical and dental services, facilities, and personnel
3. To suggest and test hypotheses and to provide other aids to medical research
4. To provide information relevant to consideration of military and civilian manpower needs and capabilities

5. To facilitate estimation of needs for medications and medical appliances

6. To provide statistics for public health education programs

The National Health Survey is in fact an extensive program of different surveys, organized within the National Center for Health Statistics. It has three major components:

1. *The Health Interview Survey.* This is a continuous survey in which individuals in some 40,000 different households (approximately 120,000 individuals) are interviewed each year [269]. The sample is selected in such a way that each week data are obtained from a small random sample of the population. Thus short-term trends can be followed closely, as illustrated in Figure 7 by data collected during the 1957 influenza epidemic.

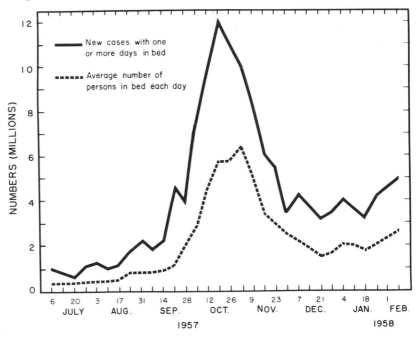

Figure 7

Weekly incidence and prevalence estimates of bed disability due to acute respiratory disease in the United States, Jul. 6, 1957, to Feb. 8, 1958. (From Linder [204].)

In addition, the data can be accumulated by month or year for more detailed tabulations. The questionnaire contains a core of questions relating to current or recent acute illness and injury, as well as questions eliciting information on chronic illness and disability. In addition to inquiries about illness per se, important information is obtained on the extent of disability associated with it. This is measured in terms of work loss, school days loss, bed disability, etc. Items of special interest, such as questions on medical x-ray exposure or smoking habits, are added from time to time.

A major limitation of the Health Interview Survey is that the diagnostic information is that given by the respondent—there is no attempt to obtain confirmation from medical sources. While this may not jeopardize use of the statistics for many purposes, it is an important restriction on their use for epidemiologic studies.

2. *The Health Examination Survey.* The Health Examination Survey was planned as a series of cycles, in each of which data would be collected on a sample of a particular segment of the population. The data comprise the historical information collected in the Health Interview Survey as well as the results of physical examination and measurements such as blood pressure, electrocardiogram, hearing and visual acuity, and blood chemistry. The first cycle, completed in 1962, covered adults 18 to 79 years of age; approximately 6700 were examined [271]. The second cycle, during 1963 to 1965, covered 7100 children between 6 and 11 years of age [272], and the third cycle, during 1966 to 1970, deals with youths 12 to 17 years of age [275]. The high levels of cooperation attained and the care taken in the standardization of methods make the data from these surveys very valuable from an epidemiologic point of view. Limitations on epidemiologic usefulness stem from the fact that prevalence, rather than incidence, is measured and that the sample sizes are such as to allow analyses for only the most frequent diseases and abnormalities.

3. *The Health Records Survey.* This was designed to supplement findings of the Health Interview and Health Examination Surveys, primarily by sampling records of institutions such as hospitals, nursing homes, and homes for the aged, since samples

for the interview and examination surveys exclude the institutional population. However, a rather broad program of surveys has developed in which vital and medical records are used and sometimes supplemented by questionnaires to patients and physicians. In addition to surveys of institutions and of patients discharged from hospital, there has been a National Natality and Mortality Survey in which mail inquiries were made of mothers of carefully selected samples of newborn infants and of infants who died. This survey has yielded national data on fertility and infant mortality in relation to socioeconomic status, education, and prior reproductive experience of the mother.

Analyses of data from the National Health Survey are published periodically in several series of monographs [280]. A flavor of the variety of these analyses is conveyed by the titles listed in Table 9. Highlights of health survey findings are frequently summarized in the *Monthly Vital Statistics Report,* and annual summaries are published in the monograph series.

*Other General Morbidity Surveys*

The recency, representativeness, and comprehensiveness of the data from the National Health Survey have reduced to primarily historical interest several previous attempts to assess morbidity in United States populations. These included studies of seven cotton-mill villages in South Carolina in 1916 [391], of Hagerstown, Maryland, between 1921 and 1923 [390], of 9000 families selected at random from all parts of the United States between 1928 and 1931 [64], of over 700,000 representative U.S. households in 1935 and 1936 [315], of the Eastern Health District of Baltimore between 1938 and 1943 [92], and surveys undertaken by the Commission on Chronic Illness in Baltimore [65] and in Hunterdon County, New Jersey [66].

In England and Wales the Social Survey was initiated in 1944 to interview random samples of the population aged 16 or over. About 3000 persons were interviewed each month and questioned as to the occurrence of illness during the previous 2 months [372]. Routine results were published in *Reports of the Ministry of Health* and in the *Quarterly Returns of the Registrar General,* and special reports appeared from time to time [341, 385]. The Social Survey was discontinued in 1952.

Limited-duration, ad hoc morbidity surveys on a national scale have also been undertaken in Canada and Denmark [281].

## Table 9
### Some publications from the U.S. National Health Survey*

| Series no.† | Publication no. | Survey and title‡ |
|---|---|---|
| 10 | — | *Health Interview Survey* |
| 10 | 52 | Current estimates from the Health Interview Survey |
| 10 | 51 | Chronic conditions causing activity limitation |
| 10 | 49 | Volume of physician visits |
| 10 | 42 | Family hospital and surgical insurance coverage |
| 10 | 41 | Family health expenses |
| 11 | — | *Health Examination Survey* |
| 11 | 31 | Hearing levels of adults by education, income and occupation |
| 11 | 30 | Monocular-binocular visual acuity of adults |
| 11 | 23 | Decayed, missing and filled teeth in adults |
| 11 | 22 | Serum cholesterol levels of adults |
| 11 | 19 | Age at menopause |
| 11 | 14 | Weight by height and age of adults |
| 12 | — | *Health Records Survey* |
| 12 | 12 | Marital status and living arrangements before admission to nursing and personal care homes |
| 12 | 9 | Charges for care in institutions for the aged and chronically ill |
| 12 | 6 | Employees in nursing and personal care homes: number, work experience, special training and wages |
| 12 | 3 | Characteristics of patients in mental hospitals |
| 13 | — | *Hospital Discharge Survey* |
| 13 | 5 | Regional utilization of short-stay hospitals |
| 22 | — | *National Natality and Mortality Surveys* |
| 22 | 9 | Socioeconomic characteristics of deceased persons |
| 22 | 5 | Medical x-ray visits and examinations during pregnancy |

* From National Center for Health Statistics [280].
† The series number identifies the source of the data and nature of the report.
‡ The title of each report specifies "United States" and the relevant dates. These have been omitted in this listing.

*Surveys of Selected Diseases*

In contrast to attempts to survey all morbidity in a population, surveys are frequently aimed at assembling data only on individual diseases or groups of diseases. Since these disease-focused surveys are frequently undertaken predominantly for research purposes, they are a valuable source of epidemiologic data.

For example, surveys of cancer morbidity in 10 metropolitan areas of the United States were conducted by the U.S. Public Health Service in 1937 and 1947 [90]; a third is in progress during 1969 to 1971 [22]. Individual investigators have published many reports of less extensive surveys, usually covering a smaller geographic area or limited to a narrower group of diseases. Two important studies of this kind in the field of mental disorder are those of Jaco on psychoses in the State of Texas [180] and of Hollingshead and Redlich [168] on psychiatrically diagnosed mental illness in New Haven, Connecticut. The technique of such surveys usually is to assemble reports of all known cases of the disease from practicing physicians, hospitals, and death records. The reports must be processed to exclude persons who are not residents of the area and to avoid duplication of reports on the same patient from different sources. The variety of sources included and their accuracy determine the completeness and value of the survey.

Diseases of which it is known that an appreciable proportion of affected individuals do not come to medical attention require special survey procedures. With some such diseases door-to-door interviewing may be conducted to ascertain undiagnosed cases. This procedure is particularly pertinent to studies in the area of mental disease, and a number of such investigations have been conducted in recent years [198, 346]. For other diseases, such as diabetes, complete ascertainment may require that biochemical tests be conducted on whole populations, and this has been attempted—usually in fairly small communities [411, 417]. For chronic diseases, prevalence, but not incidence, is usually determined by such surveys.

## DISEASE NOTIFICATION AND REGISTRATION

Certain diseases have been deemed of sufficient importance to the public health to require that their occurrence be reported to health authorities. This procedure was instituted for the control of infectious diseases. For tuberculosis and other chronic diseases the reports frequently form the basis of a registry which provides a continuous account of the prevalence of the disease in the community. Newly recognized cases are entered and maintained in the file until recovery, death, or migration from the community. Obviously it takes several years to build up such a file to completeness. Potentially these registries are sources of accurate information as to duration of disease, case fatality, incidence, prevalence, and other epidemiologic measures. This concept has been extended to other diseases, notably cancer and mental illness, in which registries have come to serve research as well as control purposes.

### Infectious Diseases

The selection of infectious diseases to be reported is mostly a local matter except for six diseases—cholera, plague, louse-borne relapsing fever, smallpox, louse-borne typhus fever, and yellow fever—the reporting of which is required by International Sanitary Regulation. In most of the United States about 40 infectious diseases are reportable. Reports are generally made by practicing physicians to local health authorities; then the reports, or tabulations prepared from them, are transmitted to state health departments and subsequently to the U.S. Public Health Service. The Public Health Service prepares weekly summaries for about 25 diseases; these are published in the *Morbidity and Mortality Weekly Report,* and annual summaries are issued as supplements to that report. On a worldwide basis, current information on notifications of infectious diseases is published by the World Health Organization [427]. The Pan American Sanitary Bureau publishes comparable information for the American continents [308].

Generally the number of cases of notifiable diseases reported is far lower than the number occurring, and the proportion varies with time and place, as well as with the disease. This deficiency may not seriously impair the value of the system for control purposes, since the beginnings of an epidemic may be apparent in a trend, even if only a small proportion of cases is being reported. However, the incompleteness seriously limits the use of such data in determining the distribution of a disease in the population.

## Cancer

A number of authorities have established continuing registries of cancer cases—some based on legally required reporting, others on voluntary reporting by hospitals or physicians. Two of these registries, in Connecticut [107] and Denmark [56], because of their early origins and completeness have provided unusually valuable information on the distribution of cancer in industrialized populations. More recently the establishment of cancer registries in Asia and Africa has pointed up the tremendous variation in the frequency of cancer of different organs in different parts of the world. Under sponsorship of the International Union Against Cancer, a summary of data from 32 cancer registries representing 24 countries was published in 1966 [85] and a second volume in 1970.

## Mental Illness

Many jurisdictions maintain central registries of patients hospitalized for mental disease. In utilizing statistics from such registries note must be taken of the types of institution included in the registration procedure, since the characteristics of patients in different types of institutions vary considerably. For example, most state data in the United States do not include patients seen in Veterans Hospitals or private institutions—groups that obviously are different from those seen in state mental hospitals. These data are also strongly influenced by administrative decisions as to what constitutes being under hospital care (for example, whether this includes patients on trial visits outside the hospital, or only those physically in the hospital), what is a first admission, and what constitutes a discharge from the hospital. With all the evident defects of data limited to institutionalized patients, centrally compiled statistics from mental institutions have nevertheless provided important information on the frequency, distribution, and changes over time of the most disabling kinds of mental illness in many populations [76, 232, 233, 302, 335, 396].

More comprehensive registries of mental illness—including, for example, all patients seen by a psychiatrist [21]—have been attempted on the basis of voluntary reporting. Such efforts are relatively recent, and their utility for epidemiologic purposes has not yet been evaluated.

### Other Diseases

The desirability of establishing registries almost inevitably enters the discussion when other diseases begin to attract public and scientific attention. The congenital malformations and stroke are in this position at the present time. A registry of congenital malformations evident at birth has been established in Sweden [185], but none yet exists for any large population in the United States. A registry of patients with stroke has been established recently in Baltimore.

Each proposal for a new registry must of course be evaluated individually, but it is necessary to keep in mind certain principles. First, a complete and accurate registry for almost any disease or group of diseases is expensive and the costs and benefits of a registry must be weighed against the costs and benefits of alternative approaches—for example, periodic surveys. Second, a small number of well-run registries in carefully selected areas is much to be preferred to numerous registries of mediocre quality. Third, the longer a registry has been in being, the more valuable are its data: the continuation of existing registries that already have accumulated accurate data over a prolonged period should take priority over the establishment of new registries. Fourth, a registry as a repository of data serves little purpose; an active and effective research program in association with a registry not only justifies the costs of the registry but also serves to maintain the quality of the data collected.

## SPECIAL POPULATIONS

Certain subgroups of the population provide opportunities for the collection of data that are either not available or less readily available for the general population. Usually, however, such subgroups have special characteristics that may limit the generalizations that can be made for the population as a whole.

### The Armed Forces

Annual reports of the Surgeons-General of the Armed Forces contain statistics on morbidity and mortality. The information is valuable because of the uniformity and generally high accuracy of diagnostic data. However, the data suffer from limitations inherent in the restriction to persons of particular age and sex groups who were able to pass an induction examination. Moreover, the practice of discharging from the population persons found to have a chronic disease likely to interfere with their subsequent performance makes interpretation of the statistics on chronic diseases difficult.

### Insured Groups

Persons holding life insurance provide opportunities for the study of mortality in relation to variables—such as height, weight, and blood pressure—that are not available for the general population. Regular reports on mortality in their insured population are published by the Metropolitan Life Insurance Company [249]. These data also have some age and sex limitations and the accuracy of some of the information obtained at the time of enrollment may be questioned. Nevertheless the data, cautiously interpreted, have provided insights into the relationship between, for example, weight and blood pressure [377].

Prepaid medical care plans, in particular such large and comprehensive plans as the Kaiser-Permanente Plan and the Health Insurance Plan of Greater New York, gather data from all the major providers of medical services for insured populations. In addition, a great deal of social and demographic information is often available for such populations. Up to now, data on such populations have been utilized primarily for specifically focused research studies [362, 365].

Similar kinds of resources are the cooperative programs established by British general practitioners under the auspices of the College of General Practice [63].

*Other Groups and Sources*

Groups enrolled in restricted medical care plans—such as those of a particular industry or educational institution—have also been used as source populations for epidemiologic data. Some hospitals publish annual reports that may be useful. This is particularly the case for maternity hospitals when the total deliveries in the hospital establishes a population that can, with caution, be used as a denominator for the computation of rates of anomalies and disorders of late pregnancy and delivery [197]. Sometimes a particular local circumstance enables estimates of morbidity from specific diseases. For example, the allocation of certain foods on the basis of medical certification of illness during the rationing of food in Great Britain enabled estimates of the prevalence of diabetes, thyrotoxicosis, tuberculosis, peptic ulcer, and other conditions according to age, sex, and geographic location [385].

## RECORD LINKAGE

*Purposes*

RECORDS OF INDIVIDUALS.    The bringing together of information from different records concerning a single individual is a well-established procedure in epidemiologic and other research. For example, it is common to search for death certificates of individuals known from some other source of information (for example, records of employment or medical treatment) to have been exposed to a suspected noxious agent. Many health departments routinely search for the birth certificates of children who die in infancy: this allows evaluation of infant mortality with respect to variables such as birth weight, legitimacy, and age and parity of mother that are present on the birth certificate but not the death certificate. Search for death certificates of persons enrolled, for example, in a cancer registry allows evaluation of survival rates by type and stage of cancer, mode of therapy, and other relevant variables.

These are ad hoc linkages—made for a specific purpose—and, generally speaking, they have been performed by hand, the searching and judgments as to whether two records do in fact pertain to a single individual being made by clerical personnel. Today the term *record linkage* is more apt to imply an ongoing procedure in which records from two or more sources are routinely searched for linkage, usually by computer mechanisms. Programs of this type are becoming commonplace in business and financial fields—probably the largest such effort is that of the U.S. Internal Revenue Service—but those in the health field are still small and experimental. Among the kinds of linkage that have been considered and that would have important epidemiologic implications are:

Different vital records (births, marriages, divorces, deaths)
Records from different hospitals
Records from different social agencies
Death certificates with records of occupation, hospitalization, etc.
Census schedules with records of hospitalization and death

It should be noted that epidemiologic purposes are by no means the sole justification for such linkages. Studies of medical care utilization, medical economics, and many other purposes would be aided.

FAMILY LINKAGES. Automatic linkages between records pertaining to different members of the same household or family have also been proposed and have been implemented in at least one area [292]. The topics on which such family linkages would provide information include family patterns of usage of medical and social agencies, patterns of concordance of disease in siblings and in spouses, and relationship of parental characteristics to fertility and patterns of mortality and morbidity in children.

*Current Studies*

In British Columbia, Canada, records of marriages, livebirths, stillbirths, and child deaths, and registrations of handicapped children from 1946 through 1965 are being linked. This program was the first major linkage study using computer methods and has yielded a great deal of genetic and epidemiologic information [293].

The Oxford Record Linkage Study was begun in 1962 primarily to study feasibility, cost, methodology, and research applications of linkages of medical records in a defined population. The population is that of Oxford, England, and surrounding areas, and the records linked include certificates of birth and death, and abstracts of records of all deliveries and all hospital inpatient treatments. The data have been used to create integrated medical records for individuals (for use in providing continuity of care, as well as for research purposes), for linking records of mother and child, and for studies of the relationships between abnormalities of pregnancy and characteristics of the fetus, between pregnancy abnormalities and infant hospitalization in the first year of life, and between different diseases in the same individual [2].

Also to be mentioned in this context is the program being conducted by the Follow-Up Agency of the National Academy of Sciences [25, 78]. Established in 1946 to exploit the large amount of medical information existing in the records of Armed Forces personnel, the Follow-Up Agency has conducted many studies involving linkages between personnel and medical records of the three Services, Veterans Administration records, death certificates, and other sources. Originally these studies related primarily to matters of military interest—for example, the follow-up of veterans invalided with head wounds [410], nerve injuries [419], or battle neurosis [33]—but matters of broader concern have also been studied—for example, cardiovascular and respiratory disease in relation to cigarette smoking habits [49], twin concordance in different forms of mental illness [325], survival following diagnosis of coronary disease [435], and the natural history of multiple sclerosis [194]. With the exception of routine linkage of death certificates to records of a roster of 15,000 twins—the roster itself having been assembled by linkage of birth certificates and military records [179]—this program does not link records on a routine basis. Rather the effort is to maintain files and resources in such a manner that linkages can be made for specific studies.

*Problems*

The interest in record linkage has been stimulated, at least in part, by the increasing amount of information that is being converted to and maintained in forms allowing computer access, and by the development of computers that make large-scale linkage mechanically feasible. The problems still to be overcome are practical, economic, ethical, and political.

The most important practical problem is that of identification of individuals—and even more so of members of the same family—from information now available on most records. The British Columbia study has demonstrated the feasibility of basing a linkage system on family names, but the population involved was relatively small and stable and the records being linked contained an unusually large amount of other information that could be used to verify preliminary matches. In the United States matching based on name has not been so successful [299, 323, 331]. Large-scale linkage operations will probably not be generally feasible until a unique identifying number has been assigned to each individual and this same number is used on all pertinent records. The problems associated with various identifying numbers that have been considered in Britain have been described by Smith [373]. In the United States the Social Security number is increasingly being used for linkage purposes outside the health field, and it would seem most advantageous to utilize it for identification of all vital and health records [282]. An account of the personal numbering systems used in three Scandinavian countries is given by Nielsen [298].

From the economic point of view there will need to be more studies such as the Oxford one to provide more complete evaluation of costs and benefits to the governmental and other agencies that must support and utilize record linkage systems.

Ethically and politically the major problems of record linkage revolve around the need to protect individuals from breach of confidentiality or misuse of the information contained in the kinds of data banks that record linkage makes possible. There are real problems in the protection of such files, but the attitudes of both public and government toward the problems, and the weight which people are willing to give to the benefits of such a program in evaluating its dangers, vary very much from country to country. The attitude in the United States seems to be among the more conservative. There has recently been considerable discussion of the general problem of confidentiality of vital and medical records in several countries [5, 129, 277, 356].

## RESOURCES FOR FOLLOW-UP

In cohort studies groups of persons are followed over time to determine whether or not they experience the outcome that is the subject of the study. In a prospective study the investigator may design his own follow-up mechanism suited to ascertainment of the particular outcome under study. However, in retrospective studies the investigator is dependent on mechanisms already existent in the community, and some knowledge of these is essential to the epidemiologist. In such studies it is usually necessary to know, as a minimum, whether the individual subjects are alive or dead and, if dead, the date of death. Frequently the cause of death as certified on the death certificate is also required.

### Population Registers

The most effective single follow-up resource, in countries where such are maintained, are population registers. These are registers of the population that are continuously updated through reports of births, deaths, marriages, and changes of name or address. In some countries such registers are the basis of population estimates. They may, in addition, be used for follow-up, population sampling, and other epidemiologic purposes. No such registers exist in the United States.

Related to the population register is the Japanese Koseki system in which each family has a permanent address. Copies of vital records are forwarded to the jurisdiction in which the permanent address is located and form a permanent family file which is accessible for follow-up purposes. This system has been used by the Atomic Bomb Casualty Commission in its follow-up studies [24].

### Death Certificate Search

In most areas alphabetic indexes of death certificates are maintained that allow searches to be made to determine whether a death certificate is on file for any person that an investigator wishes to trace. The finding of a death certificate, identified by appropriate matching criteria, may be taken as reasonable evidence that the individual is dead; the problem is in determining to what extent failure to locate a death certificate can be taken as evidence that he is alive. In any large file there are clerical and other errors, and the searching process itself may have defects which lead to failure to locate certificates that actually exist in the file. In addition, deaths of persons who migrate out of the population to which the file relates will not be identified.

In the United States the decentralization of death registration in more than 50 states and cities and the mobility of the population pose particular problems in this respect. It is never practical to search for deaths in all 50 jurisdictions and, in fact, except for routine searches within the study area and perhaps the two or three areas with the highest rates of immigration from the study area, it is usually necessary to know when and where a person died before being able to locate his death certificate. This is not always an insuperable problem. For example, in one follow-up study of Massachusetts residents with gastric ulcer, search of Massachusetts death certificates identified 76 (92 percent) of the 83 persons that intensive follow-up revealed had died [164]. This level of ascertainment may be adequate for many purposes. However, the level of ascertainment will vary with the location of the study and the age, sex, and other characteristics of the study population. The formation of a national death index which would allow search of names in all registration areas has been recommended on several occasions [282, 332] but not yet implemented.

## Social Security Administration

Records of employment, payments, and claims stemming from deaths of enrolled employees have been maintained by the Social Security Administration since 1937. These have been used in studies of occupational groups, both as a source of rosters of persons employed in certain occupations and to determine the occurrence of deaths among them [108, 235, 392]. In most cases cause of death data cannot be obtained from SSA records, and death certificates must be obtained from the registration areas. As the proportion of the population eligible for Social Security benefits increases, and as the benefits themselves are broadened—particularly, for example, with the location of responsibility for administration of the Medicare program in the Social Security Administration—this resource should become increasingly useful for follow-up purposes. At the present time, limitations of such use stem from the confidentiality of the material as well as from practical matters resulting from the fact that the files are not designed or maintained primarily for research purposes. Some specific difficulties are described by Myers [266].

## City Directories

R. L. Polk and Company publishes annually some 5500 directories of cities and towns in the United States and Canada [322]. These contain alphabetic listings by name of the head of household, as well as street listings. Telephone directories are available in most areas, and may be available in street-listing order. In many New England towns directories are prepared which list by street all inhabitants over a certain age (usually 20 or 21 years) and often include age and occupation as well as name. Individuals may be located in such directories as of a particular year and followed through subsequent editions so that at least the approximate date of their moving can be judged. Where alphabetic directories exist, the person may conceivably be located if the move has involved only change of address within the same area. Except in the case of the New England town directories, which are reasonably accurate in this respect, the listing of an individual in a directory does not necessarily indicate that he is alive. For example, a widow may maintain a telephone listing in her former husband's name after his death.

## Other Resources

In most states, applications for driver's licenses are public records and can be searched for particular names. The Post Office maintains change-of-address files for 2 years and has a Correction of Mailing List service which can be useful if the individual's move is a recent one. Use of the Retail Credit Bureau is expensive and usually resorted to only when virtually complete ascertainment is desired. Many other sources—records of former employment, health and welfare agencies, utility companies, unions, professional societies, alumni associations, etc.—may be considered in particular instances.

For a recent account of the use of these resources and of their relative productivity, the reader is referred to the study by Redmond et al. [337] of 59,072 steelworkers known to have been employed in 1953. The status (alive or dead) as of Dec. 21, 1961 was ascertained for all but 97 (0.2 percent) of the original cohort.

## POPULATION DATA

A description of sources of epidemiologic data should not be closed without a reminder that the accuracy and comparability of rates are affected by problems in their denominators as well as in their numerators, even though an extended discussion of the sources and accuracy of population data is beyond the scope of this text. Population data are most frequently derived from national censuses, usually undertaken at decennial or quinquennial intervals, and national census agencies usually make estimates for intercensal periods by extrapolation or by consideration of births, deaths, immigrations, and emigrations in the postcensal period. For the United States a useful publication [40] gives estimates of the total population by age, color, and sex for each year from 1900 to 1959. Subsequent to 1960, estimates for the country as a whole and for individual states appear in *Current Population Reports* [42]. For the world, valuable compilations of census and vital data for many countries were published in the *United Nations Demographic Yearbooks* for 1962, 1963, and 1964 [401].

Discussions of the accuracy of population data appear in textbooks of demography [181, 378, 389] and in technical reports of national census agencies [41]. In addition to comment in the *Demographic Yearbooks*, the United Nations has published an account of census methods in many countries and their implications for accuracy of the data [404].

# 7

Characteristics of Persons

In assembling information on the types of people affected with a disease and the various circumstances in which a disease occurs, the epidemiologist commonly uses those descriptive variables around which large amounts of data on morbidity, mortality, and population are routinely assembled by various agencies for their own purposes. The variables discussed in this chapter include age, sex, marital condition, and measures related to ethnic group and socioeconomic status. They are spoken of here as characteristics of persons only for convenience and not because associations in connection with them are deemed necessarily to reflect etiologic factors intrinsic within the individual.

## AGE

Age is a variable that must always be considered in epidemiologic studies. In most diseases the variations in frequency that occur between different ages are greater than those found with any other variable. Knowledge of age associations is important for two reasons: first, study of variation in the frequency of a disease with age may assist understanding the factors responsible for its development; and, second, associations between age and disease frequency are so strong that age may produce indirect effects that must be taken account of in examination of differences in disease rates related to other variables. Differences in disease rates between populations or subgroups of populations cannot be interpreted unless consideration has first been given to the relevance of possible age differences between the two populations.

Association of disease frequency with age is usually measured by relating the number of cases of the disease in each age group to the population in the same age group, and deriving a succession of age-specific incidence or prevalence rates.

Frequently, and particularly in the examination of material collected from clinical sources, it is possible to present the distribution of a series of patients by age, but information is lacking as to the age distribution of the population from which the patients came. Statements such as "this disease is most common between the ages of 50 and 60" may be made on the basis of such a frequency distribution. While they have meaning to the clinician or the administrator insofar as they indicate that more of the patients seen are in this age group than in any other, such statements do not, of course, indicate that the greatest risk of the disease lies in this age group. Even diseases for which risk increases with age throughout life will show decreasing numbers of cases in the highest age groups because the population itself decreases rapidly with increasing age after about age 55. Thus Figure 8 shows that the largest number of cases of rectal cancer have clinical onset in the age groups between 55 and 65, but the highest *rates* are noted in the oldest age groups. Although the necessity of distinguishing numbers of cases from rates is frequently overlooked in the context of age associations, the point will not be labored here in view of the discussion already presented in Chapter 5.

## Interpretation of Age Associations

Innumerable factors determine the shape of the age association for a given disease. Only a few of them are understood.

At the most superficial level, there are a number of circumstances which have little to do with age per se, but which may nevertheless affect the shape of an age-incidence graph. One of these is variation in accuracy of diagnosis according to age, a factor particularly likely to affect the oldest and the youngest

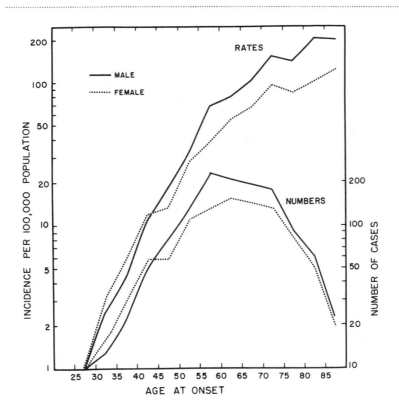

Figure 8

Numbers of new cases and incidence rates of rectal cancer by age and sex, in 10 metropolitan areas of the United States, 1947. (Data from Dorn and Cutler [90].)

age groups. There is in many clinical situations less concern over establishing an exact cause of death for an 80-year-old than for a 40-year-old person. This tends to reduce age-specific rates in the oldest age groups for diseases of difficult diagnosis and to exaggerate rates in the same age groups for "wastebasket" diagnoses. In addition, basic population data may be inaccurate for the oldest age groups, leading to further distortions. The latter situation applies in the United States particularly to the nonwhite population. At the other end of life, specific causes of death are notoriously difficult to determine in many cases of fetal and perinatal death.

The shape of an age-risk curve will also depend on whether it is based on rates of incidence, prevalence, or mortality. For example, in a fatal disease in which the interval between onset and death increases with age, the mortality age curve will be less steep than the incidence curve. Or, in a chronic disease of long duration, the peak in prevalence rate will be at a substantially later age than the peak in the incidence rate. An illustration of differences among age curves based on incidence, prevalence, and mortality is shown for multiple sclerosis in Figure 9.

Bimodality—that is, the occurrence of two separate peaks—in an age-incidence curve of a disease is always of interest. It indicates, first of all, that the material is not homogeneous—that the entity under examination might properly be divided into two. Even when a causal, rather than a manifestational, entity is being examined, bimodality suggests the existence of causal differences other than that on which classification of the disease is

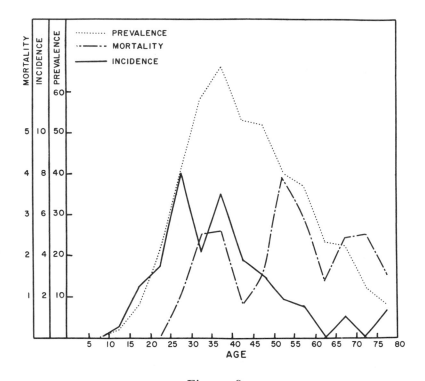

Figure 9

Rates of incidence, prevalence, and mortality of multiple sclerosis in males; Boston, 1939 to 1948. Annual rates per 100,000. (Data from Ipsen [177].)

based. For example, age curves for tuberculosis are bimodal, showing one mode in the 0 to 4 age group and a second in the 20 to 29 age group. Tuberculosis is defined in terms of experience with the tubercle bacillus, so that both these modes affect the same "disease." The existence of the two modes suggests, however, that two distinct sets of ancillary experiences must be taken into account to explain the age distribution.

Age-incidence curves for the manifestational entity Hodgkin's disease are also distinctly bimodal, showing one peak in early adult life and a second in old age (Fig. 10). Probably, therefore, parts of two distinct causal entities are contained in this manifestational entity. This hypothesis is supported by the demonstration that the disease in persons under 40 years of age differs from that in persons over that age with respect to sex ratio, racial, religious, and geographic distribution, and duration of illness [62, 221]. Such evidence should lead to reexamination of clinical and pathologic findings in the light of the epidemiologic differentiation. Thus histologic differences have recently been

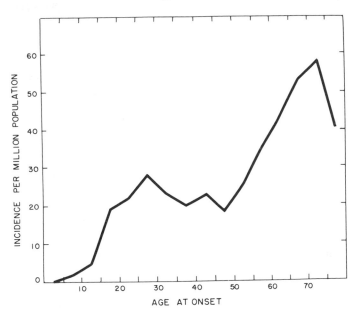

Figure 10

Incidence rates of Hodgkin's disease by age; Brooklyn, white population, 1943 to 1952. (From MacMahon [219].)

reported between Hodgkin's disease manifested in young adults and in the elderly [295].

A common type of age curve is that exhibited by the so-called degenerative diseases in which incidence rates increase progressively throughout the life span. Understanding of the mechanisms responsible for this type of age curve is a problem which is only in part epidemiologic. At present it seems likely that fundamental studies of an experimental type have most to offer in understanding those bodily changes which occur with age and which lead to increasing rates for so many different diseases. Probably the explanations of such associations are as numerous as the diseases which exhibit them. Certainly change in no single factor is likely to be responsible for incidence changes in so many fundamentally different disorders.

Huxley [176] has offered a genetic explanation for the rise with age in incidence of neoplastic disease, suggesting that it results from genetic selection against persons whose genotypes destined them to develop tumors during their reproductive years. On the other hand, Hueper [170] has supported the view that the shape of the age curve in neoplastic diseases is determined largely by the length of the latent period between encounter with carcinogenic agents and manifestation of the neoplasm, by the age at which such exposure first takes place, and by the intensity of the exposure. The long latent periods found in human neoplastic disorders following exposure to known carcinogenic agents make it inevitable that such neoplasms should occur in the older ages, even if exposure was first effective at birth. Hueper points out that the age distribution of scrotal cancer and other occupational neoplasms varies according to the age at first exposure to the carcinogenic agent. In addition, there is no experimental evidence that the latent period between initiation of exposure and development of neoplasia is any longer for young than for old experimental animals. There is, therefore, a good deal of support for Hueper's point of view.

It is not known whether there are truly endogenous changes with age which affect susceptibility to disease—that is, changes which are the inevitable consequences of the passage of time and which are completely independent of environmental circumstances to which the individual is exposed during that time. Actually the type of explanation offered by Hueper is not so different as it might seem from the hypothesis that tissue susceptibility changes inevitably with age. Aging, as a characteristic of any individual, by definition necessitates the passage of time and this must inevitably be accompanied by exposure to environmental situations which alter body chemistry and physiology. In some instances the alterations may result from avoidable exposure to a toxic agent, but in others they are a necessary concomitant of such essential life functions as the intake of food and respiration. Between these extremes are situations in which environmental circumstances may be separated to a greater or lesser degree from aging. For example, it may be that some component of the incidence of human leukemia can be attributed to exposure to ionizing radiation from natural sources. At present, aging is necessarily accompanied by cumulative exposure to background radiation, and the relationship between age and this component of leukemia incidence may, under this hypothesis, be regarded as a fairly inevitable one. However, if methods of protection were devised such that only artificial sources of radiation contributed to the total radiation experience, leukemia incidence as influenced by background radiation might be regarded as independent of age.

Whether or not there is a truly endogenous aging process (a "biological clock") resulting in increased disease susceptibility, the evidence assembled by Hueper indicates that there are certainly many alterable situations, separable from age, which contribute to the shape of age-incidence curves. The existence of a progressive association with age should not necessarily be regarded as evidence of endogenous causation and thus as grounds for pessimism with regard to preventive possibilities. Practically, effort should be concentrated on the elucidation of those deleterious environmental exposures which accompany but are nevertheless separable from age.

### SEX

As with other descriptive variables, associations between sex and a disease are most convincingly evidenced in a difference in disease *rates*—that is, through the comparison of the disease rate among males to that among females. At times, deviations of the percentage of males from 50 percent of the total cases are interpreted as evidence of a sex difference in disease rates, under the assumption that the percentage of males in the population from which the affected came is also 50 percent. This assumption may be incorrect. For example, in the 1965 Massachusetts population 70 or more years of age the male percentage was only 40 percent. Calculation and comparison of sex-specific rates are therefore preferable because they involve one fewer assumption in the interpretation of findings.

In most populations the two sexes have different age distributions, the mean age of females commonly being higher than that of males. Small differences in sex-specific rates must therefore be viewed with caution until the possible effect of age differences has been taken into account.

## Sex Distribution of Disease

More males are born alive than females, in a ratio of about 106:100. Except in areas where obstetrical care is poor, death rates are higher for males than for females at all ages. The disparity between male and female death rates in the white United States population at various ages is shown in Table 10; of inter-

## Table 10
Sex-specific mortality rates in broad age groups in the white population of the United States, 1967*

| Age (years) | Mortality rates† | | | Ratio of male rate to female rate |
|---|---|---|---|---|
| | Total | Male | Female | |
| Under 1 | 19.6 | 22.4 | 16.7 | 1.3 |
| 1–4 | 0.8 | 0.8 | 0.7 | 1.1 |
| 5–14 | 0.4 | 0.5 | 0.3 | 1.7 |
| 15–39 | 1.3 | 1.8 | 0.8 | 2.3 |
| 40–64 | 8.9 | 12.3 | 5.9 | 2.1 |
| 65+ | 60.5 | 75.0 | 49.6 | 1.5 |
| All ages‡ | 9.0 | 11.5 | 6.9 | 1.7 |

* Data from *Vital Statistics of the United States* [278].
† Annual rates per 1000 population.
‡ For "all ages" and within each broad age group the rates are standardized by the direct method to the age distribution in 5-year age groups of the total United States population in 1967.

est is the fact that the death rates of males are highest relative to those of females during the ages at which males are most active as breadwinners.

In the United States the mortality disparity between the sexes has been increasing. Illustrative data for 1933 and 1967 are presented in Table 11. Comparison of age-standardized mortality

### Table 11

Mortality rates for males and females of the white
population of the United States, 1933* and 1967

| Year | Mortality rates† | | Ratio of male rate to female rate |
|------|------|--------|------|
|      | Male | Female | |
| 1933 | 14.6 | 12.1 | 1.2 |
| 1967 | 11.5 | 6.9 | 1.7 |

* Data from *Vital Statistics of the United States* [278]. 1933 is chosen for comparison because it is the first year in which data for the whole United States are available.

† Annual rates per 1000 population, age-standardized as in Table 10.

rates in the two years indicates that rates for both sexes fell, but those for females fell more rapidly than those for males.

The higher over-all male death rate is the result of serious disadvantage in most of the assigned causes of death (Table 12). Although considerable variation in sex pattern is evident between assigned causes, death rates among males exceeded those among females for the majority of the causes listed, commonly by as much as 1.5 times or more, and in one instance (respiratory cancer) by 6.0 times. When deaths assigned specifically to diseases of the sex organs are excluded from consideration, only diabetes mellitus and hypertensive heart disease showed higher death rates among females than among males.

A finding in surveys of morbidity that seems paradoxical in the context of findings from mortality studies is that illness rates are higher among females than males. Illustrative data are shown in Table 13. With respect to all the several definitions of illness and incapacity used, rates for females are higher than those for males. This indicates either that females admit to ill-

## Table 12
Mortality rates from selected common causes for males
and females in the United States, 1967*

| Cause | Mortality rates† | | | Ratio of male rate to female rate |
|---|---|---|---|---|
| | Total | Male | Female | |
| Respiratory cancer | 29.2 | 53.6 | 9.0 | 6.0 |
| Homicide | 6.8 | 10.7 | 3.1 | 3.5 |
| Syphilis | 1.2 | 1.9 | 0.6 | 3.2 |
| Tuberculosis | 3.5 | 5.6 | 1.8 | 3.1 |
| Peptic ulcer | 4.9 | 7.7 | 2.7 | 2.9 |
| Motor vehicle accidents | 26.8 | 40.2 | 14.4 | 2.8 |
| Suicide | 10.8 | 16.2 | 5.9 | 2.7 |
| Urinary cancer | 7.4 | 11.1 | 4.5 | 2.5 |
| Accidents other than motor vehicle | 30.5 | 42.7 | 18.8 | 2.3 |
| Arteriosclerotic heart disease | 289.2 | 395.9 | 200.5 | 2.0 |
| Cirrhosis of liver | 14.0 | 19.2 | 9.4 | 2.0 |
| Digestive cancer | 48.0 | 58.2 | 39.8 | 1.5 |
| Vascular lesions of the central nervous system | 102.2 | 110.3 | 95.6 | 1.2 |
| Hypertensive heart disease | 25.2 | 24.9 | 25.2 | 1.0 |
| Diabetes mellitus | 17.7 | 16.4 | 18.6 | 0.9 |
| Genital cancer | 20.4 | 20.5 | 21.5 | — |

* Data from *Vital Statistics of the United States* [278].
† Annual rates per 100,000 population, age-standardized as in Table 10.

ness more readily than males or that they experience a higher
incidence of illnesses which, in view of the preceding mortality
data, must presumably be less lethal than those experienced by
males. In observing and attempting to explain this phenomenon
some 300 years ago, John Graunt noted [134]:

. . . there were fourteen men to thirteen women (christened)
and . . . they die in the same proportion. . . . Yet I have heard
physicians say that they have two women patients to one man.
. . . Now from this it should follow that more women should die

## Table 13

Selected measures of morbidity in males and females,
United States, 1967*

| Measure | Rate per 100 persons per year | |
|---|---|---|
| | Males | Females |
| Incidence of acute conditions | 183 | 197 |
| Days of restricted activity | 685 | 815 |
| Days lost from work | 329 | 370 |
| Discharges from short-stay hospitals | 10 | 14 |
| Physician visits | 378 | 477 |
| Days of bed disability | | |
| All ages | 284 | 346 |
| Ages under 6 | 375 | 343 |
| Ages 6–16 | 317 | 346 |
| Ages 17–44 | 247 | 367 |
| Ages 45 and older | 261 | 321 |

* From *Current Estimates,* National Center for Health Statistics [416].

than men, if the number of burials answered in proportion to that of sicknesses. But this must be salved (reconciled) either by alledging that the physicians cure those sicknesses, so as few more die than if none were sick; or else that men, being more intemperate than women, die as much by reason of their vices as the women do by the infirmity of their sex. . . .

The sex differential in morbidity is evident in all gradations of socioeconomic status, in urban and rural areas, and when examination is restricted to gainfully employed persons [6, 416]. When separate causes of illness are considered, women have higher morbidity rates than men for the majority of chronic diseases. Many chronic conditions are strikingly more common in women—for example, thyrotoxicosis, diabetes mellitus, cholecystitis and biliary calculi, obesity, arthritis, psychoneurosis, and many benign tumors. Only a few illnesses appear to be predominantly diseases of males when examined in morbidity data; these include peptic ulcer, inguinal hernia, accidents, arteriosclerotic heart disease, and respiratory cancer.

## ETHNIC GROUP

A variety of terms might be used to denote groups of persons who have a greater degree of homogeneity than the population at large with respect to present-day customs and/or biologic inheritance. While the uses of the word *race* extend from a "permanent or fixed variety" of persons on the one hand to groups with as little common background as "the race of doctors" on the other [132], the term is so much more often equated with the former than the latter usage that we prefer *ethnic group* as conveying more clearly the concept that is most useful for epidemiologic purposes.

From an epidemiologic point of view any group whose members have lived together for a sufficient length of time to have acquired common characteristics, whether by biologic or by social mechanisms, is of interest. In practice, such groups are identified by certain commonly applied descriptive terms. These include race (in its restricted sense), nativity, religion, and the names of local reproductive and social units, such as tribes and geographically or socially isolated groups.

### Race

Much epidemiologic work has been done in comparing disease rates of such "racial" groups as Caucasian, Negroid, and Mongoloid. In particular, in the United States differences between the white and Negro populations have been extensively studied. Published mortality data from this country contain a great deal of information, and extensive tabulations are available showing rates for whites and nonwhites. Although the data for the nonwhite population are frequently not further subdivided, the rates for nonwhites, when the United States is taken as a whole, can be considered to reflect the rates for Negroes with some accuracy since approximately 92 percent of the nonwhite population of the United States is Negro. The same confidence in this assumption cannot always be maintained, however, when specific areas within the United States are considered. For example, in the Census Bureau's West Region, which includes Hawaii and Alaska as well as the western continental states, only 49 percent of the nonwhite population is Negro. Furthermore, even when the United States is considered as a whole, a highly different rate in some nonwhite racial group other than the Negro—for example, American Indians or Asiatics—could result in only a small difference between nonwhite and white rates.

A large difference between rates specific for color in the United States is commonly observed, clearly indicating an overall disadvantage for the nonwhite population. For example, the mortality rate from all causes among nonwhites seen in Table 14

## Table 14

Mortality rates from selected causes and from all causes, for whites and nonwhites, in the United States, 1967*

| Cause | Mortality rates† | | Ratio of nonwhite rate to white rate |
|---|---|---|---|
| | White | Nonwhite | |
| Homicide | 3.5 | 32.3 | 9.2 |
| Tuberculosis | 2.5 | 9.6 | 3.8 |
| Hypertensive heart disease | 21.1 | 68.6 | 3.3 |
| Syphilis | 1.0 | 3.0 | 3.0 |
| Diabetes mellitus | 16.6 | 28.9 | 1.7 |
| Genital cancer | 19.2 | 32.4 | 1.7 |
| Pneumonia | 26.0 | 42.4 | 1.6 |
| Accidents other than motor vehicle | 28.6 | 43.9 | 1.5 |
| Vascular lesions of the central nervous system | 97.7 | 150.1 | 1.5 |
| Cirrhosis of liver | 13.2 | 19.9 | 1.5 |
| Digestive cancer | 47.0 | 58.2 | 1.2 |
| Motor vehicle accidents | 26.5 | 29.8 | 1.1 |
| Respiratory cancer | 28.9 | 32.2 | 1.1 |
| Peptic ulcer | 4.9 | 4.9 | 1.0 |
| Urinary cancer | 7.4 | 7.1 | 1.0 |
| Arteriosclerotic heart disease | 292.9 | 247.1 | 0.8 |
| Leukemia | 7.4 | 5.5 | 0.7 |
| Suicide | 11.3 | 5.7 | 0.5 |
| *All causes* | 904.1 | 1192.7 | 1.3 |

* Data from *Vital Statistics of the United States* [278].
† Annual rates per 100,000 population, age-standardized as in Table 10.

is 1.3 times that among whites. With respect to the selected causes listed, the higher death rate in nonwhites from several infectious diseases, notably tuberculosis, syphilis, and pneumonia, have already stimulated considerable epidemiologic interest. The tremendously higher rate of death from homicide in nonwhites deserves similar concern.

## Nativity

When people migrate from their country of birth, patterns of diet, occupation, recreation, and so on tend to be maintained for a variable length of time in the new country. Country of birth is therefore a valuable objective characteristic which can be used to distinguish within the same community groups whose environmental patterns and inherited characteristics may differ from those of other immigrant groups and from the nativeborn. Certain of these environmental characteristics may be maintained in more or less altered form for one or more subsequent generations, so that nativity of parents or of grandparents may also be used to distinguish groups with different environmental experiences.

In addition, foreignborn persons constitute a group which has necessarily encountered the stress of exposure to a new environment. Although they naturally form inviting groups for epidemiologic studies on this account, the specifics of the stressful exposure are, unfortunately, difficult to elucidate.

Much of the epidemiologic work with respect to place of birth has required special studies which provide greater detail than is found in routinely reported data. A well-known example of such a special study is the demonstration by Zinsser [434] that cases of typhus occurring in New York City between 1910 and 1933 were almost exclusively limited to persons born in Eastern Europe where typhus was endemic. This observation led to the concept of typhus occurring as the recrudescence of a long-latent infection. Another example is the study by Malzberg [232] of rates of admission to mental hospitals in relation to country of birth for the population of New York State. Admission rates were higher among foreignborn than among nativeborn persons, and were higher for those born in Ireland or Scandinavia than for the three other large foreignborn groups (Italian, German, and English). There were striking differences in this pattern between the several major diagnostic groups of mental illness. This study was made possible by the provision of special census data on the age distribution of the foreignborn population.

*Religion*

Cultural background and religious belief are so strongly correlated that religion sometimes serves as an indicator of ethnic group. For example, persons of Irish and Italian ancestry in the United States are predominantly Catholic, and those of British and Scandinavian ancestry predominantly Protestant. The more recent the ancestral migration, the stronger is this association. In most American communities, however, both Catholic and Protestant groups include such a variety of ethnic backgrounds that these religions may be of little practical use for identifying groups that have any special degree of ethnic or cultural homogeneity. The Jewish religion, on the other hand, does at present appear to identify a group that is more homogeneous than the population at large with respect to some characteristics—for example, circumcision, moderate use of alcohol, and possibly genotype.

While religion may be the classificatory item used to identify population groups, it is clear that explanations for observed differences in disease rates between religious groups may or may not be found in a feature of the religious practice. Specific methods of birth control, circumcision, and abstinence from tobacco are features respectively of Catholics, Jews, and Seventh Day Adventists that may be thought of as part of religious practice. On the other hand, prior to the study of Zinsser mentioned in the discussion of nativity, typhus in New York City was thought of as a disease of Jews. It had no more to do with the Jewish religion than the circumstance that the majority of the immigrants from Eastern Europe to New York City at that particular time were Jewish.

A great deal of interest in religious differences has focused in the field of cancer, in part because of the well-known rarity of cancer of the cervix among Jewish women in many different countries and economic groups. However, a study of mortality rates from cancer in New York City according to religion showed that cervical cancer was not the only form of cancer to show striking differences according to religion (Table 15).

Table 15

Estimated death rates from selected malignant neoplasms in three religious groups in New York City, 1953 to 1958*†

| Neoplasm site | Males | | | Females | | |
|---|---|---|---|---|---|---|
| | Catholic | Jewish | Protestant | Catholic | Jewish | Protestant |
| Cervix uteri | — | — | — | 22.0 | 9.0 | 24.3 |
| Tongue | 8.7 | 2.5 | 7.8 | 1.2 | 1.5 | 1.3 |
| Pharynx | 8.4 | 2.6 | 7.9 | 1.3 | 0.8 | 1.5 |
| Esophagus | 21.9 | 12.3 | 20.5 | 3.9 | 6.0 | 5.4 |
| Larynx | 14.9 | 6.2 | 15.7 | 1.1 | 0.7 | 0.8 |
| Lung | 50.0 | 34.0 | 60.0 | 4.8 | 7.0 | 5.0 |
| Stomach | 64.8 | 74.1 | 72.7 | 39.9 | 50.1 | 40.7 |
| Rectum | 43.2 | 39.8 | 40.5 | 27.2 | 26.3 | 25.0 |
| Prostate | 40.0 | 33.0 | 51.3 | — | — | — |
| Bladder | 24.8 | 24.5 | 28.5 | 9.2 | 7.3 | 11.0 |
| Ovary | — | — | — | 25.4 | 33.5 | 28.9 |
| Lymphosarcoma | 6.0 | 10.6 | 6.3 | 4.2 | 8.4 | 4.5 |
| Leukemia | 15.1 | 22.7 | 16.7 | 10.2 | 18.4 | 11.2 |
| Brain | 5.1 | 8.2 | 6.1 | 3.2 | 5.6 | 3.2 |
| Kidney | 9.7 | 17.8 | 12.6 | 5.8 | 8.5 | 5.6 |
| Pancreas | 28.6 | 35.8 | 31.0 | 19.7 | 25.2 | 19.9 |
| Large intestine | 59.1 | 81.4 | 59.8 | 59.9 | 74.5 | 60.2 |
| *All malignant neoplasms* | 578.1 | 572.3 | 623.0 | 430.3 | 516.0 | 450.7 |

* From Newill [296].
† Annual rates per 100,000 white population aged 45 years and over.

There are few appreciable differences between the rates for Catholics and Protestants evident in the table. As noted, these religions contain a variety of ethnic groups, and an unusual cancer experience of one group might not be revealed in such an examination. However, the Jewish group shows comparatively high rates for lymphosarcoma and leukemia, and for cancers of the brain, kidney, pancreas, and large intestine, and low rates for neoplasms of the tongue, upper respiratory tract, esophagus, and prostate, as well as for cervical cancer.

## Local Reproductive and Social Units

Small local populations that have maintained some degree of genetic homogeneity through inbreeding and have also maintained environmental constancy have been the subject of intensive anthropologic study. Populations of this type have so far not received a great deal of epidemiologic attention, perhaps because of the great variability in rates of disease which could be expected in groups of such small size. Nevertheless, the addition of accurate medical data to anthropologic studies has produced some interesting findings. The identification of the probable role of cannibalism in the dissemination of kuru in the Fore people of New Guinea [242], and indeed the entire story of the elucidation of the etiology of this disease, provides a good example of the usefulness of combining epidemiologic and anthropologic information. Investigations of certain North American Indian tribes show disease patterns so strikingly different from those of North American whites that closer study seems indicated [143, 374].

Within the white populations of Europe and the United States a few such localized groups have also been studied. For example, there have been several investigations of specific disease rates among isolated inbreeding Alpine populations [152]. Most of these studies have been interpreted with particular reference to genetic hypotheses. Religious belief is also occasionally associated with the formation of local groups which maintain varying degrees of inbreeding. One of the most extreme of such groups is the Hutterites, who have maintained an almost completely isolated genetic and social unit for three centuries. There are only fifteen family names in the entire sect. The unique characteristics of this group have been utilized in a study of the frequency and nature of mental disorders among them [101].

## MARITAL STATUS

Marital status is a descriptive variable which appears on medical and civil records almost as regularly as age and sex. Stratification into groups (single, married, widowed, and so forth) is usually not a difficult problem.

While marital status appears routinely on death certificates and in census records, data on deaths in relation to marital status are not published routinely in this country. They were, however, the subject of special reports of the National Office of Vital Statistics for the years surrounding the censuses of 1940 and 1950 [287, 289]. Age-standardized rates for 1949 to 1951 are shown in Table 16. They demonstrate a characteristic relation-

## Table 16

Mortality rates related to marital status in the white population aged 20 or more, United States, 1949 to 1951*†

| Marital status | Total | Male | Female |
|---|---|---|---|
| Single | 15.6 | 20.6 | 10.8 |
| Married | 11.3 | 13.1 | 8.7 |
| Widowed | 14.2 | 21.4 | 12.1 |
| Divorced | 22.5 | 26.7 | 13.7 |
| *Total* | 12.6 | 15.1 | 12.4 |

\* From *Vital Statistics Special Reports* [289].

† Average annual rates per 1000 population. Standardization is to the age distribution of the total United States population aged 20 and over in 1950.

ship—the lowest mortality is for married persons and the highest for widowed and divorced. This relationship is seen for both sexes.

Table 17, also calculated from age-specific rates given in the 1950 report, shows that rates for the single are higher than those for the married for most of the major causes of death. Three major explanations of this relationship are as follows:

1. Persons in poor health, or in the presymptomatic stages of ill health, tend to remain single.

2. Persons who "live dangerously," and are consequently exposed to a wide variety of disease-producing agents and situations, tend to remain single.

## Table 17

Mortality rates from selected causes in single and married white persons aged 20 and over, United States, 1949 to 1951*†

| Cause of death | Males | | Females | |
|---|---|---|---|---|
| | Single | Married | Single | Married |
| Respiratory tuberculosis | 96.7 | 22.7 | 25.0 | 11.4 |
| Tuberculosis, other forms | 3.4 | 1.3 | 1.8 | 0.8 |
| Syphilis | 14.8 | 6.6 | 2.0 | 2.2 |
| Malignant neoplasms | | | | |
|   Buccal and pharynx | 13.7 | 7.0 | 1.6 | 1.8 |
|   Digestive organs | 115.7 | 87.6 | 73.0 | 65.5 |
|   Respiratory system | 44.5 | 33.5 | 7.8 | 7.2 |
|   Breast | 0.7 | 0.4 | 54.0 | 33.2 |
|   Genital organs | 23.7 | 25.0 | 40.0 | 38.2 |
|   Urinary system | 15.5 | 13.3 | 6.6 | 5.8 |
|   Leukemia | 8.0 | 8.8 | 5.6 | 5.8 |
| Diabetes mellitus | 21.9 | 18.3 | 16.5 | 29.0 |
| Vascular lesions of CNS | 182.1 | 138.9 | 136.6 | 124.7 |
| Rheumatic heart disease | 28.7 | 18.6 | 23.8 | 17.4 |
| Arteriosclerotic heart disease | 525.6 | 409.9 | 212.0 | 179.1 |
| Chronic nephritis | 33.0 | 23.1 | 20.2 | 18.4 |
| Influenza and pneumonia | 73.5 | 27.0 | 34.1 | 18.3 |
| Peptic ulcer | 21.5 | 11.8 | 3.8 | 2.4 |
| Motor vehicle accidents | 61.9 | 33.7 | 11.0 | 10.8 |
| Other accidents | 99.2 | 46.1 | 36.4 | 21.1 |
| Suicide | 43.7 | 20.5 | 7.7 | 6.2 |

\* From *Vital Statistics Special Reports* [289].
† Average annual rates per 100,000 population, standardized as in Table 16.

3. There are differences in the ways of life of single and married persons that are causally related to certain diseases.

All three explanations may play a role in one or another of the observed associations.

As a specific illustration, prevalence rates of persons in United States mental hospitals are shown in Figure 11. The most striking difference seen is that between the rates for single and married persons. In addition to the magnitude of the difference, there is an interesting reversal of the sex pattern between the

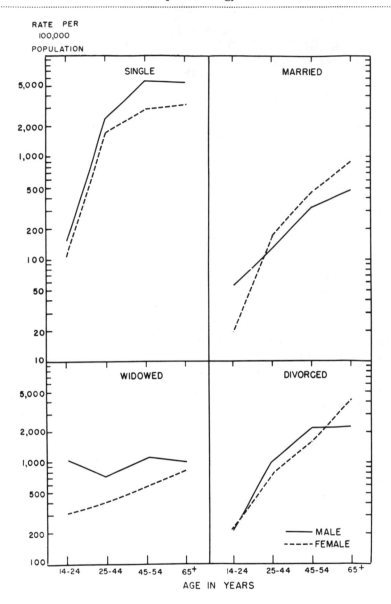

Figure 11

Point-prevalence of patients in mental hospitals per 100,000 population, by age, sex, and marital status; United States, 1950. (From Pugh and Mac-Mahon [335].)

two marital status groups. Among single persons, rates for males are higher than for females, yet among married persons the converse is true for all age groups except the youngest (14 to 24 years). Similar relations can be demonstrated in incidence (first admission) data. If the explanation of the differences is that persons with manifest or incipient mental disorders tend to remain single, then the effect of this selection must be greater for males than for females. On the other hand, there may be etiologic influences which affect single males and married females differentially. An observation that is difficult to explain on the basis of self-selection of marital status is the generally higher rates of mental disorders for widowed than for married persons, particularly in the younger age groups. The most likely explanation of this relationship seems to be that the stress of bereavement or widowhood has a causal relationship to the manifestation of mental disorder. Other explanations of the observed differences by marital status have to do with the use of mental hospital data to estimate the frequency of mental disorder. It is possible that the actual frequencies of mental disorder do not differ by marital status, but that single persons are hospitalized more frequently than married persons because of the absence of alternative care. Again, however, the high rates for widowed persons do not seem explicable on this basis, since it is difficult to believe that alternative accommodation would be less readily available to young than to old widows and widowers.

Self-selection of marital status applies not only at the time of a person's first marriage, but also to the probability of a person remaining widowed or divorced following the break-up of a first marriage. For example, low rates of suicide in married persons might be accounted for in part by a tendency for suicide-prone individuals to remain widowed or divorced once they had achieved that status, whereas the less suicide-prone might more frequently remarry. The approach of comparing "ever married" (that is, married, widowed, divorced, and separated persons as one group) with "never married" (single) is useful in overcoming the selective factors that operate after marriage [433], but it does not eliminate those associated with the original marriage.

One approach to the problem of self-selection of marital status—particularly as it relates to the possible stressful effects of widowhood—is to look for clustering of onset of the disease in relation to the time of becoming widowed. For example, the fact that suicides in widowed persons tend to cluster within the year following the bereavement points more to a causative effect of the bereavement than to the operation of selective factors [227]. This approach has not, however, been utilized to any great extent.

*Concordance Between Marital Partners*

Another use of information on marital status in epidemiologic studies is in investigations dealing with the possible influence of a common environment on the health of marital partners. It has been shown that there are a greater than expected number of instances in which both husband and wife have died from tuberculosis, pneumonia, heart disease, or cancer [54]. In morbidity data Downes found [91] that pairs of husbands and wives both had a chronic disease significantly more frequently than would be expected by chance; there was a significant association of the same illness in both spouses for hypertensive vascular disease and arthritis. Such studies are useful in pointing to disorders in which causal environmental circumstances may be sought in experiences that are common to husbands and wives. The possibility that marital partners are consciously or unconsciously selected with respect to characteristics that will determine the development of similar diseases (e.g., ethnic group or physical attributes) must of course be given consideration.

## OCCUPATION

Occupation, like marital status, appears on many routinely collected records and is used as a descriptive epidemiologic variable for a number of rather different purposes. These include the following:

1. Measurement of social or economic status. Occupation is one of the basic ways of measuring "socioeconomic status."

2. Identification of specific risks associated with exposure to noxious agents peculiar to certain occupations. This is the classic epidemiologic use of occupation that has resulted in the identification of the detrimental effects of soot, lead, benzene, aniline derivatives, ionizing radiation, and numerous other chemical and physical agents.

3. Indication of the general conditions under which an occu-

pational group works—for example, the amount of physical exercise, mental stress, or disturbance of routine associated with a particular kind of job. These general conditions may play a part in determining disease experience and yet they are not specific to any particular occupation. While association of disease rates with such general conditions may be less strong than those dependent on specific chemical or physical risks, they may be of even greater epidemiologic interest because of their relevance to circumstances outside particular occupational groups.

By far the largest body of data relating to occupation and disease derives from the analyses of the Registrar General for England and Wales, in which deaths in census and adjacent years have been related to the occupational distribution of the population as determined by the census. These analyses have been undertaken periodically since 1851, the latest and most comprehensive reports being for the years 1930 to 1932 and 1949 to 1953 [339, 342]. The reports covered both occupied and retired males aged 16 and over, and, beginning with the reports for 1930 to 1932, also gave analyses for single occupied women and for married women classified according to the occupations of their husband.

Occupations were divided into five broad classes—Professional (I), Intermediate (II), Skilled (III), Partly Skilled (IV), and Unskilled (V). In the report for 1949–1953 certain subclasses of classes III, IV, and V were also examined. In the analysis of this material considerable use has been made of the standard mortality ratio (the number of deaths, either total or cause-specific, in a given occupational group expressed as a percentage of the number of deaths that would have been expected in that occupational group if the age-and-sex-specific rates in the general population had obtained). These ratios for death from all causes and for certain causes that manifest marked socioeconomic gradients are shown in Table 18. Mortality generally increases with decreasing social class. However, quite divergent trends are seen for different diseases.

Comparable analyses for the United States, based on deaths in 1950, have been published by the National Center for Health Statistics [139].

# Table 18

Standard mortality ratios for males aged 20 to 64 in five occupational ("social") classes, England and Wales*

| Occupational class | All causes | | | 1949–1953 | | | | |
|---|---|---|---|---|---|---|---|---|
| | 1921–1923 | 1930–1932 | 1949–1953 | Tuber-culosis | Bron-chitis | Gastric ulcer | Coronary heart disease | Leu-kemia |
| I (Professional) | 82 | 90 | 98 | 59 | 34 | 53 | 147 | 123 |
| II (Intermediate) | 94 | 94 | 86 | 64 | 53 | 71 | 110 | 98 |
| III (Skilled) | 95 | 97 | 101 | 101 | 98 | 98 | 105 | 104 |
| IV (Partly skilled) | 101 | 102 | 94 | 95 | 101 | 104 | 79 | 93 |
| V (Unskilled) | 125 | 111 | 118 | 141 | 171 | 144 | 89 | 89 |

* From the Registrar General's Decennial Supplements [339, 342].

Occupation of father can be used to classify infants according to socioeconomic status. Infant mortality rates derived in this way are shown in Table 19. Infant mortality increases sharply

Table 19

Infant mortality rates per thousand livebirths, related to occupational class of father, legitimate infants, England and Wales*

| | Aged less than 1 year | | | 1949–1953 | |
| Occupational class of father | 1921–1923 | 1930–1932 | 1949–1953 | Aged under 4 weeks | Aged 4 weeks to 1 year |
|---|---|---|---|---|---|
| I (Professional) | 38.4 | 32.7 | 17.9 | 14.0 | 4.7 |
| II (Intermediate) | 55.5 | 45.0 | 22.2 | 15.6 | 6.0 |
| III (Skilled) | 76.8 | 57.6 | 28.1 | 18.3 | 10.4 |
| IV (Partly skilled) | 89.4 | 66.8 | 33.7 | 20.7 | 13.7 |
| V (Unskilled) | 97.0 | 77.1 | 40.7 | 22.8 | 18.0 |
| *Total* | 79.1 | 61.6 | 29.3 | 18.6 | 11.0 |

* From the Registrar General's Decennial Supplements [339, 342].

with decreasing socioeconomic status, and although in Britain total rates fell markedly between 1920 and 1950 the relative disparity between socioeconomic groups did not change.

Standard mortality ratios for specific occupations have given valuable leads in the identification of specific risks that might be associated with the physical and chemical exposures of certain occupations. There have also, of course, been many special studies of occupational risks. The methods are in general similar to those of cohort studies of other special groups exposed to supposedly noxious circumstances; these are dealt with later (see Chap. 11).

The variations in conditions of work that occur both between and within occupations have received increasing attention. For example, Morris and his colleagues [263] have shown that the comparative frequencies of coronary artery disease in several occupations suggest lower frequencies and less severe disease in active than in sedentary occupations. Persons in different levels of authority in the same industry have been compared with respect to hypertension and arteriosclerosis and to neurosis. Friedman et al. [120] have studied the blood cholesterol levels of accountants during periods of occupational stress, noting significant increases during such periods. Cairns and Stewart [43] have related tuberculosis rates to conditions of work within a section of the British shoe industry.

## SOCIOECONOMIC STATUS

Socioeconomic status is a theoretical concept still awaiting clear definition. So many variables, such as occupation, family income, living conditions, social prestige, and so on, are encompassed in the concept that in practice a single variable which can be objectively defined is commonly used as an indirect indicator for epidemiologic purposes. Since each variable may measure a different component of the socioeconomic complex, it is not surprising that associations may differ according to which measure is used. Associations with a single variable—for example, income—should be thought of as associations with that particular variable, rather than with the general concept of which the selected variable is only a part.

The use of occupation in this context has already been described. As noted, in addition to stratifying the wage earners themselves, this variable can be used to classify retired persons on the basis of their past occupations and married women and children on the basis of the occupation of the family wage earner.

Income might be thought of as a more direct measure of socioeconomic status than is occupation. However, the use of this variable is limited by deficiencies in both availability and comparability of data. Although data on income are collected for the population in the decennial censuses, they are not so generally available for ill persons as are data on occupation. Furthermore, even when income data are available for ill persons, as, for example, they may be in hospital records, it is questionable whether the method of ascertainment is sufficiently similar to that of census data to allow rates to be computed using numerators and denominators from such different sources. Family income has been most satisfactorily used in morbidity surveys, when data on income and other general characteristics can be assembled for the population at the same time that its health status is being ascertained. Data from the National Health Survey are shown in Figure 12. For both sexes the average number of days of bed disability decreases regularly and strikingly with increasing income, being particularly high in the lowest income group.

For most cities, census data are available that allow classification of census tracts or other small administrative units of the city according to some measure of socioeconomic status. Thus census tracts may be classified according to the median income of their populations, the percentage of the population with incomes below a certain level, the percentage of the population in certain occupational categories, or measures of housing standards such as rental or degree of crowding. Disease frequency rates may be computed and compared for residents of areas classified according to these indices. It is important to note that in this method socioeconomic status is not known for the individu-

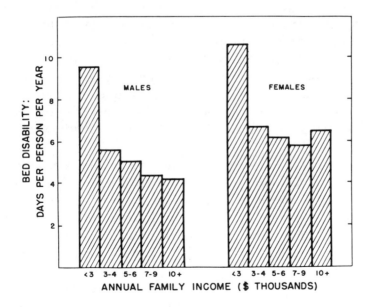

Figure 12

Average days of bed disability per person per year, by sex and family income; United States, 1965 to 1966. (Data from the National Health Survey [274].)

als concerned but is inferred from their place of residence. The reliability of the method varies greatly from one city to another and may vary also within the same city from time to time. While there is no question as to the tendency for the residences of persons of low and high economic status to cluster in certain parts of cities, the administrative areas for which the necessary census data are available may not be small enough to discriminate clearly between such clusters. If differential disease rates are demonstrated by this method, then (subject to the usual precautions) a socioeconomic association can probably be assumed. On the other hand, if no association is demonstrated, two alternative explanations must be considered: (1) that the disease is not associated with socioeconomic status, or (2) that the classification of areas is not sufficiently discriminating to detect a socioeconomic disease association which in fact exists. For example, it was noted [241] that the correlation between certain indices of overcrowding and infant mortality in the 29 boroughs of London was very high at the beginning of this century, but was virtually nonexistent in the years 1950 to 1952. Since other indices, such as father's occupation (see Table 19), suggest that the correlation between infant mortality and socioeconomic status was as high in 1950 as it had been in 1920, it is likely that the decline in the association between infant mortality and socioeconomic status measured by area of residence was due to a change in the characteristics of the London boroughs, rather than to a decline in the strength of the association of infant mortality with socioeconomic status.

Occasionally an investigator will devise an index combining a number of variables by an arbitrary formula to fit in with his concept of socioeconomic status. The index might be based on a weighted combination of such items as income, rental, family size, occupation, education, and residence. The last three, for example, were used by Hollingshead and Redlich in their study of mental disorders [168]. While such an index has usefulness in an individual study, it has the disadvantage of rarely being used in the same form by other investigators, and therefore hindering comparisons of results between studies.

A more detailed discussion of ways of measuring social class and of its relevance to illness is given by Susser and Watson

[388]. Petras and Curtis, in reviewing the literature on the relationship between social class and mental illness [316], illustrate the variety of ways in which social class has been measured and the problems that arise in the interpretation of observed associations.

## INTERPRETATION

Associations between disease risk and characteristics of persons are sought as a part of epidemiologic routine directed at stimulating the development of hypotheses concerning disease causation. The objectives in interpreting the associations that are uncovered are to suggest a variety of explanations, and to evaluate the various explanations in the light of other things that are known about the disease.

As noted in Chapter 3, substantial hypotheses rarely come from knowledge of an association with one variable. But if associations with two or three variables have been uncovered, each of which has a number of explanations, strong hypotheses may be derived by noting which explanations are common to several of the observations.

In seeking explanations of descriptive associations, it may be useful to consider the kinds of explanation indicated in the following list. (This is a check list rather than a classification, since a particular explanation might well appear in several of the categories.)

1. Errors of measurement
2. Differences in more directly associated variables
3. Differences in environment
4. Differences in bodily constitution
5. Differences in genetic constitution

The same categories of explanation apply to variables descriptive of place, as well as those descriptive of persons, and most of them may also be relevant to changes occurring with time. So as to give a series of examples having some degree of continuity, the list will be discussed in the context of disease associations with sex and ethnic group.

ERRORS OF MEASUREMENT. Measurement errors may result in apparent associations at several levels. For example, there may be differences between groups in access to medical care and hence diagnosis. Minor illnesses may be more frequently diagnosed in certain groups of males than in females because of ready access to occupationally based medical care facilities. United States national statistics indicate lower rates of congenital malformation for Negroes than for whites, but a considerably greater proportion of deliveries of Negro infants occurs in rural areas of the South where medical care (and hence observation) is inadequate. Even when facilities are equally available to all groups, there may be differences in utilization. For example, women are more reluctant than men to undergo physical examination. Even in the same medical care plan, utilization rates tend to be lower for Negroes than for whites, and for Catholics and Protestants than for Jews (in the United States).

Even if access to and utilization of medical care can be considered equal, differences in precision of diagnosis must also be considered. Thus venereal disease is more difficult to diagnose in the female than in the male. Certain skin rashes may be more difficult to diagnose in Negroes than in whites. Even if precision of diagnosis is equal, the reporting of it may vary. For example, in morbidity surveys in which anamnestic data are sought by household interview it is most commonly a female who is interviewed, and the reporting of data for females in such households is therefore likely to be more complete than that for males. Differences in reporting frequencies also may occur between ethnic groups; for example, in connection with the reporting of minor degrees of mental disturbance.

DIFFERENCES IN MORE DIRECTLY ASSOCIATED VARIABLES. Differences between groups with respect to one descriptive variable may be more directly accounted for by a difference between the groups with respect to another variable. For example, as noted at the outset of this chapter, age variation in disease rates is usually so marked that it is hazardous to examine associations with other variables unless the data are adequate to eliminate the possible effect of age differences between the compared groups. This may be done by examination of age-specific rates for the compared groups or by the use of "standardized" rates, which are summary rates adjusted to allow for age differences. The methods of standardization are described in textbooks of biostatistics [162].

In addition to differing in age, sex and ethnic origin, groups may differ with respect to almost any other descriptive variable. Thus ethnic groups in the same community often differ with respect to socioeconomic status and occupation. Similar procedures to those used to eliminate the effect of age may be applied. Thus, if a difference between whites and Negroes is observed, it would be logical to compare whites and Negroes within restricted ranges of socioeconomic status and/or within restricted categories of occupation. If the differences between whites and Negroes persist within such restricted subgroups, it is unlikely that differences in socioeconomic status explain the observed ethnic differences. Conversely, if a difference between occupational or socioeconomic status is observed, it might be desirable to determine whether these differences persist in comparisons of persons of similar ethnic backgrounds. Similar standardization techniques to those used for age may be applied to obtain summary rates after elimination of the effect of one or the other variable.

The desirability of identifying the descriptive variable that most closely localizes differences between groups in disease rates frequently arises in interpreting differences between ethnic groups. The use of migrant populations to determine whether a difference in disease incidence is associated with the particular circumstances under which the ethnic group is living at the time of observation, or whether it is a more permanent feature of the ethnic group, is discussed in Chapter 10.

DIFFERENCES IN ENVIRONMENT. Differences in environment between sex or ethnic groups may be exemplified by differences in personal customs, habits, and recreational patterns. For example, ethnic differences in quantity and quality of alcohol used are well known (at least at the anecdotal level), and differences in tobacco use are probably no less striking. Such differences exist also between males and females; they are entirely capable of explaining the sex difference in lung cancer rates, and are suspected of association with sex variation in cancer of the upper respiratory and digestive tracts. Sexual practices, including contraception, show ethnic variation and may be related to ethnic differences in diseases of the reproductive organs. Likewise, a specified sexual practice or experience may affect the health of one sex differently from the other.

Dietary differences between ethnic groups have received considerable attention through attempts to relate levels of arteriosclerotic heart disease in various ethnic groups to levels of intake of fat and other dietary constituents. Ethnic differences in vitamin deficiency diseases, notably pellagra, have also been shown to be due to differences in dietary patterns. Dietary differences, of an as-yet-unidentified nature, are also suspected of being related to ethnic variation in stomach cancer. Dietary differences also exist between the sexes and have a bearing on the higher frequency of obesity in females than in males.

DIFFERENCES IN BODILY CONSTITUTION. Constitutional differences associated with variation in disease rates include anatomic, physiologic, and mental (attitude) differences. Anatomic features are perhaps more important in connection with sex than with ethnic differences. Apart from the obvious differences in organs with specifically sexual functions, many more subtle anatomic differences between the sexes may have pertinence to differences in disease incidence. For example, the higher frequency of arthritis of the hip and pelvic joints in females has been attributed to skeletal differences and consequent differences in the lines of stress imposed by weight bearing. Although less common, such differences do occur between ethnic groups. For example, the protection against the sun's rays conferred by skin coloring presumably is associated with differences noted between ethnic groups in skin cancer frequency.

Physiologic differences between males and females are illustrated by hormonal differences, suspected of association with several important diseases including atherosclerosis and several forms of neoplasm. More obviously, specific diseases of the endocrine glands (e.g., the thyroid gland) are likely to be influenced by the total hormonal environment in which the gland is operating. Again, physiologic differences between ethnic groups are less obvious than those between the sexes. The level of immunity at the time of challenge with organisms is one type of physiologic characteristic which varies between ethnic groups. For example, the low frequency of paralytic poliomyelitis in Negroes in the United States, noted at a time preceding the introduction of poliomyelitis vaccine, was attributed to frequent early exposure (associated with overcrowding and other features of low socioeconomic status) at an age when paralysis is rare, resulting in subsequent high levels of immunity.

Mental or attitude differences as explanatory of differences in disease rates between sex and ethnic groups are most obvious with respect to the several forms of disability due to violence (Fig. 13). Here again, quite different explanations may be sought for the existence of the attitude differences in the first place. Levels of disease perception, as illustrated by sex and ethnic differences in pain tolerance, may also be thought of as part of the contribution of attitude differences to disease rates.

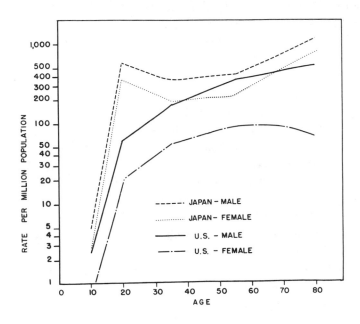

Figure 13

Death rates from suicide, by age and sex; Japan and United States whites, 1954 to 1956. (Data from the WHO *Epidemiological and Vital Statistics Reports* [424].)

DIFFERENCES IN GENETIC CONSTITUTION. Genetic differences may account for differences in disease rates between groups insofar as genetic constitution determines many of the more directly associated attributes mentioned above, such as, for example, skin color or the presence of the reproductive organs of one sex or the other. In addition, single major genes (that is, single genes which under suitable circumstances are associated with a demonstrable characteristic of the persons carrying them) may be transmitted in association either with sex or with ethnic group. In the case of transmission of such genes in a particular sex pattern, the pattern is attributable to disease-associated genes being located on the same chromosome pair that determines sex (sex linkage). Examples include hemophilia, certain forms of muscular dystrophy, and red-green color blindness. Sex-linked diseases are usually readily identifiable when major genes of a high degree of manifestation are involved.

Ethnic concentration of genetically determined disorders, on the other hand, is usually due to limitation of mating to the particular ethnic group over many generations, and the consequent limitation to that ethnic group of genetic material which originally arose as new mutations in that group or was introduced to it by immigrants. When major genes are involved, as in the case of sickle cell anemia, thalassemia, and Tay-Sachs disease, genetic analysis will usually identify this type of ethnic concentration. However, greater difficulty arises either when manifestation of a major gene is weak and dependent on other unknown factors, or when many minor genes are involved, none of which alone has a demonstrable effect. Evidence for this type of determination of ethnic differences is difficult to obtain. Simultaneous consideration should be given to collateral evidence of genetic determination within ethnic groups (familial incidence, twin studies, etc.), showing that the characteristic rate (whether high or low) is a stable feature of the ethnic group and demonstration that other types of explanations are not sufficient to explain noted differences.

# 8

---

## *Place*

Variation in the frequency of different disease manifestations from place to place has long been recognized. Knowledge of the geographic distribution of disease has obvious utility for administrative purposes and has contributed importantly to many hypotheses of etiology.

### TYPES OF COMPARISONS

Early knowledge of the geographic distribution of disease was entirely qualitative, and derived from the sporadically published observations of medical practitioners. Hirsch's three-volume *Handbook of Geographical and Historical Pathology,* translated into English in 1883 [166], is a gargantuan accumulation of such observations and represents the full flowering of anecdotal epidemiology.

The quantitative knowledge of present-day epidemiology is based in part on routinely collected and published vital data and in part on special surveys. The use of routinely collected statistics on causes of death and notifications of disease has the advantage of allowing exploratory examinations to determine the likelihood of significant geographic variation. However, routine data have a number of disadvantages. First, there are difficulties due to variations that exist from place to place in standards of medical care, diagnosis, and reporting of illness or death. Second, there is the limited number of diseases—primarily the infectious diseases and disorders that are reported as causes of death—for which data are available. Third, the regions for which data are available are usually administratively defined, and the geographic factors influential as determinants of disease frequency may only fortuitously be congruent with administrative boundaries; consequently, failure to demonstrate geographic differences in the distribution of a disease with routine data does not exclude the possibility that place indeed plays a role in its occurrence.

When probable differences are recognized in routine data, special surveys may be instituted. Special surveys are expensive and are unlikely to be undertaken unless routine data suggest specific hypotheses which need testing.

## International Comparisons

Data relating to causes of death and notifications of infectious diseases in many nations are collected and published by the World Health Organization [427]. Although the published data are restricted to those countries from which reporting is believed to be adequate, differences in accuracy and completeness of diagnosis and reporting pose serious difficulties. Uncertainty whether even gross differences in disease rates may be due to such artifacts is felt particularly when they are found in underdeveloped countries. Nevertheless, the large differences that have been demonstrated, and even those that are less striking, should not be ignored simply because of this uncertainty. They may at least merit special studies to test their validity. Considerable efforts are being made by the World Health Organization and other agencies to improve sources of data so that broader and more reliable international comparisons of disease rates can be conducted.

For certain diseases—for example, the major parasitic and bacterial diseases—the fact that they are epidemic in some areas and virtually absent in others is immediately obvious from review of either clinical opinion or statistical material. The international differences observed for the noninfectious diseases are generally smaller than those seen in infectious diseases. Nevertheless, these differences may be even more important from an investigative point of view, since most of them concern diseases of unknown etiology, and the international differences are in many instances the most striking feature of the descriptive epidemiology of the disease. Japan, for example, with relatively low rates of death from coronary artery disease, has very high rates of hypertension and cerebrovascular accidents; unusually high death rates from stomach cancer exist in Germany and Iceland, as well as in Japan; Britain has higher rates of lung cancer than any other nation, although the United States is not far behind. If the United States needs honors, it has them for coronary artery disease. Perhaps the main value of statistical data such as these is to provide a basis for the broad classification of countries into those with probably high, probably average, and probably low rates of a disease. Most of the data are too fragile to support finer classifications at the present time.

In evaluating differences between nations in disease rates—indeed, in making any geographic comparisons—the observer does well to assess the possible effects not only of differences in disease reporting but also of peculiarities in census data which might play a part in determining the relative rates.

Special studies undertaken to test the validity of international differences seen in routine data are well illustrated by those which have correlated coronary artery disease frequencies with dietary constituents in various countries. Special clinical studies have been made among groups of people in areas selected because of observed dietary patterns [357]. Valuable information on the distribution of atherosclerosis and on the levels of serum cholesterol has been obtained, although there is still no consensus as to which dietary constituents are most closely correlated with the variation in coronary disease frequency [431].

In many international studies of this type, information on both the suspected causes (such as diet) and health or disease is obtained for the same person. In this type of study the fact that the individuals observed may not be representative of the population residing in the area is not crucial. However, if disease rates based on special study groups are to be compared with dietary or other environmental characteristics derived from the general population of the area, the selection of a representative sample in the special study group does become critical and considerably increases the technical difficulties of the study.

*Variation Within Countries*

Death statistics and notifications of infectious diseases are also the major sources of data for comparisons within countries. Again, use must be made of the administrative areas for which deaths and populations bases are enumerated. Within limits, the smaller the geographic boundaries of the areas examined, the more accurately the boundaries of areas of high or low disease frequency can be drawn, provided that the individual areas have populations large enough to yield reliable rates.

For example, Figure 14 shows standard mortality ratios (SMRs) for deaths from leukemia in each state of the contiguous United States, while Figure 15 shows SMRs calculated for individual economic subregions, the latter being smaller geographic units that incorporate several contiguous counties within states. At a glance, the impressions obtained from the two figures are similar—both, for example, indicate low frequencies in the Southeast and a pocket of high frequency in the North Central part of the country. When examined more closely, however, the maps show significant dissimilarities. For example, Figure 14 suggests that rates are very high in Minnesota and that an area of high rates extends across Wisconsin to the shore of Lake Michigan. But in Figure 15 it is seen that the highest frequencies actually are found in Western Minnesota, extending into parts of the Dakotas. Similarly, Figure 15 shows that the high rate for New York State compared with surrounding states (seen in Fig. 14) is in fact a characteristic of the New York metropolitan area, but not of upstate New York.

Detailed geographic delineation of disease frequencies may not always be required. There may, for example, be interest primarily in the question of whether there is a difference in frequency between the northern and the southern parts of a country. Even so, an examination of data for small administrative units will help to clarify whether a difference noted between the north and the south (when examined as two large units) reflects a difference of the areas in general or is due to the presence

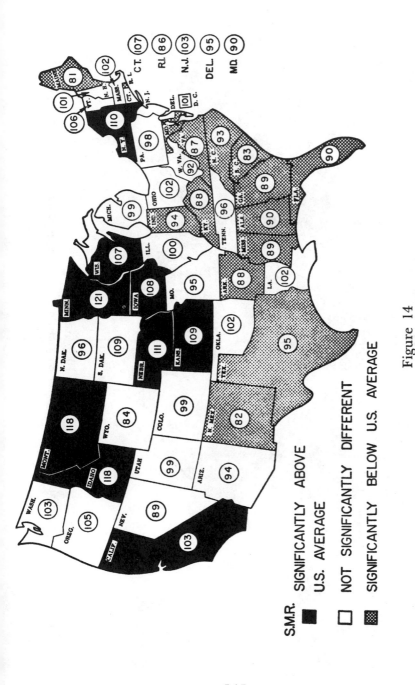

Figure 14

Standard mortality ratios (SMRs) for deaths from leukemia in 48 states; 1949 to 1955. (From Gilliam [127].)

S.M.R.
■ SIGNIFICANTLY ABOVE U.S. AVERAGE

□ NOT SIGNIFICANTLY DIFFERENT

▨ SIGNIFICANTLY BELOW U.S. AVERAGE

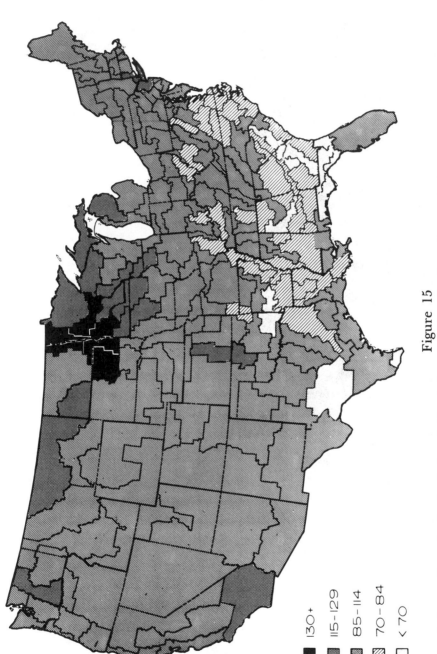

Figure 15

Standard mortality ratios for deaths from leukemia for economic subregions of the United States, 1949 to 1951. (From Gilliam [127].)

130+
115-129
85-114
70-84
< 70

within one or the other of geographic localizations of very high or low frequency. The presence of a few pockets of high frequency in one half of a country obviously requires a different interpretation from the finding of a widespread higher frequency in one half compared to the other.

The association with place within a country need not be based on spatial contiguity. For example, it may be desirable to compare counties or states having large agricultural populations with those that are largely urban. The same possibility—that one or the other category might show a high disease frequency because it includes one or two areas of very high frequency—can be examined by comparison of areas classified according to several levels of the relevant variable rather than according to a simple dichotomy, or by arranging varieties of areas into those having rates above and below average levels of disease frequency.

The examination of geographic variation may extend to the development and exploration of hypotheses attempting to explain the noted variation in terms of other known characteristics of the regions. This usually involves comparison of the disease frequencies in various areas with the frequencies of those characteristics suspected of being relevant. An example is the work of Dean and others [77] (Fig. 16) in the identification of fluoride content of drinking water as a major determinant of the geographic variation in frequency of dental caries. Communities with low levels of fluoride in the drinking water had low levels of fluorosis and high rates of dental caries, while those with high fluoride levels had high rates of fluorosis and low levels of caries. The trends suggest 1.0 ppm of fluoride as the optimum level; increasing fluoride concentration to this point was associated with only a small increase in fluorosis rates but a sharp decline in caries rates; higher concentrations were associated with only a small decline in caries rates but a substantial increase in fluorosis rates.

Information such as this is usually not derived from routine data but from special surveys designed to examine specific hypotheses. Special surveys both of animals and of man are frequently undertaken to develop an understanding of the distribution of infectious diseases. In man such surveys may involve

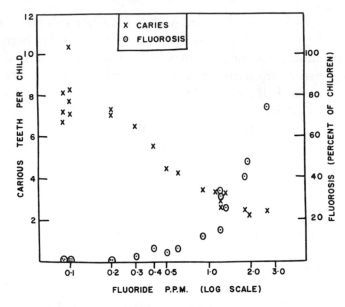

Figure 16

Fluoride content of drinking water (parts per million) correlated with dental caries experience (carious teeth per child) and with evidence of any degree of dental fluorosis; white children, aged 12 to 14 years, in 21 U.S. cities. (Data from Dean [77].)

search for existing cases of the disease. Frequently, however, they are concerned mainly with evidences of residua of infections—for example, the presence of antibodies in the serum, trachoma scars, or splenomegaly due to malaria. Clearly, examination of populations for scars and other residua of past infections is more rewarding from the standpoint of numbers found than is a search for current cases. It should be noted, however, that the information derived yields a peculiar form of prevalence—the frequency of having had and survived a past infection. The evaluation of such a rate is necessarily difficult.

A social phenomenon that involved the clinical examination of certain age groups of men from all over the United States and was useful to the geographically minded epidemiologist was the mobilization of the Armed Forces during World War II. For example, several studies [100] of the prevalence of dental caries in relation to area of residence of inductees were undertaken. Similarly, Gentry et al. [123] used data from the same source to examine the area of residence of inductees with sarcoidosis. This study provides a good example of the relationship between ethnic group and geography. Since sarcoidosis occurs much more frequently among Negroes, the finding that most cases came from the southeastern part of the United States was, at first sight, not surprising. However, even when allowance was made for the geographic distribution of the Negro population, there still appears to have been an excessive concentration of the disease in this area and in certain smaller areas within the Southeast.

## Urban-Rural Comparisons

A special type of intracountry comparison that does not involve classification into contiguous areas is the examination of differences in disease frequency according to degree of urbanization. Increasing use of this variable has demonstrated that economic and industrial development is not an unmitigated blessing.

Both the U.S. National Center for Health Statistics and the Registrar General for England and Wales publish tabulations of deaths by cause according to urban or rural residence. In the United States the division is along county lines (except in New England states, where towns and cities are the units), counties being classified according to whether they lie within one of the Standard Metropolitan Statistical Areas (SMSAs) established by the Bureau of the Census (metropolitan counties), or not (nonmetropolitan counties). Special tabulations, undertaken in connection with the Air Pollution Medical Program of the U.S Public Health Service, provide death rates by cause for each SMSA for the years 1949 to 1951 [236] and 1959 to 1961 [94]. The 1949 to 1951 tabulations, in addition to allowing comparisons of individual SMSAs, allow comparison of the metropolitan with the nonmetropolitan counties. A distinction is also drawn between counties with a central city in an SMSA and counties that do not include a large city although still included in an SMSA. The latter are presumably less urbanized than the former.

Data for England and Wales published by the Registrar General provide even more detail for study of urban-rural differences. Tabulations of deaths by cause, age, and sex are given for six large conurbations (coalescenses of major towns), for urban areas outside the conurbations divided into three groups according to population size, and for rural areas.

Table 20 illustrates urban-rural comparisons for selected causes of death in the white population of the United States. Death rates are generally higher for urban than for rural areas, both for all causes of death and for many individual causes. The data for deaths from "symptoms, senility, and ill-defined conditions" indicate that diagnostic and reporting difficulties may enter into these comparisons, although—at least in the United States and Great Britain—the effect of such differences is small. The most striking excess in urban as compared with rural populations is seen for arteriosclerotic heart disease, tuberculosis, and cirrhosis of the liver. The excess rural death rates from nephritis and vascular lesions of the central nervous system, although small, are of interest because they are contrary to the general trend.

Urban-rural comparisons are also frequently made during the course of special studies. For example, in the infectious diseases, inferences regarding mechanisms of spread have been made from comparisons of urban and rural areas with respect to frequency, age distribution, and rapidity of spread of the disease. Diseases spread by contact and respiratory infections are acquired later in life and often less frequently in the country than in the city. On the other hand, many diseases transmitted from animals to man have greater opportunity to affect human beings in rural areas.

Results of two cancer morbidity studies, one a special survey in Iowa and the other of data from the Danish Cancer Registry, are shown in Table 21. Minor differences in this table must be interpreted with caution since diagnostic standards may well be somewhat higher in urban than in rural areas, even within these two limited geographic regions. However, strikingly higher rates for urban areas are seen in both studies for cancers of the pharynx, esophagus, lung, urinary bladder, and cervix.

## Local Distributions

The preparation of maps showing the distribution of cases of a disease within the local community is a long-established epide-

# Table 20

Mortality rates for selected causes of death, by degree of urbanization, United States, white population, 1949 to 1951*†

| | Males | | | Females | | |
|---|---|---|---|---|---|---|
| | Metropolitan counties | | Non-metropolitan counties | Metropolitan counties | | Non-metropolitan counties |
| Cause of death | With central city | Without central city | | With central city | Without central city | |
| All causes | 1161 | 1061 | 1049 | 777 | 743 | 722 |
| Arteriosclerotic heart disease | 338 | 306 | 246 | 165 | 152 | 113 |
| Cancer (all sites) | 166 | 156 | 123 | 139 | 136 | 118 |
| Vascular lesions of CNS | 98 | 96 | 107 | 92 | 93 | 98 |
| Accidents | 74 | 71 | 99 | 32 | 31 | 38 |
| Hypertension | 60 | 56 | 53 | 60 | 60 | 52 |
| Tuberculosis | 30 | 19 | 21 | 11 | 8 | 12 |
| Other infectious diseases | 14 | 13 | 19 | 8 | 8 | 14 |
| Nephritis | 16 | 16 | 20 | 12 | 13 | 17 |
| Diabetes mellitus | 14 | 13 | 12 | 21 | 21 | 17 |
| Cirrhosis of liver | 17 | 13 | 8 | 8 | 7 | 4 |
| Peptic ulcer | 10 | 9 | 7 | 2 | 2 | 1 |
| Symptoms, senility, and ill-defined conditions | 9 | 8 | 18 | 5 | 5 | 12 |

* From Manos [236].
† Average annual rates per 100,000 population, standardized to the age distribution of the total population of the United States in 1950.

## Table 21
Urban-rural differences in incidence of cancer of selected sites, Denmark, 1948 to 1952, and Iowa, 1950*†

| Site and sex | Denmark | | | Iowa | |
|---|---|---|---|---|---|
| | Copen-hagen | Provincial towns | Rural areas | Urban area | Rural areas |
| Lip (M) | 2.9 | 4.7 | 8.1 | 17.3 | 15.7 |
| Tongue (M) | 1.4 | 1.0 | 0.3 | 1.6 | 1.1 |
| Pharynx (M) | 1.9 | 0.8 | 0.3 | 4.3 | 1.5 |
| Esophagus (M) | 8.0 | 5.1 | 3.8 | 3.9 | 2.1 |
| Stomach (M) | 37.0 | 43.4 | 41.8 | 24.7 | 24.7 |
| Stomach (F) | 23.6 | 26.7 | 29.8 | 13.1 | 14.1 |
| Rectum (M) | 25.2 | 22.5 | 17.4 | 16.3 | 12.4 |
| Rectum (F) | 13.9 | 12.2 | 11.2 | 10.0 | 11.0 |
| Lung (M) | 43.6 | 15.3 | 8.3 | 29.0 | 10.2 |
| Kidney (M) | 8.8 | 4.4 | 3.7 | 4.8 | 3.5 |
| Kidney (F) | 5.2 | 3.0 | 3.4 | 3.3 | 2.8 |
| Bladder (M) | 15.3 | 7.7 | 5.6 | 20.2 | 12.9 |
| Bladder (F) | 4.1 | 2.4 | 2.1 | 6.6 | 3.2 |
| Leukemia‡ (M) | 8.4 | 7.0 | 6.6 | 14.4 | 11.4 |
| Leukemia‡ (F) | 6.0 | 5.0 | 4.5 | 10.9 | 7.2 |
| Cervix uteri (F) | 38.4 | 34.9 | 20.2 | 43.4 | 23.6 |
| Corpus uteri (F) | 14.4 | 10.9 | 7.9 | 11.0 | 10.9 |
| Breast (F) | 57.4 | 49.3 | 40.9 | 78.0 | 62.4 |
| All sites (M) | 284.8 | 224.7 | 185.7 | 350.6 | 250.2 |
| All sites (F) | 272.5 | 241.5 | 208.6 | 351.6 | 261.5 |

* From Clemmesen and Nielsen [57] and Haenszel et al. [146].

† Annual incidence rates per 100,000, standardized to the age distribution of the total United States population in 1950.

‡ For Iowa, these rates include other cancers of the hemopoietic system.

miologic procedure. A classic example, Snow's investigation [376] of the outbreak of cholera in the Golden Square area of London in August and September of 1854, is illustrated in Figure 17. The identification by Snow of the place where each patient was attacked enabled him to center attention on the pump in Broad Street (*A*), available to the general public as a source of water. He noted that the outbreak centered around this pump and that the number of cases was small in areas that were

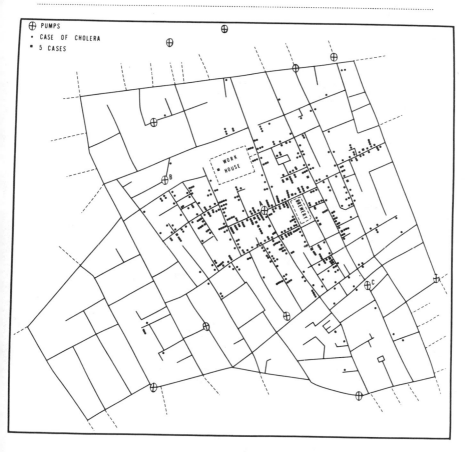

**Figure 17**

Street map of the districts of Golden Square, St. James and Berwick St.,
London, showing the distribution of cholera cases in the outbreak of August
and September, 1854. (From Snow [376].)

closer to some other source of water. The localization of cases
around the Broad Street pump became still more striking to
Snow when he noted that, although there were several cases in
the vicinity of the pump in Marlborough Street (B), the water
from this pump, being obviously polluted, was avoided by residents of the area who preferred to walk the additional distance
to the pump in Broad Street. In addition, he noted that while
several cases seemed to be quite close to the pump in Rupert
Street (C) these patients actually had to walk a considerable

distance to that pump because of the configuration of the streets in the area.

While formal reference to the population at risk is usually not included in such a map, knowledge of the distribution of the population is essential to interpretation. An area of the map may be free of cases merely because it is not populated. For example, the 5 cases shown in the workhouse on Snow's map mean little unless it is known that the institution had 535 inhabitants. By contrast, a percussion-cap factory in Broad Street had 18 cases among approximately 200 workers. The workers in the factory used water from the Broad Street pump, but the workhouse had its own well on the grounds. Similarly, the absence of cases among workers in the brewery in Broad Street becomes significant when it is known that 70 men were employed there. This feature gave support to Snow's hypothesis when, inquiring of Mr. Huggins, the proprietor, he ascertained that: "The men are allowed a certain quantity of malt liquor, and Mr. Huggins believes they do not drink water at all; and he is quite certain that the workmen never obtained water from the pump in the street. There is a deep well in the brewery" [376].

The making of a spot map such as this is commonly the first procedure in the investigation of a localized outbreak of disease. As noted, inferences from such a map depend on the assumption that the population at risk of developing the disease is fairly evenly distributed over the area, or at least that heterogeneities are known and can be considered in interpreting the map. When the space clustering is less striking than that shown in Figure 17, there may be uncertainty as to whether or not variations in the population distribution account for the disease clustering. If populations of the subsections of the affected area are known and are sufficiently large, it may be possible to compute rates for the subsections. However, this is often not possible for small areas that are of interest.

Another approach was illustrated in a study of 233 cases of breast cancer in Boston in 1965 [350]. It was noted that in this series there were 23 instances, involving 67 cases, of more than one case being resident on a single street. Even though there was no reason to suspect the existence of space clustering in this disease, 67 out of 233 cases seemed an unduly high proportion. To assess the likelihood of this occurrence being due to population variation, seven random samples, each the same size as the breast cancer series, were drawn from the female population aged 35 or older, and these were also examined for multiple residences on the same street. After exclusion of certain streets which traversed almost the entire city (no account was taken of house number in this study), the numbers of instances in which there was more than one woman resident on the same street in the seven random samples were 17, 21, 19, 20, 17, 20, and 22. The mean for the seven samples was 19.4 and the comparable count for the breast cancer cases was 21. Values similar in the random samples and the breast cancer series were also obtained for the numbers of voting precincts and census tracts represented by more than two women in a single series. There was, therefore, no evidence that breast cancer cases tended to cluster within the city other than the clustering that would be expected to follow from the distribution of the population of appropriate age and sex. This method is, of course, feasible only when population registries, detailed maps, or other resources for selecting random samples of the population of the area, exist or can be created.

As with larger geographic units, routine data or clinical impressions suggesting localization of disease in small areas may lead to special surveys to define more adequately the boundaries and patterns of the distribution. Clinical impressions of very high frequencies of severe chronic nephropathy in certain villages located along the Sava River in Yugoslavia and the Danube in Bulgaria and Rumania have led to systematic surveys, some of which are described by Gaon [122]. The impression of striking place-localization of the disease has been confirmed, but so far not explained.

## INTERPRETATION

The demonstration of association of a disease with place implies either that the inhabitants of the particular place possess characteristics of etiologic importance in the disease and different from those of the inhabitants of other places, or that etiologic factors are present in the biologic, chemical and physical, or social environments of the people inhabiting the affected places, or that both these types of explanation apply.

## Characteristics of Inhabitants

Characteristics of persons that produce associations with place include some of the demographic characteristics discussed in Chapter 7. Age, for example, is so obvious a confounding factor that allowance for age differences between the populations of different places should form part of the method of the comparison and not need to enter into interpretative considerations. Mention has already been made of ethnic differences as determinants of geographic patterns. Religious groups also tend to be geographically clustered—for example, it is likely that the low death rates from lung cancer in the State of Utah can be attributed to the abstinence from tobacco that is characteristic of the large Mormon population.

On the other hand, the personal characteristics involved may be more subtle and not identifiable through use of gross demographic variables. An example of disease variation from place to place that may be attributable to genetic differences is the variation in frequency of sickle cell anemia in Africa. The sickle cell trait, which does not usually cause anemia, occurs in persons heterozygous for the gene which in homozygous form is associated with sickle cell anemia. Within East and West Africa, the sickle cell trait tends to be most frequent in areas in which malaria rates are highest. Allison [9] has shown that persons who are heterozygous for the sickling gene, although as frequently infected by the malaria parasite, are more resistant to it. It seems likely, therefore, that selection in favor of persons with the sickling trait is at least partly responsible for the occurrence of high sickling rates in districts with high malaria rates [206]. On the other hand, it is also likely that the present distribution of the sickling gene accounts for some geographic variation in the distribution of malaria as a disease manifestation, since prevalence rates of the sickling trait between 20 and 30 percent are fairly frequent among West African tribes.

Another kind of genetic explanation of place variation in disease rates is based on variations in the degree of inbreeding present in different areas. For example, Hewitt [159], noting a decline in rates of spina bifida as one proceeds westwards across North America, suggested that this might be due to greater outbreeding among inhabitants of the Western areas. A similar kind of mechanism is discussed in Chapter 9 in connection with time changes.

## Characteristics Peculiar to Place

That a noted geographic association may be explained in terms of characteristics inherent to the place of occurrence of a disease is suggested by any of the following criteria:

1. High frequency rates are observed in all ethnic groups inhabiting the area.
2. High frequency rates are not observed in persons of similar ethnic groups inhabiting other areas.
3. Healthy persons entering the area become ill with a frequency similar to the indigenous inhabitants.
4. Inhabitants who have left the area do not show high rates.
5. Other species than man inhabiting the same area show similar manifestations.

The more of these criteria that a disease satisfies, the more probably the frequency of the disease is in fact determined by a characteristic (or characteristics) directly related to place. The role of studies of migrant populations in clarifying these relationships is discussed later (Chap. 10). The fact that one or several of the criteria are not satisfied does not rule out the possibility that strong etiologic agents peculiar to the locality are operative in the genesis of a disease. For example, criterion 4 may be inappropriate if the disease is one with a lengthy preclinical phase or is associated with progressive and irreversible pathologic change; or criteria 1 and 5 may not pertain in the presence of genetic or other additional causal factors.

It is worth noting parenthetically that differences in observed geographic distributions may lead to erroneous as well as to enlightening conclusions when additional associations are present. For example, an important argument used against the hypothesis of an etiologic similarity between syphilis and general paralysis of the insane was that general paralysis was quite rare in many countries where syphilis was very common [192].

If the evidence that a particular place or type of place exercises an etiologic influence on a disease seems reasonably convincing, it is possible to seek responsible mechanisms among several of the broad (and not mutually exclusive) features which make up our concept of place.

BIOLOGIC ENVIRONMENT. Best understood of the disease-determining features of place are the climatic and ecologic characteristics that determine the animal and vegetable environment. Such characteristics influence disease patterns by providing temperature, humidity, and other conditions appropriate for the survival of parasites outside the body (for example, the cercariae of schistosomiasis, the larval stages of some intestinal parasitic worms, and the various leptospira); by providing conditions suitable for the reproduction of animal vectors (for example, mosquitoes, tsetse flies, ticks, and various ectoparasites of man and other animals); and by determining the size and kind of animal populations available either as hosts for stages of the parasites or as reservoirs of infection (for example, mollusks in schistosomiasis and the mammalian reservoirs of plague, rabies, trypanosomiasis and yellow fever).

The vegetable environment, in addition to influencing the animal environment, may have a direct role, as illustrated by the geographic distribution of such prosaic diseases as poison ivy dermatitis and such exotic ones as ergotism.

CHEMICAL AND PHYSICAL ENVIRONMENTS. The chemical constituents of at least two components of the human environment —drinking water and inspired air—vary from place to place in a way that may influence health. The classic example of a place-related disease is perhaps endemic goiter. That it was associated with certain places was recognized long before it was known to be caused by iodine-deficient soil. Swayback in sheep is also the result of a deficiency, in this instance of copper. With respect to high levels of certain chemicals in certain places, dental fluorosis was recognized as a place disease long before its etiology was understood—indeed almost as soon as it was recognized as a clinical entity. McKay and Black, in 1916, wrote: "The remarkable thing about the lesion is that it is practically . . . limited . . . to certain well-defined geographical areas, in which it occurs in the teeth of only those individuals who were either born and lived continuously in any of these areas during the years of enamel formation; or in those who, although being born elsewhere, were brought into such districts for a continuous residence during the years of enamel formation" [213].

Surveys of "blackfoot disease" (peripheral vascular disease with gangrene) and skin lesions in a small area of Taiwan have revealed an etiologic syndrome consisting of blackfoot disease, hyperpigmentation, keratosis, and skin cancer, apparently due to chronic arsenic poisoning from high levels of arsenic in drinking water from deep artesian wells [400].

The inhalation of toxic chemicals peculiar to certain localities was well illustrated by the acute effects of the London fog shown in Figure 1 (p. 4). It seems likely, though not fully established, that atmospheric pollution also has long-term effects on human health, including a possible role in the etiology of lung cancer. Such an association may explain the unenviable position of Great Britain with respect to death rates from lung cancer.

Physical environment plays an obvious role in diseases and disabilities directly connected with exposure to heat, cold, or high altitude. In the last context, a congenital malformation of the cardiovascular system—patent ductus arteriosus—appears to be unduly frequent among infants born in areas of high altitude, a feature that may be explicable in terms of exposure to low oxygen tension at a critical stage of development [310]. There has been interest in the identification of possible geographic variations in rates of diseases known to be associated with exposure to ionizing radiation—for example, leukemia and bone cancer—according to variation in the levels of background radioactivity. In part because of the relatively small populations that reside in areas of very high background radioactivity, this possibility has not yet been adequately explored.

SOCIAL ENVIRONMENT. Social arrangements peculiar to specified places are major determinants of the biologic, chemical, and physical environments to which the inhabitants are exposed. These arrangements appear to be the main forces in control of the nature and quantity of animal and vegetable species sharing the environment, the frequency and diversity of interpersonal contact, the presence of reservoirs and vectors for spread of infection, and the degree and kind of physical and chemical additions to the air and water.

Social conditions determining preferences, availability, and distribution of food are known to be responsible for geographic patterns in the distribution of such disorders as beriberi, pellagra, and obesity. In addition, the less tangible factor of social climate peculiar to a time and place may be productive of manifestations that members of other social systems may view as disease, although unfortunately the evidence so far remains largely anecdotal. Hirsch [166], for example, noted that: "Methodist evangelizing . . . spread like a pestilence from Ohio through Tennessee, Virginia, Kentucky and the Carolinas, affecting hundreds of thousands; the victims were known by various names, according to the form their enthusiasm took. . . ." And Panum [309], during his well-known investigation of an outbreak of measles on the Faroe Islands in 1846, having taken the opportunity to observe many other facets of life in the region, concluded that both the physical characteristics of the islands and the religious attitudes of the people led to a type of mental disorder which was distinct from disorders he had seen in other areas.

In descriptive epidemiology there is nowhere a more obvious need for the development of quantitative measures than in the consideration of social arrangements and relationships.

# 9

## *Time*

The pervasiveness of the changes associated with the passage of time necessitates the consideration of this variable in any analysis of factors associated with place or person. Further, time is a necessary element in the definition of every epidemiologic measure and a basic component of the concept of cause. It is in only a limited context, therefore, that time can be considered separately in this chapter as an epidemiologic variable useful in the localization of disease.

### CALENDAR TIME

Time may be measured in whatever units we wish—instants or eons. When marked changes in disease frequency are noted over a period of time that seems very short relative to the total experience of the observer, explanations are often easier than when the changes evolve more slowly.

### Point Epidemics

Large and fleeting excesses in disease frequency often result from what are called point epidemics—the response of a group of people to a source of infection or contamination to which they were exposed almost simultaneously. The same episode of cholera for which localization by place was shown in Figure 17 is illustrated in Figure 18 according to its localization in time.

Such sharp localization in both place and time is particularly helpful in revealing etiologic factors, since it suggests that a single exposure was involved and that the interval between exposure and onset was short. The latter supposition is based on the knowledge that there is always some variation around the mean interval between exposure and onset of disease. For such variation to be encompassed within a few days is a strong indication that the mean interval itself is quite short. Both this supposition and the likelihood that a single exposure was involved make search for the causal mechanism a less formidable prospect.

Marked increases in disease frequency in a short period of time have regularly been found to be associated with sudden

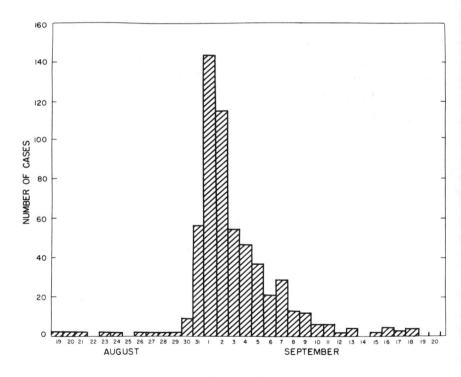

Figure 18

The outbreak of cholera in the Golden Square area of London, August and September, 1854. (Data from Snow [376].)

encounters with microbiologic organisms or chemical agents, via air, food, water, or skin contact. The rise and fall of epidemics are necessarily slower when engendered by forces that are introduced into a population more gradually. However, if time is measured in larger units and a more distant perspective taken, fluctuations in disease frequency that appeared gradual when small time units were used may present a pattern similar to that of a point epidemic. The greater difficulty in identifying such relatively long-term epidemics is due in considerable part to the changing social scene that insures that consistent data are seldom available over prolonged periods.

### Secular Change

Secular change refers to changes that occur gradually over long periods of time; in epidemiology the term usually implies changes in disease frequency encompassing several decades.

Death certificate data are the major source of information on secular changes. Morbidity data adequately reflecting secular changes are still limited to certain geographic areas, to notifications of occurrences of infectious diseases, or to use of mental hospitals. Clinical impressions, although valuable in the detection of large or rapid changes, are not dependable in detecting more subtle ones.

As judged by death certificate data, no disease has retained a constant frequency during the past 50 years. The first question in the evaluation of secular changes noted in such data is whether the change is due to variation in diagnosis, reporting, case fatality, or some circumstance other than a true change of incidence. Changes due to altered procedure in assigning causes of death were discussed in Chapter 6; they are usually readily identifiable because of their abruptness and coincidence with known alterations in procedures. Change in case fatality rates is an obvious factor that has influence on secular trends in death rates. Inconstancy of the characteristics of the population must also be considered. Change in age distribution, for example, is an obvious and readily identifiable source of secular change. As with geographic variation, consideration of the effects of changes in the age distribution of a population should properly be part of the analysis, rather than of the interpretation, of a disease trend. Other changes, such as fluctuating proportions of various ethnic groups in a population, may not be so readily identifiable, or, if identified, may not be so readily investigated because of absence of population or other data necessary for the computation of group-specific rates.

The component of the over-all question of epidemiologic relevance that is most difficult to answer relates to the effects of changes in clinical diagnosis, concepts, and terminology. This problem is difficult to attack because such changes evolve gradually and, while it is frequently possible to state with confidence that diagnosis of a particular condition is more complete now than it was 20 years ago, it rarely is possible to estimate how much more complete and to judge to what extent the observed changes in disease frequency may be attributed to the greater completeness. Attempts to estimate how many cases of a particular disease diagnosed at the present time would have been diagnosed with the knowledge and facilities available at some time in the past are usually unrewarding.

The following procedures may assist in forming an opinion on the role of changes in diagnostic capacity as a factor in disease trends:

1. Comparison of trends for the disease under investigation with trends for other diseases judged equally susceptible to increased diagnostic capability. For example, in Figure 19 death rates from lung cancer in England and Wales during the period 1911 to 1965 are compared with death rates from cancers of other internal sites. While lung cancer is by no means the only site that showed an increase, the data leave little doubt that something happened for lung cancer that did not happen for cancers of other internal sites. If this was of a diagnostic nature, it betrays a past ignorance that was remarkably localized from an anatomic point of view. Reasoning of this type can only be suggestive because such an anatomically localized oversight is not inconceivable, and because it is usually not possible to find two disorders in which improvement in diagnostic procedures advanced at an exactly equal rate.

2. Comparison of the frequency with which a disorder is present at autopsies performed at different periods of the observed

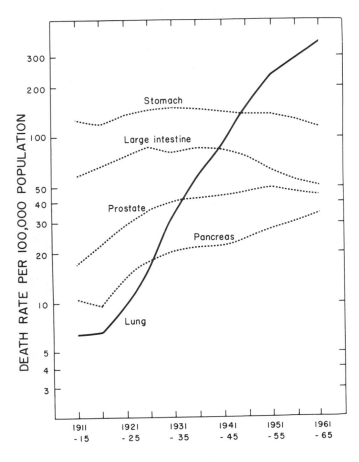

Figure 19

Equivalent average annual death rates from selected sites of cancer in males aged 50 to 74, England and Wales, 1911 to 1965. Rates shown are the averages of those for each of the 5-year age groups between 50 and 74. (Data from Case and Pearson [47].)

secular change. This procedure will be more satisfactory the less fatal the disease under investigation, or, in other words, the greater the probability that the patients autopsied died of some other cause. In a nonfatal disease, the number of patients in whom the disease is found at autopsy is a measure of the prevalence of that disease at the age at which the patients died. The number can be related to the number of autopsies to derive a prevalence rate. In a highly fatal disease, although the measure will be more directly related to incidence—in the sense that mortality is a form of incidence—it will usually not be possible to derive rates because of inability to relate the autopsies to any defined population. The restriction of the method to institutions where, throughout the period under consideration, a high proportion of deceased persons underwent autopsy reduces error resulting from changing patterns in the selection of deaths for autopsy. However, this does not eliminate the possible effect of secular changes in the types of patients admitted to the institution.

3. Examination of the extent to which the apparent trend might result from secular change in the proportion of cases receiving other diagnoses, with assessment of the reasonableness of the assumptions necessary to account for the observed trend. This method was followed by Gilliam [126] in the examination of the effect on the trend in lung cancer death rates if various proportions of patients who died in earlier years had erroneously been certified as dying from other respiratory diseases when in fact they had lung cancer. Because the number of deaths attributed to other respiratory diseases was much larger than the number attributed to lung cancer, particularly in the earlier years of this century, a small proportion of them, if they had actually been diagnosed as lung cancer cases, would have made a substantial addition to the number of deaths certified as due to lung cancer. The apparent trend in lung cancer death rates would therefore be substantially reduced. However, the proportion of misdiagnosed cases necessary to eliminate the trend entirely was so large that the assumptions did not seem reasonable when considered in conjunction with available data from autopsy material.

There are also a number of general arguments that can be applied to the assessment of the epidemiologic significance of an apparent secular trend. Thus trends that are markedly different for different age, sex, or ethnic groups living in the same community are less likely to be artifacts than if they were not so localized within subgroups. Also it may be illuminating to ask

—for example, in the case of lung cancer—whether diagnostic ability became more sophisticated between, say, 1950 and 1970 at the same rate as it did during earlier years when such diagnostic aids as x-ray and bronchoscopy were being developed. Such a question is meaningful in light of the fact that lung cancer rates have continued to increase at as fast a rate in the later as in the earlier period.

There is no doubt that lung cancer has undergone a real and substantial increase during the last half century. However, secular trends of this magnitude are unusual in the noninfectious diseases. Much more frequently, as in the apparent increases in death rates from coronary artery disease, peptic ulcer, leukemia, and pancreatic and ovarian cancer, the question whether the apparent secular change reflects a real change in disease frequency remains in doubt, in spite of use of all the procedures and arguments mentioned. Although this uncertainty regarding the actual mechanism of the secular change must be given consideration in the formulation of hypotheses of etiology, denial of the *possibility* that the change may be of real etiologic significance serves no purpose. It is more reasonable to consider that such changes might have occurred and to evaluate causal hypotheses in the light of this possibility. Usually the secular change will not form any large part of the direct evidence that must be assembled to test the causal hypotheses more formally.

### Interpretations

The type and magnitude of social, biologic, physical, and chemical changes that occur with the passage of time are as infinite as time itself. Discussion of circumstances related to the occurrence of place-related diseases (Chap. 8) is equally relevant to a consideration of the role of time, but will not be repeated here.

Certain interpretations—for example, those having to do with variation in adequacy of diagnosis or reporting—are less easily eliminated from consideration in time associations than in place associations. This is because the conditions prevailing during earlier times often cannot be subjected to the special surveys that can be conducted to test a hypothesis of association with place. On the other hand, interpretations invoking genetic differences in populations are usually more easily ruled out as productive of time associations, although changes in the genetic structure of the population of an area can indeed occur in a relatively short time. One obvious mechanism is through population migration; such a possibility is usually readily detected. Another mechanism is by the breakdown of genetic isolates, a process that has been proceeding rapidly and on a significant scale during the present century. An increase in marriages between members of groups that had previously been strongly inbred will lead to reduction in the frequency of diseases in which recessive autosomal genes play an etiologic role if the relevant gene is present in only one of the groups, since predisposition to such a condition depends on receiving the gene from both parents. Again, however, the occurrence of such a demographic change will usually be detected readily if it occurs on a scale sufficient to account for any substantial secular change.

It has been noted previously that changes occurring over a relatively short time are more productive of hypotheses than those occurring over decades. This is true even when the changes do not have the abruptness of a point epidemic. The example of Snow's observation of a change in the incidence of cholera in the customers of the Lambeth Water Company over a 5-year period was referred to in Chapter 1. The importance of the observation of the rapidity of the change lies in the relatively short period that must be examined to identify conditions that may be causally related to the change. A more recent example is illustrated in Figure 20, which shows a striking increase between 1941 and 1945 in the incidence of first admission to U.S. mental hospitals for males between the ages of 15 and 34, the greatest increase being for the age group 20 to 24. The pattern suggests that the stresses of military life during World War II may have been psychotogenic. An alternative hypothesis is that induction into the service acted as a case-finding mechanism for this age and sex group, and hence led to increased rates of hospitalization. This may be partially correct, but it seems unlikely to be a complete explanation, since the trend persisted until 1945, while the number of persons being inducted and examined declined markedly after 1943.

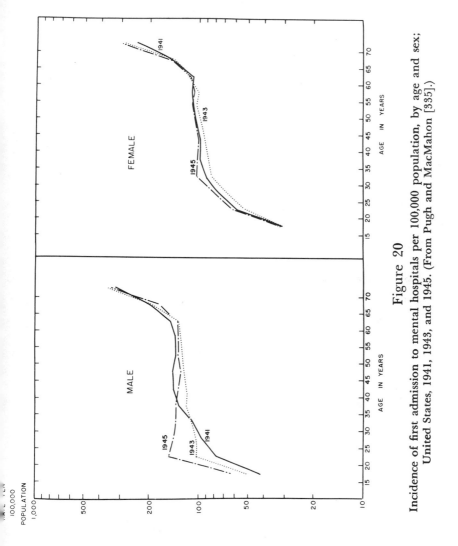

Figure 20

Incidence of first admission to mental hospitals per 100,000 population, by age and sex;
United States, 1941, 1943, and 1945. (From Pugh and MacMahon [335].)

## CYCLIC FLUCTUATIONS

Cyclic variation in disease frequency has been of great interest to epidemiologists. Seasonal fluctuations, for example, are among the most striking epidemiologic features of many infectious diseases and have received much attention.

The study methods commonly used are relatively simple. Cases are plotted by time of onset according to a conventional time unit. In detection of seasonal fluctuations, months or quarter-years are generally used (Fig. 21). Use of a reference population and the calculation of a series of rates are usually unnecessary refinements, unless periodic changes in the size of

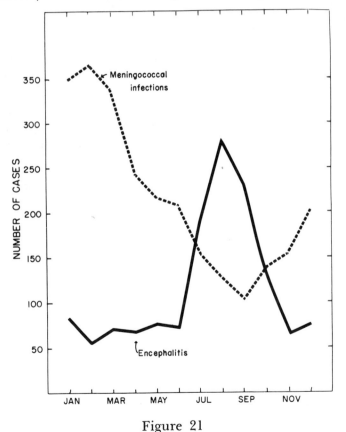

Figure 21

Reported cases of meningococcal infections and of primary encephalitis, by month; United States, 1968. (From *Morbidity and Mortality Weekly Report* [283].)

the population are likely, as in a vacation resort or military training area.

More efficient methods for detecting cyclic changes have been proposed by a number of workers. Edwards [104] has suggested a useful method in which, as applied to seasonal variation, the year is considered as a circle divided into twelve segments corresponding to months. The "center of gravity" of the cases is then estimated. In the absence of seasonal variation, the expected center of gravity of a series of cases would be in the center of the circle. Any excess or deficit of cases in particular segments will cause a shift toward or away from those segments. The position of the actual center of gravity indicates the month of highest incidence, and its distance from the center of the circle indicates the relative strength of the seasonal variation. Thus, in Figure 22, births of children with cleft lip are shown as having a strong seasonal trend with a peak in March, while the trend for cleft palate is less striking and centers in December.

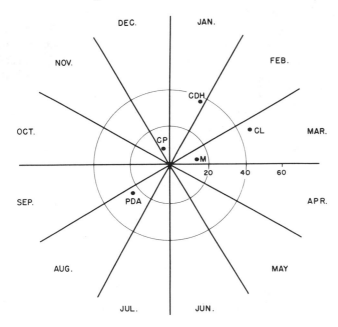

Figure 22

Seasonal variation in the births of children with congenital dislocation of the hip (CDH), cleft lip and palate (CL), cleft palate (CP), mongolism (M), and patent ductus arteriosus (PDA). (From Edwards [105].)

The mathematical procedures involved in this method, in particular those relating to the estimation of the variances of the centers of gravity, are conceptually difficult for the nonmathematician and computationally fairly complex. Perhaps for these reasons, the method has not been extensively used. However, the method may demonstrate cyclic fluctuations of a lower order of magnitude than would appear significant in a simple $\chi^2$ test. It should be noted that the efficiency of this test depends on the underlying model of a condition with a single high and a single low period of risk. Conditions with more than one seasonal peak —as has, for example, coarctation of the aorta [254]—would not be analyzed appropriately by this method.

### Interpretation of Seasonal Variations

Seasonal variation in the flora and fauna of the environment has a profound effect on many human diseases, and this area is one in which considerable investigation has been undertaken in attempts to explain periodic variation in disease rates. Investigations have ranged from the study of pollens concerned in hay fever to the search for insect vectors with relevant seasonal patterns of reproduction or feeding. For example, in the Western United States diseases contracted from ticks, such as Rocky Mountain spotted fever, show marked seasonal localization in spring and early summer, corresponding to the period of feeding activity of adult ticks. The mosquito-borne encephalitides, on the other hand, are localized in late summer and early fall.

Seasonal fluctuations in occupational or recreational activities may also account for variation in exposure to sources of infection. Thus the marked concentration of human leptospirosis during the summer months is accounted for by increased exposure to infected waters in the course of bathing and fishing. Increased crowding during cold weather leads to conditions conducive to the spread of epidemic typhus.

Seasonal variations in the acute infectious diseases of childhood pose some of the major unsolved problems of infectious disease epidemiology. In spite of the consistent occurrence and striking magnitude of these variations, they remain largely unexplained. There appears to be no seasonal variation in the secondary attack rates of measles, chickenpox, or mumps, once an infection has been introduced into a household [371]. Variation in the characteristics of the viruses does not therefore seem a likely explanation of the seasonal variation in the nonfamilial cases. An understanding of the seasonal variation of the common infectious diseases might have great preventive potential. For example, if the factors governing the seasonal distribution of poliomyelitis had been known and had proved manipulable, some degree of prevention of the disease might have antedated that brought about by the vaccine.

Seasonal circumstances that are entirely manmade may play a part in seasonal disease patterns. Thus Friedman et al. [120] showed rises in serum cholesterol levels of accountants corresponding to critical dates in the tax calendar. If this is a real effect, it is unlikely that it is limited to accountants.

For diseases of early life, variation in risk by season of birth may point to the existence of environmental influences acting during intrauterine or very early postnatal life and give hints as to their nature. One relationship of this type is that between intelligence and season of birth. Children born in the summer months achieve a significantly higher mean score on intelligence tests than those born in the winter [321]. In addition, risk of admission to a state school for the mentally retarded was shown by Knobloch and Pasamanick [188] to be highest for children born in February and lowest for those born in August. A number of hypotheses have been developed as a result of this observation, one of which relates mental retardation to unidentified nutritional disturbances in early pregnancy, these disturbances being caused by changes in maternal diet during the hot summer months. In investigating this hypothesis further, Knobloch and Pasamanick compared admission rates for mental retardation for children whose critical stage of intrauterine development (in this case, supposed to be the third month) occurred during summers in which the temperature was high with those born following summers in which the temperature was low. Admission rates were significantly higher for the former group than for the latter [188].

## CLUSTERING IN TIME

The descriptive studies discussed so far have all been based on the comparison of rates that depend on knowledge of the size and distribution of populations at risk. Comparisons are sometimes made on the basis of numbers of cases, but in such studies it is assumed that the population base remained the same throughout. Knowledge of the relative sizes of compared populations is therefore implicit.

However, hypotheses of etiology are sometimes derived from the clustering of certain events simply along the time axis in the histories of affected individuals, without inferences being made as to the population at risk and without comparisons with unaffected groups. This type of time clustering is most readily observed in diseases in which the interval between the precipitating event and onset of illness can be measured with precision.

For example, Aycock and Luther [20] obtained histories of tonsillectomy from a series of patients with poliomyelitis. They noted that among 36 cases of poliomyelitis that occurred within 12 months of tonsillectomy, there were 16 in which poliomyelitis followed within 1 month of the operation. All 16 of these cases occurred within 7 to 18 days of tonsillectomy, a period the authors considered compatible with the incubation period of poliomyelitis. Even though no data were available to determine how many children selected at random might have given a history of tonsillectomy within 7 to 18 days, the marked clustering of tonsillectomies within the month prior to onset strongly suggested a causal relationship between tonsillectomy and the poliomyelitis.

Similarly, data of Tetlow [395] on 67 patients in whom mental disorder occurred during pregnancy or the puerperium showed a marked clustering of cases with onset of symptoms in the 4 weeks after delivery (Fig. 23). Within the group of patients with onset in the 4 weeks after delivery there was additional clustering, nearly half of this group becoming ill in the week immediately following delivery. Such clustering suggests the presence of psychotogenic factors operative around the time of delivery.

A more sophisticated approach to this question is by measurement of the interval between the suspected causal event and onset of the disease in a series of cases, and determination of the mean and variance of this interval. The variance of the interval should be smaller if the measurement is taken from the date of

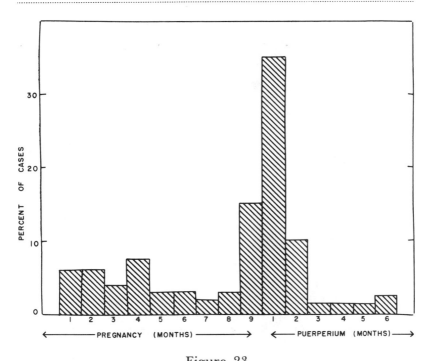

Figure 23

Distribution by time of onset of symptoms of 67 patients with mental disorder associated with pregnancy and the puerperium. (From Tetlow [395].)

occurrence of a causally related event than if taken from points in time having less direct causal connection to the disease. This method was used in an investigation of the possible relationship of jaundice among service personnel to yellow fever vaccination [353]. In this study it was not useful to compare affected and unaffected individuals with respect to frequency of yellow fever vaccination, since practically all the military personnel under observation had been vaccinated. Investigation of the time relationships, however, showed that the interval between vaccination and onset of the disease was less variable than the date of onset. The standard deviation of the date of onset for the 5917 cases in California, around the mean of June 1, was 5.7 weeks, whereas the standard deviation of the interval between vaccination and onset of jaundice, around a mean of 14.6 weeks, was only 3.5 weeks (Fig. 24).

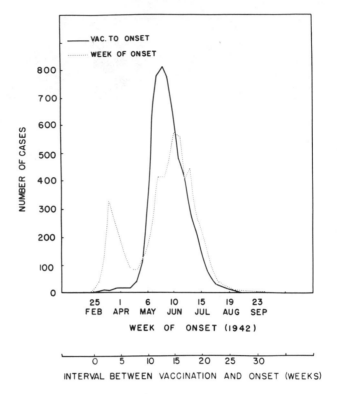

Figure 24

Distribution according to week of onset and according to interval between yellow fever vaccination and onset of jaundice, for 5917 cases of jaundice in U.S. military units in California, 1942. (From Sawyer et al. [353].)

A more formal comparison than simple inspection of such variances may be desired. A statistical procedure for testing the significance of the difference between correlated variances is given by Snedecor and Cochran [375].

Clustering of causal events along the time axis in the histories of affected individuals will be less apparent when the interval between cause and effect is variable, and will be additionally less apparent if there is a consistent change in this interval during the period of observation. For example, if the interval between exposure and onset decreases as an epidemic progresses (as may be the case in an outbreak of staphylococcal food poisoning), it is possible that the actual dates of times of onset of cases may be more closely grouped about their mean than the intervals between exposure and onset are about theirs. Consequently, the fact that the variance of the interval dated from a certain event is not smaller than the variance of, for example, the date of onset does not necessarily indicate a lack of causal connection between the event and the disease.

It should also be noted that while clustering in time does indicate that a certain preceding event and the onset of a certain disease are associated in time, the same reservations about the causal nature of such an association must be made as are made about associations based on relative frequency of concordance of two events.

# 10

Some Combinations of Person, Place,
and Time

All epidemiologic analyses require awareness of the interactions between person, place, and time in the causation of disease. However, in certain kinds of study this interaction is particularly evident. Studies of migrant populations, for example, are aimed primarily toward the separation of factors associated with place from those that are characteristic of persons. In addition to studies of migrants, this chapter will deal with analyses designed to clarify relationships between age and time, and with the detection of disease clustering in time and place.

## MIGRANT POPULATIONS

Migrant populations are of epidemiologic interest from several points of view. They may play important roles in the spread of infectious disease. They may also be exposed to or relieved from stressful situations which static populations do not experience so frequently or so intensely. Finally, they provide opportunities for clarification of the mechanisms underlying unusual disease patterns noted in particular places or particular ethnic groups.

### Person or Place

In theory, studies of migrant populations should provide powerful tools for distinguishing disease patterns associated with particular places from those associated with the characteristics of persons inhabiting those places, since they enable comparison of similar persons living in different places and of different persons living in the same place. In practice, it is difficult to formulate generalizations that can be made from observation of disease rates in migrant populations. This difficulty stems in part from the fact that relatively few substantial studies of migrants have been completed to date, and in part from the variety of interpretations that can be put on the results of the studies that have been completed. The circumstances of specific migrations are often unique, the migrants are frequently not representative of the population of the land from which they migrate, and the extent to which specific environments characteristic of the homeland are retained by migrants is quite variable.

For example, many migrations of Jews, in both the remote and the immediate past, have led to the establishment of large Jewish populations in many areas of the world. It might be thought that the circumstances of life of these populations are so varied that any disease or characteristic manifested by all or most of them must have its basis in a common genetic inheritance. Indeed, there are genetic factors that are responsible for high rates of certain diseases—for example, Tay-Sachs disease—in Jewish populations. However, at least one feature of a strictly environmental nature has been retained by Jews throughout these many centuries of migration and has been suspected of significance in their disease experience. This is circumcision of the male infant. On the other hand, physical and biologic environment—exposure to air and water pollution or to infectious disease, for example—are circumstances that would be expected to change rapidly and rather substantially on migration. Between these extremes are environmental factors—diet, for example—that change slowly and with varying degrees of speed from those characteristic of the homeland to those of the host country, but of which vestiges frequently remain several generations after the migration.

In spite of the difficulties which such variations pose in specific interpretations, studies of migrant populations have been of value. They have been used: (1) to determine whether high rates of certain diseases noted in certain countries are intrinsic to the inhabitants of that country, (2) to demonstrate that certain places do possess characteristics of significance in the etiology of certain diseases, independent of the people who inhabit those places, and (3) to assess the significance—from the point of view of risk of a particular disease—of the years spent in the homeland, prior to migration, relative to those spent in the host country.

CHANGES IN DISEASE RATES IN MIGRANT POPULATIONS.   A number of important studies have been and are being conducted on the population that migrated from Japan to the United States between 1890 and 1924. Relative to that of the United States, the pattern of causes of death observed in Japan is very unusual. While death from arteriosclerotic heart disease occurs with only about one-quarter the frequency of that in the United States, deaths from intracranial vascular lesions are between two and three times as common. Marked differences in cancer mortality, which are seen in incidence as well as mortality data, include a frequency of stomach cancer more than five times that of the United States, but almost exactly the inverse situation prevails for cancer of the intestine. Cancer of the breast and of the prostate are relatively infrequent in Japan, but cancer of the cervix is more than twice as common as in the United States.

The question immediately comes to mind whether these differences in disease rates are due to differences in the Japanese and American environments and ways of life, or to more intrinsic—for example, genetic—differences between the two populations.

Table 22 shows standard mortality ratios for U.S. whites and for the U.S. population of Japanese ancestry, expressed relative to an arbitrary value of 100 for the same cause of death and the same sex in Japan. For the U.S. Japanese, the rates are shown separately for those born in the United States and those not. The nativeborn are predominantly first-generation Americans —that is, born of parents who were born in Japan—and most of the foreignborn were born in Japan.

For several of the conditions listed—for example, intracranial vascular lesions and cancer of the cervix—the U.S. Japanese, even those born in Japan, show rates similar to those of U.S.

## Table 22
Standard mortality ratios* for selected causes of death
in Japan, in Americans of Japanese ancestry, and in
U.S. whites, 1959 to 1962†

| | | U.S. of Japanese ancestry | | |
| | | Not U.S.- | U.S.- | U.S. |
| Cause and sex | Japan | born | born | whites |
|---|---|---|---|---|
| Cancer | | | | |
|   Esophagus (M) | 100 | 132 | 51 | 47 |
|   Stomach (M) | 100 | 72 | 38 | 17 |
|   Stomach (F) | 100 | 55 | 48 | 18 |
|   Intestine (M) | 100 | 374 | 288 | 489 |
|   Intestine (F) | 100 | 218 | 209 | 483 |
|   Breast (F) | 100 | 166 | 136 | 591 |
|   Cervix uteri (F) | 100 | 52 | 33 | 48 |
| Intracranial vascular lesions (M) | 100 | 32 | 24 | 37 |
| Intracranial vascular lesions (F) | 100 | 40 | 43 | 48 |
| Arteriosclerotic heart disease (M) | 100 | 226 | 165 | 481 |
| Arteriosclerotic heart disease (F) | 100 | 196 | 38 | 348 |

\* SMRs relative to a death rate of 100 in Japan.
† From Haenszel and Kurihara [145].

whites, and quite different from those of Japanese in Japan. That such a change in disease experience could come about within the lifetime of the migrant population is almost unequivocal evidence that some features of the Japanese environment are responsible for the high rates of these diseases in Japan, and it indicates further that these are not features of the Japanese environment that migrants take with them. This conclusion does not imply that genetic factors are irrelevant in these diseases, but simply that such factors do not explain the differences in rates between Japan and the United States.

For some other causes of death—notably cancer of the stomach and of the intestine—rates for the U.S. Japanese are intermediate between those for Japan and those for U.S. whites. Again, the significance of environmental factors is suggested. Intermediate rates among Japanese-born Americans might be explained by a long induction period for the disease, long duration prior to death, some retention of the relevant environment, or

*178*

other mechanisms. However, the fact that even those Americans of Japanese ancestry who were born in the United States had rates substantially different from those of U.S. whites indicates either that the responsible environmental factor is retained for a considerable period in the host country and is passed on to generations born in the host country—as dietary customs might be, for example—or that more intrinsic features—for example, genes—play a role in addition to the changing environment.

For one of the conditions listed in Table 22—cancer of the breast—the death rate for the Japanese Americans is much more similar to that of Japanese in Japan than to that of U.S whites. Such an observation is of course compatible with the hypothesis that the U.S.-Japan difference in this disease has a genetic basis. However, even if such an observation were made over several generations of the migrant population, the example of circumcision of Jewish male infants is a reminder that some environmental factor firmly bound to the migrant culture might be responsible. In addition, it is worth noting that the particular observation in the table is, so far, limited to a single generation born in the host country. If a disease were dependent in part on, for example, diet in childhood, it is not at all inconceivable that the first generation of migrants born in the host country would experience rates more characteristic of the home than of the host country.

Most studies of international migrants have, like the study from which the above data derived, been based on mortality data. The background and design of studies of British and Norwegian migrants to the United States that incorporate morbidity information and a great deal of information on personal habits and other data possibly explanatory of the disease patterns observed are described by Reid and others [344, 345]. These studies are designed to explore the differences noted between Britain, Norway, and the United States in rates of cardiovascular and chronic respiratory disease.

SIBLING STUDIES.    One difficulty in interpreting the results of studies of migrants is that migrants may not be representative of the population of their homelands. Both the desire and the opportunity to migrate may differentially affect different ethnic groups within the country, different socioeconomic classes, persons in different states of health, or persons of unusual physical or psychological constitution.

To overcome the effects of this selection—at least partially—a few investigators have compared migrants with their siblings who remained in the home country. For example, migrants from Ireland to the United States have been compared with siblings who remained in Ireland [34, 399]. The focus of this study is the low rate of atherosclerosis in Ireland relative to that in the United States. However, study of the effects of migration from an area of high atherosclerosis rates to one of lower rates might conceivably have greater implications for preventive programs. An opportunity for this is provided by the recent migration of several thousands of North Americans to Israel. Sibling pairs, in which one sibling migrated to Israel and one remained in the United States, are being studied to determine the effect of migration on blood pressure, serum cholesterol, and other factors associated with increased risk of coronary artery disease [358]. A limitation of the application of such studies is suggested by noting that both these investigations are concerned with risk factors in coronary heart disease—the number of migrant-nonmigrant sibling pairs that can be identified is sufficiently small that only the most common conditions can be studied by this method.

The use of siblings does reduce the problems of selection involved in migrant studies. Siblings would, for example, tend to be genetically and socioeconomically more similar than the migrant and nonmigrant populations as a whole. However, these problems are by no means eliminated. It is possible that, even within sibling pairs, it is the stronger, weaker, more intelligent, or more unstable individual who migrates. Since these studies usually require the collection of special data from the siblings themselves, information to examine such possibilities can be assembled in the course of the study.

AGE AT MIGRATION. It has been suggested that when a migrant population carries its disease risk with it, but their offspring born in the host country have disease risks characteristic of the host country—as seems to be the case for multiple sclerosis, for example [10]—investigation of the age at migration that is associated with adoption of the host country's disease risk might assist in pinpointing the age at which etiologic factors are operative. For example, with respect to multiple sclerosis, migrants from Europe to Israel go from a high-risk to a low-risk area, and they experience a high risk of the disease even in Israel. On the other hand, migrants to Israel from Asia and Africa travel from one low-risk area to another, and in Israel they experience rates similar to those of nativeborn Israelis. The relationship to age at migration was studied by Alter et al. [11]; the results are shown in Table 23. Taken at face value, the inci-

### Table 23

Incidence of multiple sclerosis among European, African, and Asian immigrants to Israel, by age at immigration*

| Age at immigration (years) | Number of patients | | Person-years resident in Israel | | Annual incidence per 100,000 | |
|---|---|---|---|---|---|---|
| | European | African and Asian | European | African and Asian | European | African and Asian |
| <15 | 4 | 4 | 530,000 | 890,000 | 0.76 | 0.65 |
| 15–29 | 28 | 7 | 790,000 | 1,750,000 | 3.54 | 0.40 |
| 30–34 | 21 | 3 | 1,560,000 | 1,178,000 | 1.35 | 0.26 |

* From Alter et al. [11].

dence rates indicate that the higher rates for immigrants from Europe are essentially restricted to persons who migrated after the age of 15 years. This suggests that the etiologic factors that presumably operated in their homelands prior to migration had their influence prior to this age. Europeans who migrated prior to age 15 apparently did not experience these factors.

The authors recognize the uncertainties in these data—the numbers, particularly of migrants under 15 years of age, are very small, and it is not clear the compared groups were of similar age distribution. Thus it is conceivable that the lack of risk difference for the migrants under 15 is a function of lack of ethnic difference in risk in the younger age groups rather than in age at migration per se. Presumably time will resolve this question if the population continues to be followed. Even with these uncertainties, the data are suggestive and the method a potentially valuable one.

## Stresses of Migration

Quite apart from their exposure to disease risks that are unusually high in either their homeland or their host country, the fact of migration itself seems to carry certain risks, some of which have been documented. However, few have been satisfactorily explained, other than in terms of the risks associated with entering an area of high exposure to biologic or chemical agents.

Several studies in this field illustrate the effects of intranational, as well as international, migration. In the infectious diseases, for example, Wheelis' work [413] demonstrating a relationship between recent entry into the U.S. Navy and high rates of communicable disease is pertinent.

Hospitalization for psychotic disorders appears to be more frequent among some migrant groups. An early study was that of Ødegaard [302, 303], who showed high rates of mental hospitalization among the Norwegian-born population of Minnesota. The studies of Malzberg [234] on admission rates among the foreignborn in New York State were referred to in Chapter 7 (p. 116). Interestingly, more recent studies [335] have not shown appreciable differences between admission rates for nativeborn and foreignborn U.S. populations.

A similar situation exists with respect to migration within the United States. A question in the 1940 census asked: "Where were you 5 years ago (Apr. 1, 1935)?" This denominator enabled Malzberg and Lee [234] to derive rates of psychosis among persons known to have made a recent move and compare them with rates among those not known to have made a recent move. The findings, summarized in Table 24, show higher rates for migrants for both sexes, both racial groups, and for each category of psychosis. Ten years later, in Ohio and Massachusetts, no difference was found in admission rates for those born elsewhere [335]. Similarly, in a survey of residents of Texas seeking care for psychotic disorders in 1951 to 1952, no unusual risk was found for migrants to the state from other parts of the United States [180]. In Manhattan, rates of mental impairment among the noninstitutionalized population were similar for the native-

## Table 24

First admission rates for psychoses among "five-year migrants" and "nonmigrants," New York State, 1939–1941*†

| Color and sex | Manic depressive | | Schizophrenia | | Other psychoses | | All psychoses | |
|---|---|---|---|---|---|---|---|---|
| | Migrant‡ | Nonmigrant‡ | Migrant | Nonmigrant | Migrant | Nonmigrant | Migrant | Nonmigrant |
| White male | 17 | 6 | 86 | 37 | 181 | 94 | 269 | 130 |
| White female | 37 | 14 | 76 | 35 | 133 | 74 | 231 | 116 |
| Nonwhite male | 10 | 6 | 261 | 74 | 804 | 267 | 1032 | 333 |
| Nonwhite female | 56 | 9 | 187 | 70 | 595 | 172 | 810 | 240 |

* From Malzberg and Lee [234].

† Average annual rates per 100,000 population, standardized to the age distribution of the New York State population aged 14 and over in 1940.

‡ "Migrants" in these data are persons living in New York State on Apr. 1, 1940 who were not living in New York State on Apr. 1, 1935; "nonmigrants" are persons resident in New York State on both dates.

born as for the foreignborn, and for native New Yorkers as for those who had migrated to New York from other parts of the United States [379].

These findings illustrate some of the difficulties in interpreting the results of studies of migrants. There are, first, the difficulties in assessing whether the unusual rates for migrants reflect factors in the selection of migrants, differences in likelihood of hospitalization or of reaching other forms of medical care, or differences in the incidence or prevalence of mental illness. Further, the discrepancies between the results of the older and of the more recent studies point to the fact that the circumstances of migrations are different. It is understandable that intra-U.S. migrations during the 1930s might exert quite different pressures on the migrants than those which have occurred in more recent times.

### Relationship to Other Demographic Variables

It has been stressed that in interpreting the results of studies of migrants, it is necessary to consider the demographic and other characteristics of the migrant populations. Similarly, in studies of diseases in which migration may be an etiologic factor, it is necessary to recall that age, socioeconomic, ethnic, and other demographic subgroups may vary with respect to migrant status. Figure 25, for example, illustrates that the rate of migration within the United States increased at a much faster rate for the nonwhite than for the white population between 1910 and 1950, although the differential decreased in the subsequent decade.

### BIRTH-COHORT ANALYSIS

We have used the term *cohort study* to describe the observation over time of one or more groups of people (cohorts) that have some common characteristic or exposure. A special type of cohort is one formed of persons born within a particular period of time—for example, a year or a five-year period. Such a cohort is referred to as a birth-cohort.

From the experience of a single birth-cohort, trends in disease

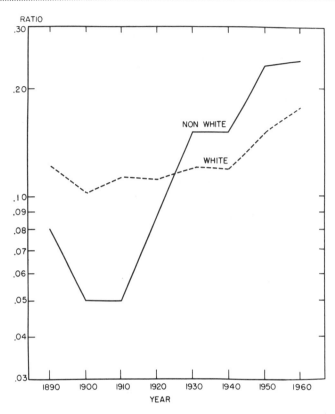

RATIO

YEAR

Figure 25

Ratios of the number of persons living in regions different from their region
of birth to the number living in the region of birth; United States, 1890 to
1960. (Data from U.S. Census Reports [37, 38, 39].)

rates with age cannot be distinguished from those with time,
since age is defined in terms of the passage of time. For example,
if we had available only the experience of the birth-cohort of
1880, we would be unable to determine whether the fact that
the members of this cohort had a higher death rate when they
were aged 80 than when they were aged 10 was the result of
higher rates for older persons or of higher death rates prevailing
in 1960 than in 1890. The fact that we have the experience of
several birth-cohorts at hand allows us to compare the death
rates for persons belonging to different birth-cohorts at the same
age (which they will achieve at different times), and for persons
belonging to different cohorts at the same point in time (at

which they will have different ages), and so evaluate to what extent changes are associated with different calendar times and to what extent with different ages.

The disease rate manifested by a particular age group at a particular point in time may be determined by:

1. Factors characteristic of the persons in the age group—for example, the high rates of pregnancy in certain age groups are a function primarily of age, in that they have been seen in these age groups in all time periods.
2. Factors characteristic of the time—for example, an acute epidemic which affects persons of all age groups alive at that time.
3. Experiences that the birth-cohort occupying that age group at that time has undergone at some earlier point during its journey from its birth-year to the year of observation.

Factors of the first and second type were considered in Chapters 7 and 9, respectively. The third category of experiences is considered here. Recognition of the significance of such determinants of disease rates is important in evaluating the shape of graphs depicting the association of disease risk with age, in interpreting trends in age-specific rates over time, in identifying unusual patterns of disease occurrence that lead to hypotheses as to the age at which etiologic factors are operative, and in assisting in predicting trends in disease occurrence.

*Patterns of Age Association*

The association of a disease with age may be described in two ways:

1. An age curve based on the age-specific rates observed in a cross section of a population at one point in time. An example was given in Figure 8 (p. 105), which showed age-specific incidence rates of rectal cancer in the population of ten selected areas of the United States in 1947. The populations on which the rates in the different age groups were based belonged to quite different birth-cohorts. Thus, the rate for the age group 30 to 34 was based on persons born between 1913 and 1917, and

that for the age group 60 to 64 on persons born between 1883 and 1887. This type of curve is known as a current or cross-sectional age curve.

2. A curve based on age-specific rates for a particular birth-cohort observed at successive points in time as it grew older. In this case, for persons born in 1890 the incidence rate at age 30 to 34 would be based on data for the years 1920 to 1924, and, in the same curve, the rate for age 60 to 64 would be based on data for that age group in 1950 to 1954. This type of age curve is known as a generation or birth-cohort age curve.

If there has been no secular change in disease rates, the shapes of age curves drawn from cross-sectional and birth-cohort data will be identical. However, if there has been a change and the distinction between the two methods is not kept in mind, misleading interpretations may result. For example, the censuses of New South Wales, Australia, include counts of persons who are deaf (Table 25). An observer of the census of 1933, noting the

## Table 25

Number of deaf-mutes enumerated in three censuses
of New South Wales, Australia*

| Age | 1911 | 1921 | 1933 |
|---|---|---|---|
| 0–4 | 16 | 17 | 11 |
| 5–9 | 59 | 72 | 95 |
| 10–14 | *111* | 86 | 89 |
| 15–19 | 64 | 57 | 141 |
| 20–24 | 65 | *115* | 98 |
| 25–29 | 60 | 59 | 69 |
| 30–34 | 54 | 67 | *140* |
| 35–39 | 57 | 62 | 71 |
| 40–44 | 36 | 47 | 59 |
| 45–49 | 32 | 50 | 52 |
| 50–54 | 28 | 26 | 47 |
| 55–59 | 14 | 24 | 40 |
| 60 + | 38 | 76 | 68 |
| Unknown | 6 | 3 | 2 |
| *Total* | 640 | 761 | 982 |

* From Lancaster [195].

peak of deaf-mutes aged 30 to 34 and having satisfied himself that this did not result from an unusually large total population at risk in this age group, might incautiously conclude that there were factors operative around age 30 to 34 which predispose to deafness. An observer of the census of 1921 might reach the same conclusion, but with respect to the age group 20 to 24. It is, of course, possible that the factors responsible for deafness were most highly concentrated in the age group 20 to 24 in 1921 and at 30 to 34 in 1933. A more acceptable interpretation, however, is that a particular birth-cohort with a high prevalence of deafness happened to occupy these particular age groups at the time of the two censuses. The birth-cohort born in 1899 was, in fact, identified as one exposed to a particularly severe epidemic of rubella while in utero [195]. The age distribution of deafness at a particular census was, therefore, indicative of an etiologic factor occurring many years earlier rather than of age variation in the operation of etiologic factors.

A more complex example is provided by the comparison of cross-sectional and birth-cohort age curves for cancer of the lung by Dorn and Cutler [90] (Fig. 26). Cross-sectional age curves— the broken lines in the figure—suggest that rates of lung cancer increase to the 60 to 69 age group but then decline with further increase in age. This might suggest that the population's exposure to etiologic agents falls off after a certain age, and this would be somewhat surprising since there is little to suggest that exposure to cigarette smoke decreased after middle-age during the period concerned here. Certainly one would not expect the population's cumulative exposure to have declined with age. An alternative explanation of the pattern becomes evident when the same data are used to draw age curves for birth-cohorts—the solid lines in the figure. It is seen that for birth-cohorts risk continues to increase throughout life, but that at any given age rates are higher for later than for earlier birth-cohorts. Thus the fact that, in 1949 to 1950, persons aged 90 had lower lung cancer rates than persons aged 60 could be explained, not by a decline with age in risk of the disease, but by the fact that persons aged 90 belonged to an earlier birth-cohort which, probably because of less heavy cigarette smoking, had lower lung cancer rates than succeeding generations throughout its life.

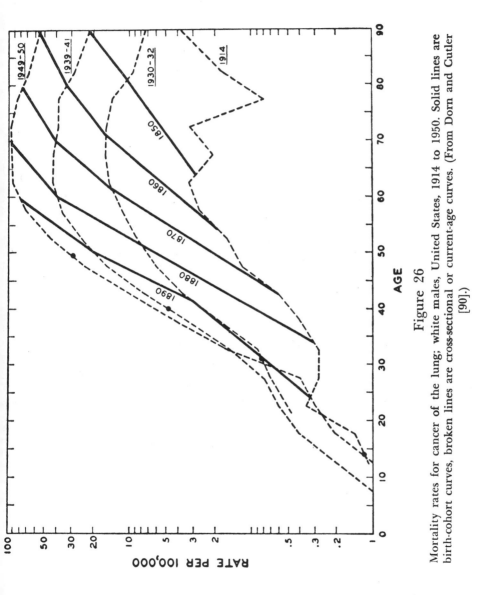

Figure 26

Mortality rates for cancer of the lung; white males, United States, 1914 to 1950. Solid lines are birth-cohort curves, broken lines are cross-sectional or current-age curves. (From Dorn and Cutler [90].)

Classic papers on the difference between cross-sectional and birth-cohort age curves are those of Andvord [14] and Frost [121] who showed that variations over a period of time in the age association of deaths from tuberculosis could be explained by lifetime differences in risk between birth-cohorts.

## Age-Specific Time Trends

In studying changes in disease rates over time, it is frequently desirable to compare trends for different age groups. Again, if incorrect interpretations are to be avoided, it is necessary to recognize that persons in different age groups at a point in time represent different birth-cohorts.

Figure 27 shows age-specific death rates from cancer of the tongue in England and Wales over a 55-year period. The trends are different in different age groups. In the youngest age groups, rates declined throughout the period, while in the oldest groups they increased slightly during the first half of the period. An investigator unaware of the long induction period for human cancer might be tempted to seek etiologic factors which diminished in force in successively older age groups at successively later time periods. An alternative explanation is suggested by arranging the same curves in such a way that a vertical line joins the values exhibited by persons of different ages belonging to the same birth-cohort rather than the values exhibited at a point in time by persons belonging to different birth-cohorts (Fig. 28). The age trends then become consistent: cohorts of persons born up until about 1860 experienced constant or increasing rates in all the age groups that can be examined in these data. Cohorts born subsequent to 1860 experienced declining rates, and the decline is seen in all the age groups that they have so far occupied.

## Relevance to Etiologic Hypotheses

For some etiologic factors it can be determined a priori whether time changes are likely to affect birth-cohorts throughout their lives—as with congenital deafness due to rubella—or all age groups at a point in time—as with an influenza epidemic. When studying diseases in which such factors are known to exist,

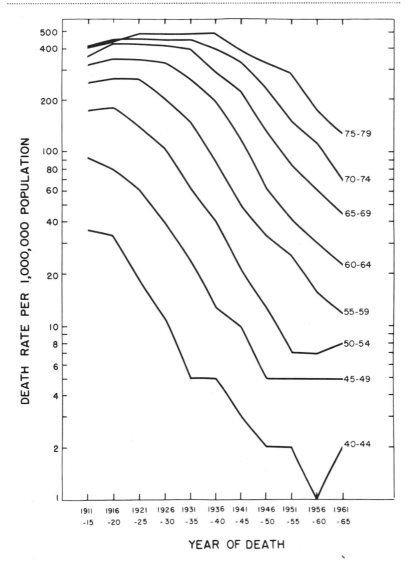

Figure 27

Age-specific average annual death rates from cancer of the tongue in males; England and Wales, 1911 to 1965. (Data from Case and Pearson [47].)

patterns of age and time trends can be examined by an appropriate method.

When dealing with a disease of unknown etiology, the possibility that the data might fit either type of pattern must be kept

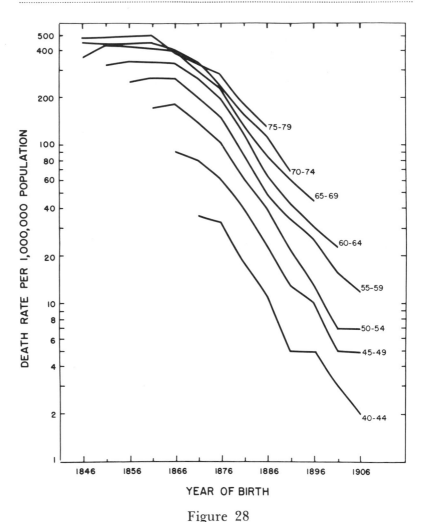

Figure 28

Data from Figure 27 rearranged to show age-specific rates for birth-cohorts of males born between 1846 and 1906.

in mind. If an age-time pattern is convincingly explained by one or the other kind of hypothesis, certain inferences follow. For example, if the data in Figures 27 and 28 are interpreted as evidence that the time trends in cancer of the tongue are characteristic of birth-cohorts, then it follows that important determinants of the disease occur early in the life of a cohort and that it is these *early* determinants that are changing with time. The early factors may not necessarily operate at birth, but they must have operated at some time before the cohort pattern becomes evident in the disease trends. In the present example, they must have operated prior to age 40. The factors also may not be those most directly related to the causation of the disease. In the instance of lung cancer, for example, if rates for this disease are characteristic of birth-cohorts, it does not necessarily imply that all lung tumors are irrevocably induced early in the life of the cohort—it may merely mean that, for example, the smoking habits of the cohort are determined early in its life. In fact, the rapid decline in lung cancer risk that follows discontinuation of smoking indicates that if lung cancer is always induced early in life, its progression to clinical manifestation may certainly be interrupted later on.

To illustrate the uses of birth-cohort analysis in forming epidemiologic hypotheses, a few examples will be given. The reader may wish to refer to the original works for a more detailed description of the procedures that were followed.

PARKINSON'S SYNDROME. Etiologic factors operating over a short time period lend themselves particularly well to elucidation by cohort analysis. For example, Poskanzer and Schwab [329] noted a gradual increase in the age of patients with Parkinson's syndrome seen at the Massachusetts General Hospital between 1915 and 1960. The mean age of patients seen in 1920 to 1924 was 32.4 years and that of patients seen in 1955 to 1959 was 59.4 years. The hypothesis was suggested that Parkinson's disease occurred predominantly in certain birth-cohorts that were aging between 1920 and 1960. Of potential significance was the fact that these cohorts were exposed to the epidemic of encephalitis lethargica that occurred around 1920 and has not reappeared since. Parkinson's syndrome was a recognized complication of the acute stage of this infection, although only a small proportion of cases of Parkinson's disease now give a history of it. If the increase in mean age of patients with Parkinson's syndrome was indeed a cohort phenomenon, the possibility was raised that subclinical episodes of encephalitis lethargica are causally related to Parkinson's disease first manifest several decades later.

An argument against the cohort hypothesis in this situation, at first glance, is the fact that the mean age of the patients increased only 27 years over a period of 35 years. However, the cohorts exposed to encephalitis lethargica did not come from a single birth-year; the clinical disease was most frequent between 20 and 40 years of age but affected most age groups between 5 and 60 years. The older members of the exposed cohorts would, in subsequent years, have higher death rates than those who were relatively young at the time of the epidemic. The mean age of the total group would, therefore, advance at a rate less than 1 year for each calendar year. The investigators computed the mean age at subsequent censuses of the population that had been between 5 and 59 years of age in 1920. The results are shown in Figure 29. The close correspondence between the increase in age of these cohorts and that of the patients with Parkinson's disease strengthens the hypothesis [329].

CHRONIC NEPHRITIS. Between 1890 and 1950, there was a large excess of deaths from chronic nephritis in young adults in New South Wales in comparison with rates in other Australian states. Henderson [157] noted that the rates followed an age-time pattern best explained by the hypothesis that certain cohorts of children were exposed to a toxin which led to death from chronic nephritis between 10 and 40 years later. The agent appeared to have entered the environment of childhood about 1870 and gradually diminished after about 1920. Direct follow-up studies [158] suggested that the agent was lead, present in house paint that was used on verandas on which the infants played.

PEPTIC ULCER. Susser and Stein [387] analyzed mortality rates from peptic ulcer in England and Wales and demonstrated convincingly that the time changes occurred in a fashion characteristic of those due to changes in birth-cohort risks. Generations born in the last quarter of the 19th century manifested the highest rates and these rates pertained throughout their lives. Both gastric and duodenal ulcer showed lower rates in subsequent birth-cohorts, the decline for gastric ulcer beginning earlier and being sharper than that for duodenal ulcer. A similar decline in

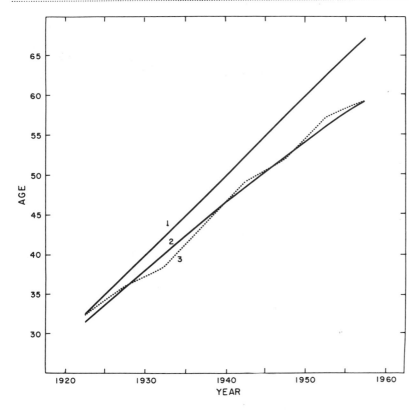

Figure 29

Mean ages at onset of Parkinson's disease in patients seen at Massachusetts General Hospital, 1920 to 1960 (line 3); mean age in census year of the cohort of persons aged 5 to 59 in 1920 (line 2); age of a cohort of persons aged 32.5 in 1920 to 1924 (line 1). (From Poskanzer and Schwab [329].)

incidence of peptic ulcer has been noted in recent birth-cohorts of physicians in Massachusetts [259].

CEREBROVASCULAR DISEASE. Yates [429] presents an interesting analysis of deaths from cerebrovascular disease, in which an attempt is made to separate the changes intrinsic to birth-cohorts from a notable but temporary decline which occurred during the Second World War and affected all adult ages simultaneously.

These examples illustrate that a clear differentiation between changes affecting birth-cohorts and those affecting populations in a cross-sectional way can often be made when either a time-limited exposure is involved—as in Parkinson's disease and chronic nephritis—or the direction of a secular trend is reversed during the period of observation—as in cancer of the tongue and peptic ulcer—so that a peak or nadir in age-specific rates can be examined to determine whether it seems more a characteristic of birth-cohorts or of current time. The lack of these features in many diseases limits the number of situations in which this type of analysis can clarify etiologic mechanisms.

## Prediction of Time Trends

It is often useful for administrative purposes to predict trends in disease rates or in expected numbers of cases, either for a particular disease or group of diseases or for all diseases. Recognition of whether past trends are characteristic of birth-cohorts or of current time will increase the accuracy of such predictions.

Perhaps the most important consideration is that the size of the population in particular age groups is very much determined by the size of the relevant birth-cohorts. If a large deficit or excess of births occurs in a particular period—as during the years of the economic depression or after World War II (see Fig. 6, p. 83)—these will be reflected in the age composition of the population for the duration of life of the cohorts. In predicting numbers of cases of a disease of which rates vary with age, it may be necessary to take such changes in the age structure of the population into account. For example, young adults 20 to 40 years of age admitted to mental institutions for psychosis provide the majority of very long-term patients in such institutions, many of them growing old there. As a consequence of the high birth rate in the years after World War II the number of persons in these age groups is now expanding rapidly and will continue to do so. For example, between 1965 and 1980, the population of Massachusetts aged 25 to 34 is expected to grow from 575,000 to 950,000. Predictions of the future needs for mental hospital beds must take this phenomenon into consideration [334].

As well as the size of the population in a given age group, its demographic characteristics influence its disease experience. Those demographic characteristics that do not change with age —race, nativity, etc.—can also be predicted from consideration of the expected age of particular birth-cohorts. For example, in the absence of any further waves of immigration or emigration, the age distribution of the foreignborn population of the United States can be predicted with reasonable accuracy from knowledge of its present distribution and of expected death rates. The aging and progressive decrement of the cohort of foreignborn persons who were present in Massachusetts in 1930 is illustrated in Figure 30.

In addition, if there is evidence that changes in *disease rates* are characteristic of birth-cohorts, more accurate estimates of the trends in specific diseases may be made. For example, if the cohort hypothesis for Parkinson's syndrome referred to earlier is

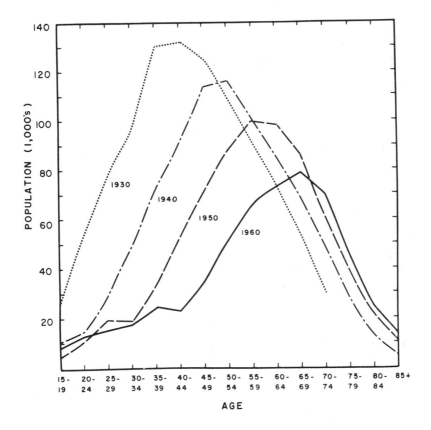

Figure 30

Foreignborn population of Massachusetts by age, at the censuses of 1930 to 1960. (Data from U.S. Census Reports)

correct, it can be predicted that the number of cases of the disease diagnosed each year in Massachusetts will decline from 15,600 in 1960 to 13,300 in 1970 and 3900 in 1980 [329]. In this instance, since the cohort hypothesis is not universally accepted, prediction of the precipitous drop between 1970 and 1980 may serve less for planning purposes than as a test of the hypothesis itself.

Similarly, incidence rates of cancer of the breast have been fairly constant or have increased slightly during the last few decades. Any prediction that this trend is likely to continue must be hedged by observation of sharp increases in rates for young women. In Connecticut, for example, rates for women under 55 years of age increased by 45 percent between 1930 and 1965 [113]. Since rates in these age groups are small relative to those in older women, the increases in young women have so far had only a small effect on the over-all rates for all ages combined. However, if the increases in rates in young women are characteristic of the cohorts of women who are now under 55—and there is some evidence that they might be [220]—the total rates can be expected to increase rather sharply as these cohorts come to occupy the ages of higher breast cancer risk.

In the forecasting of trends in general death rates, there has been considerable controversy as to whether rates should be extrapolated for birth-cohorts or in a cross-sectional manner [324]. The problem is an empiric rather than a theoretical one, and can be decided only by examination of past data to determine whether trends are or are not occurring in a way that suggests cohort types of change. Actually, in so complicated a series of events as the determinants of the total death rate, it is quite clear that a variety of mechanisms of both cohort and cross-sectional types are operative, and predictions are correspondingly uncertain. In individual diseases more simple patterns may be evident and form the basis for predictions in which somewhat more confidence can be placed.

## TIME-PLACE CLUSTERING

Variation of disease frequency in time was described in Chapter 9 and clustering by place in Chapter 8. Actually, fluctuations in disease rates by time and place are almost always interdependent; concentration of disease in a particular place is generally characteristic of a particular time and time changes are more marked in certain places than in others. In fact, local clustering of disease in time and place can occur without evidence of variation in the over-all distributions by either time or place when large temporal or geographic units are analyzed. Consider, for example, an epidemic which progresses regularly from one side of a country to the other, affecting a constant proportion of the population as it proceeds. At any point in time, the disease will show marked aggregation within a few districts, and any single district will exhibit a marked time trend as the disease passes through it. However, if rates for the country as a whole are looked at for a time span corresponding to that of the epidemic, it could appear that all areas of the country were equally affected and that an equal number of cases occurred in each time interval. Such a circumstance, while theoretically possible, is unlikely—a marked time-place clustering will usually be accompanied by observable variation in either time or place alone. However, the interaction may be more important than is suggested by separate examination of either of the variables alone, and low levels of epidemicity may not be identified by examination of time or geographic variation alone.

Time-place interaction is, of course, characteristic of infectious diseases, usually being so obvious that no special methods are required to detect it. However, from time to time, reports appear of isolated time-place clusters in diseases of unknown etiology, such as leukemia [155] and Down's syndrome [386], raising the question whether infectious mechanisms may be involved in such diseases also. Of course, one can always unearth apparent clusters—of diseases as well as of other misfortunes; the problem is to know whether these clusters occur more frequently than would be expected by chance. In the diseases of interest—for example, certain congenital malformations and leukemia and other malignant diseases—clusters are sufficiently infrequent that the determination of whether their frequency exceeds chance expectation requires special statistical methods.

## Methods

The objective of time-place analysis is to determine whether "clusters" of two or more cases that occur close together in time also tend to occur in the same geographic area. There are several problems involved in determining the number of instances in which cases occur close together—either in time or geographic distance—even if the investigator has defined what is meant by close. One approach which might be considered, for example, is to compute the distances between adjacent cases and use these distances as the measure of closeness. In respect to time, this approach is feasible, since the cases can be arranged in order of occurrence and the intervals between successive cases computed. However, in respect to geographic distance, there is no such arbitrary way of ordering cases scattered over a map, and the distribution of distances between cases will vary according to how the investigator selects "adjacent" cases.

Another approach would be to divide the total space (time or geographic) into small segments (e.g., months or years, blocks or towns). Those cases falling into the same segment could then be considered close and it can be determined whether the cases that share segments of time tend also to occupy similar geographic segments. This method will detect marked clustering, but when less obvious clustering is to be detected the selection of the sizes of the geographic or time segments presents considerable difficulty. For the method to be efficient, the size of the segments must have relevance to intervals that are biologically meaningful. Unfortunately, however, the search for time-place clustering is most appropriate in situations in which the meaningful intervals are not known. If small time segments or geographic areas are used, many pairs or clusters of cases will be missed that are close together but happen to fall on opposite sides of the boundaries of the segments. If the segments are large, they may conceal clustering occurring in smaller segments (e.g., weeks, or blocks) within the larger units (e.g., years, or towns) being used in the analysis.

METHOD OF ALL POSSIBLE PAIRS. The device of computing the temporal and geographic distances between all possible pairs of cases in a study series was suggested by Knox [189, 190]. In a series of $n$ cases, there will be $n(n-1)/2$ possible pairs. The distribution of time intervals between all these pairs will depend on the incidence of cases in the study population and on any change in incidence that may occur during the study period. Similarly, the distribution of geographic distances between pair members will depend on the frequency of the disease and the density and distribution of the population. Although neither one of the over-all distributions—by time interval or by geographic distance—can, in the absence of denominator data, be interpreted as indicating any tendency to localization of the disease other than that which would follow from localization of the population, cross-tabulation of the pairs by time interval and geographic distance will reveal whether those pairs that are close together in time also tend to be close together geographically.

Illustrative data are shown in Table 26. The residences of the mothers of 723 cases of anencephaly and/or spina bifida in Providence, Rhode Island, were located on a map and the map coordinates of each residence recorded. The cases were also identified by first day of the mother's last menstrual period, as an indicator of the date of conception. The days were numbered consecutively from the beginning to the end of the study period. The 723 cases yield 261,003 possible pairs. For each pair, both the time interval and the geographic distance between its members were computed, the time interval by subtraction of the number assigned to the day of mother's last menstrual period for the first member of the pair from that assigned to the second, and the geographic distance by application of Pythagoras' theorem to the map coordinates. Needless to say, except in a very small series, these procedures are feasible only with the aid of a computer. The distribution of the 261,003 possible pairs is shown as the observed frequencies in the table—for example, there were 5 pairs in which the members were separated by less than 0.25 km and less than 15 days. The expected values in the table are based on the assumption that the distribution of pairs by time interval is independent of that by geographic distance. Thus, the value 2.9 expected cases within 0.25 km and less than fifteen days is derived from $(882/261,003) \times 854$.

A simple descriptive comparison of the observed and expected values in such a table may be of value. There may be insufficient indication of clustering to warrant further consideration, or, conceivably, the table may reveal the presence of clustering of such a degree that tests of significance are not needed to con-

## Table 26

Distribution of all possible pairs of cases by time interval and distance. 723 cases of congenital neural tube defects in Providence, Rhode Island, 1936–1965*

| Distance (km) | Obs or Exp | 0–14 | 15–29 | 30–59 | 60–89 | 90–179 | 180–364 | 365–12087 | Total |
|---|---|---|---|---|---|---|---|---|---|
| <0.25 | Obs | 5 | 6 | 5 | 6 | 16 | 42 | 774 | 854 |
|  | Exp | 2.9 | 2.9 | 5.5 | 5.2 | 15.9 | 33.2 | 788.5 | 854.0 |
| 0.25–0.49 | Obs | 7 | 8 | 13 | 12 | 41 | 98 | 1872 | 2051 |
|  | Exp | 6.9 | 6.9 | 13.1 | 12.6 | 38.1 | 79.7 | 1893.8 | 2051.0 |
| 0.50–0.99 | Obs | 23 | 26 | 43 | 42 | 96 | 244 | 5881 | 6355 |
|  | Exp | 21.5 | 21.3 | 40.6 | 38.9 | 118.0 | 246.9 | 5867.8 | 6355.0 |
| 1.00–1.99 | Obs | 69 | 79 | 140 | 132 | 403 | 831 | 19593 | 21247 |
|  | Exp | 71.8 | 71.1 | 135.8 | 130.2 | 394.7 | 825.5 | 19618.0 | 21247.0 |
| 2.00–4.99 | Obs | 248 | 261 | 528 | 497 | 1557 | 3203 | 75135 | 81429 |
|  | Exp | 275.2 | 272.4 | 520.4 | 498.9 | 1512.5 | 3163.8 | 75185.9 | 81429.0 |
| 5.00 + | Obs | 530 | 493 | 939 | 910 | 2735 | 5723 | 137737 | 149067 |
|  | Exp | 503.7 | 498.6 | 952.7 | 913.2 | 2768.8 | 5791.8 | 137638.1 | 149067.0 |
| *Total* | Obs | 882 | 873 | 1668 | 1599 | 4848 | 10141 | 240992 | 261003 |
|  | Exp | 882.0 | 873.0 | 1668.0 | 1599.0 | 4848.0 | 10141.0 | 240992.0 | 261003.0 |

Time interval (days)

* Source: unpublished data [153].

vince the investigator that it is real. If the clustering is not of such intensity, as in the present example, it may at least suggest the geographic distances and time intervals which might be used in a subsequent study designed to test a specific hypothesis. For example, Table 26 indicates an excess of observed over expected pairs in the two cells characterized by intervals of less than 30 days and distances of less than 0.25 km.

The matter becomes complex when the investigator wishes to determine whether the clustering observed in his particular set of data is likely to be due to chance.

One statistical problem derives from the lack of independence of the individual measurements, each point being represented $(n - 1)$ times. Knox [190] pointed out that, if attention is directed to the pairs occupying the cell bordered by such small time and distance intervals that the number of pairs is small, their members will probably be independent, and the observed values can be compared with a Poisson distribution of which the mean and variance is the expected number of cases. In the particular example in Table 26, comparison of 11 (or more) observed with 5.8 expected in the two cells less than 0.25 km and 30 days gives $P \sim 0.03$ (one-tail test). David and Barton [73] have subsequently calculated the exact mean and variance of Knox's criterion and have shown the appropriateness of the Poisson model in situations similar to that with which Knox was dealing. Mantel [238] describes the procedures for computing variances by the exact permutational method in situations in which the appropriateness of the Poisson model may be in doubt.

A second group of problems stems from the lack of a priori specification, or even knowledge, of what intervals are meaningful in the context of the particular disease under investigation. A priori specification of some arbitrary intervals may satisfy certain statistical instincts but it has disadvantages. There is, of course, the necessity of convincing one's colleagues that the boundary intervals were indeed arbitrarily chosen prior to examination of the data. In addition, there is the fact that arbitrary selection of boundaries may be inefficient in that, if there is no prior knowledge leading to the selection of such boundaries, the most relevant boundaries can be identified only from the data at hand. Thus, in the data in Table 26, selection of the two cells used in the previous paragraph gives significant differences between observed and expected numbers, but selection of other boundaries would not. Procedures for dealing with this problem objectively have been developed by David and Barton [73].

The statistical problems involved in the detection of time-place interaction using the all-possible-pairs procedure have been considered by Pinkel et al. [320], David and Barton [73], Pike and Smith [318], and Mantel [238]. The proposed solutions are statistically too complex to be described here, but they have been reviewed in some detail by Mantel [238] and Mustacchi et al. [265]. However, methods for both identifying and testing the tempero-spatial localization of cases in a single body of data are not as satisfactory as the procedure of using one body of data to formulate a hypothesis that is specific as to the time and distance intervals involved in clustering, and a second body of data to test that hypothesis. For example, Pike et al. [319], in analyzing data on time-place clustering of Burkitt's tumor in Uganda, noted that clusters of cases were most marked within 180 days and 40 kilometers of each other and suggested these as a priori values to be tested in later data. Even this procedure has difficulties, in that the same geographic or temporal distance may not have the same biologic implications in a different set of circumstances—e.g., an urban versus a rural population. Attention should therefore be given to having reasonably similar populations for the derivation and the testing of the hypothesis.

ALTERNATIVE METHOD. An approach quite different from that based on all possible pairs is that used by Ederer et al. [102] to study childhood leukemia in Connecticut. The approach depends again on the a priori selection of arbitrary units of time and place; in this instance years and towns were used. The question then asked is: Given that so many cases occurred in a particular town in a 5-year period, what is the probability of occurrence of the observed distribution by individual years? Although it was shown that the method was clearly capable of identifying clustering of poliomyelitis and hepatitis, it seems likely to be less efficient in detecting clustering at very low levels of intensity than are the methods based on all possible pairs. As noted by Mantel [238], Ederer's method is sensitive to both temporal and tempero-spatial clustering, so that analyses must be undertaken to differentiate the two.

*Interpretation*

The great interest in time-place clustering in recent years lies in the fact that, if observed to occur within small place and time dimensions, it provides rather suggestive evidence of the role of infectious agents, since these are the kinds of etiologic agent that seem most likely to occupy different geographic locations at different times. There are, of course, alternative explanations of time-place clustering, but it is important to recognize some of the things that do *not* produce time-place interaction. For example, variation in diagnostic accuracy or ascertainment in different sections of a study area or over the period of a study will not produce time-place clustering unless the variation is affecting both variables simultaneously. Variations in disease rates by ethnic group or socioeconomic status will also not produce time-place clustering, even if particular ethnic groups or economic classes tend to inhabit particular locations. As Doll noted [80], in discussing the time-place clustering observed for Burkitt's tumor in Uganda [319], the essential characteristic of an explanatory factor must be movement—movement of a susceptible population from one place to another during the study period (a process that can usually readily be detected), movement of diagnostic or reporting mechanisms from one place to another as the study progresses, or movement of an etiologic agent.

In recent years time-place clustering has been studied in leukemia [102, 190, 247, 397] and in Down's syndrome [196, 381] and other congenital malformations [189]. The results have often been negative [102, 247, 381]. Even when statistically significant clustering has been detected, it has been no more striking than the level exemplified in Table 26. That is to say, only a small proportion of the cases in any series have occurred in clusters. A question that is as intriguing as why *any* cases occur in clusters is, therefore, why so *few* come in clusters if infectious agents are indeed involved. Possibilities include that the responsible organism is of low infectivity or that the proportion of persons susceptible (for example, those at a critical stage of pregnancy) is small in any one community as the organism passes through it. The *number* of clusters is not an indication of the possible significance of the agent responsible for the clustering. The clustering merely reveals a mechanism which might have much wider relevance.

Clustering does not, of course, necessarily imply that there is direct transmission of an agent from one affected individual to another. It is equally compatible with the movement of generally increased levels of infection from one area to another, and, in the diseases under consideration, the latter indeed seems the more likely mechanism.

# 11

---

## Cohort Studies

Cohort studies constitute one important form of epidemiologic investigation undertaken to test hypotheses regarding the causation of disease. The distinguishing features of cohort studies are:

1. The group or groups of persons to be studied (the cohorts) are defined in terms of characteristics manifest prior to the appearance of the disease under investigation.
2. The study groups so defined are observed over a period of time to determine the frequency of the disease among them.

In the following discussion the distinction between retrospective and prospective cohort studies, described in Chapter 3, should be kept in mind. The distinction depends on whether or not the cases of disease have occurred in the cohort at the time the study is begun. In a retrospective cohort study all the relevant events (causes *and* effects) have already occurred when the study is initiated. In a prospective study the relevant causes may or may not have occurred at the time the study is begun, but the cases of disease will not have occurred, and, following selection of the study cohort, the investigator must wait for the disease to appear in its members. The distinction between these two approaches is important, not because of any conceptual differences or differences in interpretation of findings, but because of relevance to some of the practical issues to be discussed.

## SELECTION OF STUDY COHORTS

Groups of persons may be selected for cohort studies for a variety of reasons: (1) they have undergone some unusual exposure or experience of which the effects are to be evaluated, (2) they offer some special resource that may facilitate ascertainment of their exposure, follow-up, or disease experience, (3) a cohort study is desirable and this particular study group seems as good as any, or (4) some combination of the above reasons applies.

### Special Exposure Groups

Studies of persons with unusually high levels of exposure to a particular substance are usually the first step in exploring the possible relationship of the substance to disease. Even if the substance is one to which entire populations are exposed—for example, a pesticide—groups with unusually heavy exposures, such as might be received in the manufacture or use of the chemical, would logically be studied first in order to gain information on the nature and possible ranges of risks that might have to be explored in a broader population study. Thus nearly all the information available on the risks of ionizing radiation in man comes from studies of groups heavily exposed in the course of war [256], medical therapy [70, 174, 317], or occupation [201, 209, 360].

Occupational groups have provided a prime source of cohorts of persons with unusually heavy exposures to chemical, physical, and other disease-producing agents. A classic example is the study of Case et al. [45] on urinary bladder cancer in workers in the dyestuffs industry.

As with Case's study, special-exposure cohorts can frequently be assembled retrospectively. For example, Court Brown and Doll [69] studied the occurrence of leukemia in patients given x-ray therapy for ankylosing spondylitis. The cohort consisted of 13,352 patients treated between 1934 and 1954, and the outcome evaluated was death from leukemia or aplastic anemia between 1935 and 1954. Both the exposures and the deaths had occurred at the time that the study was undertaken in 1955. A prospective component was added to this study by continuing to follow the cohort, as established in 1955, to identify deaths occurring in subsequent years [70].

The significance of a particular exposure may not be realized or facilities for studying its consequences may not become available until many years after persons were first exposed. Indeed, this is one of the reasons that so many of these studies can be done retrospectively. This may lead to difficulties in identifying the members of a study cohort. While Court Brown and Doll were able to enroll persons in the cohort as soon as they became eligible (through receiving radiotherapy), this may not always be possible. For example, Wada et al. [408] studied deaths—particularly deaths from respiratory cancer—among former employees of a mustard gas factory which was in operation from 1929 to 1945. The study was begun in 1965, and from a variety of sources it was possible to assemble a list of 2620 of the 5000 total number of employees who had worked in the factory during its operation. However, causes of death could not be ascertained prior to 1952, and it was necessary to restrict the observation period to the years 1952 to 1967. The study is therefore one of a cohort defined between 7 and 23 years after the exposure, and including only a proportion of the exposed persons. Similarly, Case and Lea [46] in 1955 wished to study mortality among military personnel exposed to mustard gas poisoning in World War I. The study cohort consisted of persons who in 1930 were receiving pensions for the effects of such exposures; mortality in the cohort was examined for the years 1930 to 1952. Thus the observations relate neither to the total number of persons exposed to mustard gas nor to the total period during which effects might have occurred.

The effect of such losses prior to the formation of the study cohort must be distinguished from the effect of losses after the cohort is defined. Losses before definition of the cohort may limit the generalizations that can be made from the results of the study. For example, negative findings in the study cohort would not exclude the possibility that excess illness occurred prior to the definition of the cohort or among persons not included in the cohort. However, such losses do not affect the validity of the findings in the cohort itself. In contrast, losses occurring after formation of the cohort *may* affect the validity of the findings, as will be discussed later.

While many studies of special exposure groups are conducted retrospectively, studies of survivors of the atomic bombings of Hiroshima and Nagasaki [24] and of lung cancer in uranium miners on the Colorado Plateau [209, 409] are examples of cohort studies of special-exposure groups which have essentially been prospective throughout. The cohorts were identified shortly after the exposure—or, in the case of the uranium miners, during the exposure—and have been followed continuously to date.

In some instances when prospective observations are required —because, for example, adequate data on outcome cannot be obtained retrospectively—and the time during which effects might be expected is very long, the period of required observation can be reduced by admitting to the study persons who are at different stages in the desired observation period. For example, Hutchison [174] wished to observe with semiannual blood counts women who had been given radiation therapy for carcinoma of the uterine cervix. Observation of the outcome of interest, leukemia, was desired over a period from 0 to 20 or more years after the radiation therapy. The approach was to admit to the study women who at any time in the past had had the radiotherapy and who were currently being followed by the clinics involved in the study. In the course of the 5-year study, observations were made on some women from 0 to 4 years after therapy, others from 1 to 5 years after therapy, and so on, including some who were more than 15 years post-therapy. Thus observations relevant to an extended period of possible risk were made during a relatively short study period. While this procedure reduces the length of follow-up necessary, it does of course correspondingly increase the number of persons that must be included in the study cohort.

## Groups Offering Special Resources

Certain groups offer advantages for cohort studies because of special facilities for follow-up or for ways of identifying particular outcomes among their members. Since such groups would only fortuitously also have special exposures of epidemiologic concern, they are most usefully studied when either the exposure of interest is a common one—for example, cigarette smoking—or the group is very large. Examples of some groups that have been studied follow.

PERSONS ENROLLED IN PREPAID MEDICAL CARE PLANS. Certain union-sponsored medical care programs and programs such as the Health Insurance Plan of Greater New York and the Kaiser-Permanente Plan provide populations large enough for many types of cohort study. The prepayment component of the plan not only makes it likely that most members will seek most of their medical care within the program—and that their records will therefore be available—but also provides, through continued membership, a mechanism for periodic follow-up.

CERTAIN OCCUPATIONAL GROUPS. To investigate the relationship between cigarette smoking and lung cancer, Doll and Hill [84] studied physicians listed in the Medical Register of the United Kingdom in 1951. Because of the legal obligation to maintain registration, the members of this group were relatively easy to identify and trace; they might also be expected to receive better than average medical care (and hence diagnosis). Doyle et al. [93] describe a cohort study of male civil service employees in Albany, New York, who because of stability of occupation and accessibility seemed a suitable group among whom to study the occurrence of heart disease. Workers in industrial plants also provide populations that are readily accessible and easily followed. However, the number of persons in any one plant is unlikely to be large enough for the study of specific diseases, unless some special risk is present in the plant.

INSURED PERSONS. The many studies of life insurance statistics might be classified as cohort studies. Persons taking out insurance policies between certain dates constitute the entering cohort, the subsequent mortality being measured by death claims. A special study utilizing such a population group is that of Dorn and others [87, 184] on the effect of smoking on mortality among holders of U.S. government life insurance. These policyholders were veterans, primarily from World War I. The cohort consisted of all such policyholders known to be alive in July, 1954. This study differs from most insurance studies in that entrance into the cohort was determined not by the time the insurance was taken out, but by virtue of its members being alive at a specified time, the insurance having been taken out at some time in the past. As was pointed out in the discussion of special-exposure cohorts (p. 209), this delayed entry to the study cohort should not affect the validity of the results as they pertain to the relationship between smoking habits in 1954 and the probability of subsequent death, even though it may well be, for example, that smokers, having higher death rates than non-smokers, were less completely represented in the cohort established in 1954 than they were among the total population that took out this form of life insurance.

OBSTETRIC POPULATIONS.   Investigations of the possible roles of prenatal experiences in the production of defect or disease noted at birth are ideally suited to the cohort type of study. In the first place, the period of follow-up is short. Secondly, the delivery and recording of outcome are frequently the responsibility of the same agency (physician or hospital) as that which undertook the measurement of exposure during pregnancy. The two circumstances, indeed, are often recorded in the same medical record.

VOLUNTEER GROUPS.   Hammond and Horn [151] assembled a cohort of 189,854 white men between the ages of 50 and 69 by asking 22,000 American Cancer Society female workers (themselves volunteers) to have a questionnaire filled out by about 10 such men "whom she knew well and would be able to trace." An attractive feature of volunteer groups such as these is the relative ease of obtaining detailed information, since willingness to supply information usually goes along with the person's agreement to enter the study. The possibility of bias resulting from the method of selection of such groups is, however, a major problem. For example, it is possible that the American Cancer Society volunteers, having suspicion that smoking was injurious to health, might have tended to select men who not only were agreeable to entering the study, but who also were heavy smokers and in lower than average states of health. Although individuals who had gross illness were excluded from the cohort, this might not eliminate the difficulty entirely. Such a bias, it may be noted, would probably have its major effect early in the follow-up.

OTHER GROUPS. There are other special circumstances and groups that may facilitate cohort studies. The program of studies utilizing the special resources available for following veterans in the United States was referred to in Chapter 6. College alumni records have provided the basis for long-term retrospective cohort studies relating experiences and characteristics manifest during the college years to mortality from certain diseases several decades later [306, 307].

*Geographically Defined Cohorts*

When a cohort study is to be done of a general population, the cohort may be defined in part on the basis of administrative or geographic boundaries, such as those of a town or county. In the selection of an appropriate area, one of the more important, though prosaic, considerations is the accessibility of the population to the investigator. In addition, characteristics of the population, such as its stability and socioeconomic status, and characteristics of the town, such as the quality of its medical care facilities, will be important considerations. Even though such an area is defined primarily in geographic terms, it will usually be necessary to restrict the study cohort to particular age, sex, or other demographic groups within the general population of the area.

For example, in the late 1940s the U.S. Public Health Service decided to follow a cohort of persons over a period of 20 years to study the occurrence of cardiovascular disease among them. In order to obtain a cross section of socioeconomic, ethnic, and other demographic subgroups in the cohort, it was decided to conduct the study in a general population rather than in any special group. The study was to be restricted to the age group 30 to 59 years, to allow observations of persons immediately prior to and entering the years of highest incidence. It was estimated that a population of 5000 persons in this age range would give approximately 1500 new cases of the disease of interest over a 20-year period—a number judged adequate to provide reliable rates. The population of the town of Framingham, Mass., was selected for the study; Framingham at that time was a community of 28,000 persons in eastern Massachusetts. It was considered sufficiently remote from metropolitan Boston to retain its identity as a separate community, but not so remote that access was difficult. The population was reasonably stable and the industry diversified. As with other Massachusetts towns (see p. 101), population lists that would facilitate sampling and follow-up were kept and updated annually. There was a single general hospital, of high quality, which would simplify surveillance of hospital admissions. The medical profession, the administration, and the population of the town were ready to cooperate. To reduce the size of the study group to the desired 5000, a random two-thirds sample of the population 30 to 59 years of age was drawn. The sample invited to participate numbered 6507 persons—a number higher than 5000, since a proportion of those invited were expected to decline to participate [74].

A somewhat similar study has been conducted in the town of Tecumseh, Mich. [119]. In this instance all 9822 persons in the town were invited to participate.

## OBTAINING DATA ON EXPOSURE

In a study of a cohort that has been defined without prior knowledge of any special exposure, information must be collected that will allow classification of the cohort members according to whether or not they have been exposed to the factor under investigation. When the cohort has been selected because of special exposure, all its members may be considered to have been exposed; nevertheless, it will usually be desirable to be able to classify individuals according to their level of exposure, at least in broad classes. At the same time that data on exposure are being obtained, information can be sought on differences between exposure categories with respect to demographic variables that might affect the frequency of the disease under investigation. Such information will be required for effective analysis, whether or not the cohort was selected in terms of some special exposure. In addition, if the disease under investigation is a very common one, it may be necessary to exclude persons who already manifest it at the time of becoming eligible for the study; this also will require collection of information on eligible persons at the time of entry into the study.

## Sources of Information

The kinds of information indicated above can be classified into four general categories related to the procedures needed to obtain it: (1) information available from records, (2) information that can be supplied by the individual members of the cohort, (3) information that can be obtained only by medical examination or other special testing of the cohort members, and (4) information that requires testing or evaluation of the environment within which the cohort members have lived or worked. Information from more than one category—or indeed from all four—may be required for a particular study.

INFORMATION FROM RECORDS. In some studies—for example, studies of groups exposed to radiotherapy or other medical procedures, or of insured or working populations—the records that are used to determine eligibility for the cohort may include sufficient data to derive crude estimates of level of exposure, as well as demographic and other pertinent information. The studies of ankylosing spondylitis patients, aniline dye workers, and soldiers exposed to mustard gas that have already been referred to, relied exclusively on recorded sources of exposure data.

In some situations records are the *only* reliable source of information. For example, Court Brown and Doll [69] were able to classify their cohort by dose of radiation received; such information would not have been available from the patient himself or any other source but the medical record. Similarly, Feinleib [112] assembled retrospectively from medical records cohorts of women who had undergone various kinds of pelvic surgery, distinguishing groups that had had no, one, or both ovaries removed. While the fact that they had undergone pelvic surgery might be known to most women who have had such procedures, the specific nature of the operation is often not known.

Recorded information has two advantages. First, it can usually be obtained for a high proportion of the cohort. Second, it allows objective classification prior to any knowledge of the outcome that is the focus of the investigation, or even before it is known that the person involved is to be included in a study group. For these reasons it is usually desirable to assemble whatever information is recorded on cohort members, even if additional sources are also required to obtain data on the exposure that is the primary focus of the study.

INFORMATION FROM COHORT MEMBERS.   A number of cohort studies have been directed toward assessment of the effects of smoking. Until recent years adequate data on smoking habits have not been routinely obtainable from most kinds of records, although the information can be provided readily by the person involved. Since cohort studies require large populations, simple and economical ways of obtaining such data are desirable. Mail questionnaires have been used in several studies. Smoking histories were obtained in this manner for British physicians by Doll and Hill [84] and for American veterans by Dorn [87]. In these two studies, response rates to the first mail questionnaire were almost identical—68 percent; Dorn increased this to 83 percent by a second questionnaire to those who failed to answer the first. A mail questionnaire was used in a study of married women in eastern Massachusetts between 25 and 50 years of age to assemble for prospective observation a cohort of women using oral contraceptives. After two mailings, information was obtained from 65 percent [153].

Little published information is available on the factors that affect response rates to mail questionnaires, at least in relation to medical inquiries. There appear to be only small differences in response rates according to length of questionnaire (within reasonable limits), extent to which the accompanying letter is personalized, or other factors pertaining to the questionnaire itself. There are, however, appreciable differences in response rates according to age of the persons to whom the questionnaires are sent, and between geographic areas [153]. Perhaps the most important consideration for the investigator who wishes to obtain high response rates is the selection, where feasible, of a study population whose members are likely to have some personal interest in the study.

INFORMATION FROM MEDICAL EXAMINATION. For some exposure characteristics of interest—for example, serum lipids, blood pressure, body build—information can be obtained only by medical examination of the cohort members. This is the case, for example, in most studies oriented toward cardiovascular disease.

INFORMATION FROM MEASURES OF THE ENVIRONMENT. In some situations adequate information on exposure levels can not be obtained from any of the above sources alone. For example, it may be necessary to measure exposure levels in the environment of various areas in a plant in which individual members of a cohort work. Insofar as present or future exposures are concerned, this may pose no great problem, but if a substantial part of the exposure being assessed has occurred prior to initiation of the study, changes in the conditions of the working environment may make retrospective evaluation quite difficult.

For example, in a study of mortality among U.S. uranium miners [209, 409], workers were considered eligible for inclusion in the cohort from the time they were first examined by a Public Health Service team. These examinations took place between 1950 and 1960, but many of the men had worked in the industry for many years previously and had accumulated a considerable radiation exposure prior to entering the study cohort. Since most of the men had worked in several mines for varying lengths of time and since radiation levels vary quite markedly between mines, an estimate of cumulative exposure could be derived only from a combination of employment records maintained by the mines, detailed employment histories taken from the men, and estimates of radiation levels in individual mines.

In such a situation there is also a need to summarize the accumulated exposure for each man. In the study just referred to, each mine was characterized as to its average Working Level—a measure translatable into physical terms of exposure to radon daughter products. The cumulative exposure was measured in Working-Level-Months (WLM); for example, work for 12 months in a mine with an average exposure of 1 Working Level contributed 12 WLM. Men were then categorized according to the total WLM accumulated during their mining experience. Measures such as this have obvious drawbacks, both in concept —they imply, for example, that effects are independent of dose rate (that is, that 12 months' exposure to 1 Working Level has the same effect as 1 month's exposure to 12 Working Levels)— and in inaccuracies in the primary measurements that enter into them. Nevertheless they do provide a basis for formation of broad categories of accumulated exposure and are an essential first step if the data are to be examined for a relationship between level of exposure and extent of risk.

### Effect of Nonresponse

When data on exposure must be obtained from the individual members of a study cohort—either by questionnaire or by examination—it is likely that information will not be obtained for some proportion. The Tecumseh study is remarkable in that 88 percent of the selected cohort underwent the initial examination [119]. However, nonresponse rates of about 30 percent are not unusual. For example, in Framingham, 4469 (69 percent) of the 6507 persons in the initial sample actually underwent the first examination [74]. Similar response rates to mail questionnaires have already been referred to. In such situations it is necessary to evaluate the effect of this nonresponse on the outcome of the study.

Some of the considerations in evaluating the effects of this loss might perhaps be discussed more appropriately in connection with the description of analysis and interpretation of cohort studies. However, since they are also relevant to decisions regarding data to be collected on the entering cohort, they will be described here.

In theory the true relationship between the exposure and outcome variables will be distorted only if the loss through inability to assign individuals to exposure categories is biased with respect to *both* exposure and outcome—for example, that persons with high cholesterol levels *and* having a high risk of coronary disease for reasons other than their cholesterol levels are more or less likely to be excluded from the study. If the loss is biased only with respect to exposure—for example, persons with high cholesterol levels fail to cooperate—an incorrect impression of the distribution of cholesterol levels in the population will be obtained, but the experience of the study cohort will accurately reflect the strength of the relationship between rates of coronary disease and cholesterol levels in the population. If the loss is biased only with respect to outcome—for example, that persons in poor health fail to respond, as indeed seems to occur in many studies [84, 150]—then disease rates in the study cohort will be lower than in the population, but the ratio of the rates of persons with high cholesterol levels to those of persons with low levels will be the same as in the population as a whole. If the loss is unbiased with respect to both exposure and outcome, then, of course, it can be safely ignored.

In practice it is often difficult to know whether the loss is selective with respect to exposure, outcome, or both. To settle this question conclusively, one would have to have the same data for the lost persons as for the cohort—and in that case the lost persons would not, of course, have been classed as lost. A number of procedures may be followed to allow an indirect assessment. While each can provide only a partial answer, the results may in sum be convincing. The procedures include:

1. More intensive efforts to obtain exposure data for a small sample of the nonrespondents, to determine whether the nonrespondents are different from the respondents in regard to exposure. By means of a second questionnaire sent, 10 years after the original inquiry, to a sample of some physicians who had previously answered and some who had not, Doll and Hill [84] showed a substantially higher proportion of moderate and heavy smokers among the earlier nonrespondents—a feature that probably contributed to the lower than expected mortality among the respondents.

2. Comparison of nonrespondents with respondents with respect to any ancillary information (e.g., age, sex, or ethnic group) that can be obtained from records or sources other than the main source of exposure information.

3. Follow-up of nonrespondents as well as respondents so that certain outcomes can be compared in the two groups. For example, if the outcome under investigation is coronary artery disease, it may not be possible to obtain for the nonrespondents the specific clinical information to be obtained for the cohort members, but it may be possible to monitor the hospital admissions or deaths in both groups.

4. Examination of disease rates in the cohort in different time periods. If differences in disease rates between exposure categories in the study cohort are due in part to selective processes, the differences in rates are likely to become smaller as the study progresses, since the effects of such biases will be strongest in the early years of the study. For example, the mortality of British physicians in the study cohort referred to was estimated to be 63 percent of that of all British physicians during the second year of the study, 85 percent during the third year, and about 93 percent between the fourth and tenth years [84]. The effect of the initial selection had apparently not entirely worn off, even 10 years later, but it was relatively small after the third year.

## Reassignment to Exposure Categories

In many cohort studies there is only one assessment of exposure—that made at the time of entry of the individual into the study cohort. However, appreciable numbers of individuals may change their exposure class during the course of a long-term study. Such studies as the one in Framingham, involving periodic interviews and examinations of members of the cohort, allow opportunities for periodic revision of exposure classes according to changes in information. Changes in exposure which occur but which are not taken into consideration will tend to make the strength of an observed association lower than that which actually existed between exposure and development of the disease. In other words, the true association will be greater than that found. The risk of introducing this kind of error seems more acceptable than that of producing false associations, as might happen if knowledge of outcome influenced the reassessment of exposure status. A conservative approach would then lead to utilization of the initially determined exposure categories throughout the study. In studies of exceptionally long duration this generalization may not be applicable. Moreover, when there is considerable interest in defining as accurately as possible the *amount* of exposure associated with a certain level of disease risk, and the exposure accumulates during the course of the study—as, for example, in the study of U.S. uranium miners—then it will be more appropriate to reassess exposure levels periodically during the study.

In studies of long duration or in instances such as the study of uranium miners, separate examination of outcome in those individuals who changed exposure groups during the course of the study is highly desirable. Such examination may assist both in detecting possible biases involved in the reassessment and in allowing an evaluation of real changes in risk associated with change of exposure category—for example, from smoker to nonsmoker.

## SELECTION OF COMPARISON GROUPS

### Internal Comparisons

In many cohort studies the comparison groups are built in, a single cohort being entered into the study and its members then classified into exposure categories. For example, the cohorts of the Framingham and Tecumseh studies were defined without any knowledge of the status of individuals with respect to causal variables. On the basis of information obtained at entry to the study, however, the individuals can be categorized into smokers or nonsmokers, according to serum cholesterol levels, and so on. No outside comparison group is required.

### Comparison with Population Rates

In other studies—particularly when a special-exposure cohort has been assembled—some basis for comparison is required to evaluate whether the outcome observed in the cohort differs from that which would be expected if the members had not been at any special risk. A common comparison is with the experience of the general population at the time the cohort is being followed.

Since most special-exposure cohorts are too small for the derivation of reliable age-, sex-, and cause-specific rates, the procedure is usually to compare the observed number of cases in the cohort with an expected number. The expected number is estimated by applying the general population rates, specific for sex, age, and cause, to the numbers in the corresponding age and sex groups in the cohort and summing the expected number of cases over all sex and age groups. It is necessary to take into account the fact that the members of the cohort age as the study progresses, and it may also be necessary to take account of changes over time in the general population rates.

In addition to considering specific items such as age and sex, the population from which the expected rates are taken should be selected so as to be generally similar to that from which the exposed cohort derived. There should be, first of all, reasonable geographic comparability. For example, in the U.S. uranium miners study, rates for white males in the four states in which most of the mining population was located—rather than for the U.S. as a whole—were used [209]. In addition, there may be selective factors within the same geographically defined population—for example, that a particular ethnic group predominates in a special-exposure group because the occupation from which the exposure group derived has a predominance of that ethnic group.

Naturally, comparisons with population rates are possible only for outcomes for which population rates are available. This has limited the method essentially to the study of conditions for which death rates can be used to evaluate risk, and to some studies of cancer incidence, hospitalization for mental illness, and other situations where special data are available.

## Comparison Cohorts

Another method of obtaining a basis for comparison is the selection and following of another special cohort, similar in demographic characteristics to the exposed group, but not exposed.

For example, in studies of industrial exposures, persons in other occupations in the same industry may be suitable. To evaluate mortality rates in a cohort of radiologists, Seltser and Sartwell [360] compared them with rates in similarly defined cohorts of internists and of ophthalmologists and otolaryngologists. In some studies of the frequency of neoplasms in children irradiated for thymus enlargement, siblings of the irradiated infants have been used as comparison groups [317, 370].

In theory, an ideal comparison cohort for the studies of patients irradiated for ankylosing spondylitis or thymic enlargement would be patients with ankylosing spondylitis or thymic enlargement who were not irradiated, since such comparison would also rule out the possibility that ankylosing spondylitis or thymic enlargement themselves were responsible for any unusual outcome noted. Such groups are rarely available, however, in nonexperimental situations.

Studies of cohorts identified at birth offer favorable opportunities for selection of comparison cohorts because of the ready identification of the related population. Thus cohorts of birth-injured children might be compared with cohorts of infants selected at random or on a paired basis from the same population of births.

## Multiple Comparisons

It may be that, for a specific cohort of exposed persons, neither general population rates nor another special group provide entirely satisfactory bases of comparison. In such situations it may be possible to strengthen the evaluation by providing for a variety of comparisons. To illustrate some of the criticisms that can be raised regarding certain comparisons and how these can be countered to some extent by multiple comparisons, the results of a retrospective cohort study of infants irradiated for thymic enlargement are shown in Table 27. In this study a comparison cohort of siblings was used, and, in addition, expected numbers of cases of the outcomes of interest, based on general population rates, were calculated for both the exposed and the unexposed cohorts [370]. Comparison with general population rates can be criticized on the basis of the variation in incidence of leukemia and thyroid cancer according to geography, ethnic group, economic group, and other variables which were not accounted for in the calculation of the expected number of cases. Several unsatisfactory features of comparison groups derived from siblings are discussed in Chapter 12 (p. 249). The fact that the observed cases of cancers other than leukemia and thyroid

## Table 27

Frequency of leukemia and thyroid cancer among children treated by x-ray in infancy for thymic enlargement*

| Disease | Irradiation (1722 children) | | No irradiation (1795 siblings) | |
|---|---|---|---|---|
| | Number observed | Number expected | Number observed | Number expected |
| Leukemia | 7 | 0.6 | 0 | 0.6 |
| Thyroid cancer | 6 | 0.1 | 0 | 0.1 |
| Other cancer | 4 | 1.9 | 5 | 2.0 |
| All cancer | 17 | 2.6 | 5 | 2.7 |

* From Simpson et al. [370].

cancer exceed the expected number of cases in both the irradiated group and their siblings might be interpreted as evidence of more thorough case-finding among the two cohorts than among the general population which furnished the rates for calculation of the expected numbers. However, the extent of this possible bias, as measured in the "other cancer" group, is by no means large enough to explain the relative excess of leukemia and thyroid cancer among the irradiated group. That the excess for leukemia and thyroid cancer is so much greater than that for other cancers—whether the basis of comparison is the siblings or the general population—supports the view that the risk of thyroid cancer and leukemia experienced by the irradiated infants is indeed increased.

Even in studies where internal categorizations or other special cohorts provide the primary basis for comparison, it is desirable also to compute expected frequencies in the study cohort or cohorts for those outcomes for which population data can be obtained.

## FOLLOW-UP

Having defined the study cohorts and obtained data on exposure and other relevant characteristics, there remains the task of determining the outcome among the groups to be compared. Generally the outcome to be ascertained will be the appearance of either morbidity or death from a certain disease or group of diseases. The procedures required will of course vary with the outcome to be determined, ranging from routine surveillance of death certificates to periodic medical examination of each member of the cohort.

Some of the resources available for following groups of persons were described in Chapter 6. It is clear that completeness of ascertainment of outcome should be equal in all exposure categories. This objective is most easily attained when the method of ascertainment or follow-up depends on a mechanism completely separate from that by which exposure was categorized. Perhaps most satisfactory is reliance on some routine procedure that is applied equally to all persons, regardless of the fact that they are members of a special study group. For example, in the studies of Doll and Hill [84] and Dorn [184] on cigarette smoking, data on exposure were obtained from the individuals constituting the cohort, but knowledge of the outcome—death, and death from particular causes—was obtained from routine records. In the former study, copies of all death certificates on which there was indication that the decedent was a physician were sent to the investigators; in the latter, claims for insurance benefits were the primary sources of information. In both studies these primary sources were supplemented by inquiry of hospitals or physicians caring for the patient prior to death.

Routine records of death requisite for the termination of a pension, those kept by industry, and those kept by treatment centers were the respective mechanisms of follow-up for the studies of mustard gas pensioners, dyestuffs workers, and patients with ankylosing spondylitis referred to earlier. For the last group, the routine records of the treatment centers were supplemented by a search of death certificates of the general population for matches between the cohort members and persons who had died of leukemia or aplastic anemia. Such methods are economical since they do not require location and interview of each individual cohort member.

To be efficient, the routine source of information utilized must be one that will reveal the great majority of the cases of disease or death that actually occur in the cohort. Many of these sources unfortunately do not provide data on those members of the cohort who, because of emigration, change of occupation, or other reasons, are no longer under the surveillance of the record-keeping agency. Under these circumstances it may not be clear how many cohort members actually are at risk of the outcomes under investigation, and the importance of assessing such uncertainties is obvious.

While satisfactory as a measure of the occurrence or nonoccurrence of such diseases as leukemia and lung cancer, death is often too crude an index of outcome. For example, in the Framingham, Albany, and Tecumseh studies already referred to, indices of heart disease are sought that can be obtained only by periodic clinical examination of individual cohort members. This procedure yields a great deal more information on the individuals examined than would the use of any routine records. However, it has two disadvantages:

1. The proportion of individuals examined decreases with the passing years and the membership of the cohort on which data are obtained becomes increasingly selected. The possible influence of such selection can be evaluated by comparing cohort members for whom clinical examinations were obtained with those for whom they were not, with respect to their demographic characteristics and crude criteria of outcome not requiring patient contact, by use of such sources of data as records of subsequent hospitalization or death.

2. As mentioned earlier (p. 220), there is some danger of diagnosis of outcome being influenced by exposure class. This risk might be reduced by such means as not permitting the diagnostician access to past records or by not permitting him to delay diagnostic appraisal. But it is difficult for a physician to remain ignorant of the antecedents of a patient he is examining, or for him to make a diagnosis in the absence of historical information. "Blind" readings, the use of objective biochemical tests, and other measures familiar to the designers of therapeutic trials should be used in such studies whenever possible.

## ANALYSIS

Basically, analysis of data from cohort studies involves derivation of rates of a specified outcome among the cohorts under study. These rates can be compared between various exposure groups of the same cohort or between exposed and nonexposed cohorts. Alternatively the number of cases of a disease observed in a special-exposure cohort can be compared with the number expected on the basis of general population rates, as outlined on p. 221. The requirement that the groups compared be similar with respect to age and other pertinent variables has been stressed.

*Person-Years of Observation*

A frequently used denominator for calculating rates of the specified outcome is person-years of observation. This denominator takes simultaneously into consideration the number of persons under observation and the duration of observation of each person. For example, if 10 persons remain in the study for 10 years, there are said to be 100 person-years of observation. The same figure would be derived if 100 persons were under observation for 1 year or 200 persons for 6 months. The practical consideration which makes the use of this concept a convenience is that a cohort may not retain the same strength during the whole of the period in which outcome is being measured:

1. Entrance dates may vary. For example, veterans answering Dorn's second mail questionnaire on smoking entered the cohort some 3 years after those answering the first. Patients with ankylosing spondylitis entered the British cohort at various times between 1935 and 1954.

2. During the course of the study certain individuals will drop out from the "under observation" category because of death, loss from the cohort, or other reasons.

In addition to changes in numbers under observation, changes in the age distribution of the cohort will necessarily occur as its members are followed in time. If the changes in numbers and age occur equally in the various exposure groups they might, for purposes of comparison between exposure groups, be ignored. However, an assumption that all groups will be equally affected is rarely sound. Separate calculations of rates which take into account differences due to both changing strength and age are indicated.

CALCULATION.    Data from the early years of the study of Doll and Hill, shown in Table 28, illustrate the person-years method.

Table 28

Number of men under observation at successive anniversaries of entering the study, by age, in a cohort study of British physicians*

| Age (years) at specified date | Number of men under observation on | | | | | | Person-years† |
|---|---|---|---|---|---|---|---|
| | Nov. 1, 1951 | Nov. 1, 1952 | Nov. 1, 1953 | Nov. 1, 1954 | Nov. 1, 1955 | Apr. 1, 1956 | |
| Under 35 | 10,140 | 9,145 | 8,232 | 7,389 | 6,281 | 5,779 | 35,489 |
| 35–44 | 8,886 | 9,149 | 9,287 | 9,414 | 9,710 | 9,796 | 41,211 |
| 45–54 | 7,117 | 7,257 | 7,381 | 7,351 | 7,215 | 7,191 | 32,156 |
| 55–64 | 4,094 | 4,212 | 4,375 | 4,601 | 5,057 | 5,243 | 19,909 |
| 65–74 | 2,694 | 2,754 | 2,823 | 2,873 | 2,902 | 2,928 | 12,462 |
| 75–84 | 1,382 | 1,433 | 1,457 | 1,485 | 1,483 | 1,513 | 6,431 |
| 85 and over | 181 | 200 | 223 | 256 | 278 | 296 | 1,028 |
| *All ages* | 34,494 | 34,150 | 33,778 | 33,369 | 32,926 | 32,746 | 148,686 |

* From Doll and Hill [83].
† See text for method of calculation.

No new physicians were admitted to the study cohort after the beginning date (Nov. 1, 1951); the changes in age distribution are therefore due solely to the aging of the cohort and the occurrence of deaths. The derivation of this table did not involve repeated censuses of the cohort, but was based on extrapolation from the known ages of its members in 1951 and on the data that were being routinely assembled on decedents.

The person-years of observation, shown in the last column, were derived as follows: In the age group under 35 years, there were 10,140 men alive on Nov. 1, 1951, and 9145 alive on Nov. 1, 1952. Therefore if death occurred evenly through the year, there were on average 9643 men alive during the first year of the study and these contributed 9643 person-years of observation. Similarly, during the second, third, and fourth years, respectively, there were an average of 8688, 7811, and 6835 men under observation. During the last period (5 months) the average number under observation was $6030 \times 5/12 = 2512$ person-years. The person-years of observation during the entire period was, therefore, $9643 + 8688 + 7811 + 6835 + 2512$ or a total of 35,489 person-years.

Such calculations can be made for each exposure category, and are shown for this study in Table 29. The summary rate (total) for all ages for each exposure group was derived by standardizing rates for each exposure group to the age distribution of the population of the United Kingdom in 1951.

Cohort studies do not, of course, necessarily require the use of person-years in the denominator of rates of outcome. For example, person-years are not ordinarily used when the period of risk is limited, as in studies of pregnancy for fetal defects, where attack rates can be expressed per individual without specification of time (see Chap. 5, p. 61).

*Persons Lost to Follow-Up*

In certain types of cohort study, particularly those in which follow-up information is obtained by periodic medical examination or other contact, a number of members of the cohort will be lost to trace at each follow-up examination. Such patients can no longer be considered under observation, and some adjustment of the denominator of the rate, whether it is persons or person-years, is required. The difficulty raised by persons lost to trace is that the probability of loss may be related to the exposure category, to the outcome being measured, or to both. Thus it is possible that cohort members who develop the disease under study may tend to migrate to some other geographic area for treatment, or on the other hand they may tend to move less than those not affected. Further, smokers, for example, may be more, or less, "restless" than nonsmokers. Since it is extremely difficult to detect all such possibilities that might have relevance in a particular study, the "only correct method of handling persons lost to follow-up is not to have any" [86]. However, this ideal is rarely achieved—at least in countries with high population mobility, such as the United States. Even if some persons are not lost—that is, their whereabouts are known and it is known that they are still alive—they may still be lost insofar as determination of outcome is concerned, if they have moved from the area of the study and specialized examination is required for ascertainment of outcome.

The consequences of having a proportion of persons lost to

## Table 29

Death rates from lung cancer according to smoking habits of British male physicians aged 35 and over, 1951 to 1956 *

| Age group (years) | Nonsmokers | | | Light smokers† | | | Moderate smokers† | | | Heavy smokers† | | |
|---|---|---|---|---|---|---|---|---|---|---|---|---|
| | Person-years | Number of deaths | Annual rate per 1000 | Person-years | Number of deaths | Annual rate per 1000 | Person-years | Number of deaths | Annual rate per 1000 | Person-years | Number of deaths | Annual rate per 1000 |
| 35–54 | 11,266 | 0 | 0.00 | 23,102 | 2 | 0.09 | 23,751 | 4 | 0.17 | 15,248 | 4 | 0.26 |
| 55–64 | 1,907 | 0 | 0.00 | 6,333 | 2 | 0.32 | 6,514 | 6 | 0.92 | 5,155 | 16 | 3.10 |
| 65–75 | 1,078 | 0 | 0.00 | 5,201 | 7 | 1.35 | 3,893 | 13 | 3.34 | 2,290 | 11 | 4.80 |
| 75 + | 856 | 1 | 1.17 | 3,950 | 11 | 2.78 | 1,931 | 4 | 2.07 | 722 | 3 | 4.16 |
| *Total*‡ | 15,107 | — | 0.07 | 38,586 | — | 0.47 | 36,089 | — | 0.86 | 23,415 | — | 1.66 |

* From Doll and Hill [83].

† Smoking categories: Light: 1 to 14 gm. daily. Moderate: 15 to 24 gm. daily. Heavy: 25 gm. or more daily.

‡ The rates for all ages are derived by applying the age-specific rates to the total United Kingdom population in 1951.

follow-up are similar to those of failure to obtain exposure information on some members of the entering cohort (see p. 218). In theory, the loss will affect the relative rates for exposure categories only if it is biased with respect to both exposure category and outcome. Losses to follow-up that are biased only with respect to exposure category—for example, that are heavier for smokers than for nonsmokers—should not affect the rates of the outcome if proper allowance is made for the loss in the analysis. Losses in follow-up that are biased with respect to outcome alone will affect the absolute levels of the rates of the outcome, but not their relative levels between different exposure categories. However, if the follow-up losses are at all substantial, they may produce considerable distortion of the actual risks and will be undesirable, even if the ratios of the risks in various exposure categories remain unaltered.

Ways of dealing with the problem of losses to follow-up in the analysis depend on the method of obtaining the outcome information:

1. When follow-up depends on a regularly scheduled examination and ascertainment of the outcome depends on detecting a change in status between one examination and the next, the most accurate procedure is to assume that persons lost to trace between two examinations were lost immediately after the first examination. The denominator will then be the number of persons actually examined on each occasion (or the number of person-years experienced between two examinations by persons having the second). The reasoning behind this procedure is that persons lost between the two examinations cannot figure in the numerator of the rate and should therefore not be included in the denominator.

2. When follow-up depends on a certain event occurring between two dates and ascertainment of the events takes place at the time of their occurrence (as, for example, when deaths are being ascertained through some reporting system), a number of alternatives are possible:

a. If the exact date at which the person leaves the cohort is known, an adjustment can be made for the length of time he was under observation.

b. If it is known only that a person disappeared at some time between the two dates, it can be assumed that he was under observation for half the period between the two dates.

c. Two denominators can be calculated, one based on the assumption that all persons were lost immediately after the last date they were known to be present, and one based on the assumption that they were all lost immediately prior to the first date on which they were known to be absent. The correct rate must lie somewhere between the rates based on the two assumptions.

By use of one or the other of these methods, it is usually possible to evaluate the effect of follow-up losses in the various exposure groups. However, the problem resulting from the possibility that loss to follow-up is biased with respect to both exposure category and outcome remains. It may be possible to make two assumptions: first, none of the persons lost to trace developed the specific outcome, and second, all the persons lost to trace developed the specific outcome. This yields an estimate of the range of rates possible in each exposure category. Unfortunately, this procedure is useful only in studies in which the proportion lost to trace is small and the frequency of specified outcome is very high—for example, in studies of case fatality in severe diseases. In most epidemiologic studies the frequency of the outcome measured is commonly smaller than the proportion of persons lost to trace, and the range between the estimates of outcome frequency will be too large to be of practical value.

### Relative and Attributable Risk

There are two commonly used measures of the association between exposure to a particular factor and risk of a certain outcome.

RELATIVE RISK. Relative risk is the ratio of the rate of the disease (usually incidence or mortality) among those exposed to the rate among those not exposed. The death rates shown in Table 30 correspond to the total rates in each exposure category in Table 29, except that the exposure categories are based only on number of cigarettes smoked—other forms of tobacco being

## Table 30

Death rates from lung cancer attributable to cigarette
smoking, British male physicians, 1951 to 1961*

| Cigarettes smoked per day (in 1951) | Annual death rate per 1000 | Attributable annual death rate† per 1000 |
|---|---|---|
| None | 0.07 | 0 |
| 1–14 | 0.57 | 0.50 |
| 15–24 | 1.39 | 1.32 |
| 25 + | 2.27 | 2.20 |
| *Total* | 0.65 | 0.58 |

* From Doll and Hill [84].
† Death rate in the particular smoking category minus the death rate in non-smokers.

ignored—and data for a 10-year period of follow-up are used. On the basis of these rates it is seen that the risk of death from lung cancer was 32 times as great for heavy smokers as for nonsmokers (2.27/0.07). Comparing these two categories, the relative risk is therefore 32.

ATTRIBUTABLE RISK. Attributable risk is the rate of the disease in exposed individuals that can be attributed to the exposure. This measure is derived by subtracting the rate (usually incidence or mortality) of the disease among nonexposed persons from the corresponding rate among exposed individuals. It is assumed that causes of the disease other than the one under examination had equal effect on the exposed and nonexposed groups. For example, the rates in Table 30 indicate that heavy smoking is associated with a risk of death from lung cancer of 2.20 (2.27 minus 0.07) per 1000 per year; this accounts for 97 percent of the total risk of death from lung cancer experienced by heavy cigarette smokers in this particular population.

Similarly an estimate can be derived of the impact that a specified exposure may have on the total population with respect to a particular outcome. For example, the lung cancer death rate for nonsmokers (0.07) may be subtracted from the lung cancer death rate in the total population (0.65); the result obtained might be termed the *population attributable risk* of lung cancer resulting from cigarette smoking. If this estimate is to be applied to some other population, it must obviously be one similar in exposure frequency to that from which the estimate was derived. The concept of population attributable risk is useful in that it provides an estimate of the amount by which a particular disease rate might be reduced if the specified exposure were removed. On the basis of the data in Table 30, one might expect that 89 percent ($[0.58/0.65] \times 100$) of deaths from lung cancer among male British physicians could be avoided if the factor of cigarette smoking were eliminated.

## Synergistic Effects

If the exposure investigated in a cohort study is found to be associated with increased risk of a particular outcome, it is of practical importance to determine whether the risk associated with this particular exposure is simply additive to that associated with any other known causes of the disease or whether individuals exposed to more than one cause experience a risk greater than the sum of the risks of those exposed to either cause alone. For example, in a study of asbestos workers [359] it was, of course, considered necessary to take account of the smoking habits of the exposed cohort in evaluating their lung cancer risk. It was found that the smoking habits of the group were not sufficiently different from those of the general population to account for any substantial part of their excess lung cancer risk. However, the risk among exposed individuals who were smokers was found to be much greater than the sum of the risks associated with asbestos and cigarette smoking alone. Thus the relative risk of lung cancer in smokers compared to nonsmokers is about 10; the relative risk associated with 20 years' exposure to asbestos dust was found to be of the same order of magnitude; but asbestos workers who smoked were estimated to have 92 times the risk of dying of bronchogenic carcinoma as men who neither smoked nor worked with asbestos. A similar synergism between cigarette smoking and another carcinogenic agent in the causation of lung cancer has been demonstrated in the study of U.S. uranium miners [209].

Opportunities for studies of such interactions between multiple known causes of the same disease have so far been few. However, they are of considerable theoretical interest and, if found, may offer guidelines for the selection and/or counseling of individuals exposed to one or the other of the toxic agents.

## INTERPRETATION

Interpretation of the results of a cohort study will generally center on two problems: (1) evaluation of the extent to which methodologic difficulties contribute to differences (or lack of differences) in outcome rates between exposure categories, and (2) whether observed differences in outcome between exposure categories are likely to reflect causal relationships between the exposure and the outcome under investigation. Considerations relevant to the first problem have been touched on throughout this chapter, and those relating to the second were dealt with in Chapter 2. Only two particular aspects will be elaborated on here.

### Dose-Response Relationship

As noted in Chapter 2 (p. 21), the existence of a dose-response relationship—that is, an increase in disease risk with increase in amount of exposure—supports the view that an association is a causal one. The strikingly consistent increase in risk of lung cancer with increase in cigarette consumption, illustrated in Figure 31, has played a major role in acceptance of this relationship as causal [333, 349].

The relationship between lung cancer risk and accumulated radiation exposure in U.S. uranium miners is illustrated in Figure 32. Again, the fact that in the higher exposure categories the risk increases with the level of exposure argues in favor of the relationship being causal. On the other hand, the fact that in the lowest three categories the relationship is not regular has been interpreted as evidence that doses of the orders received by the men in these categories do not increase their lung cancer risk and that some other component of the mining experience is responsible for the excess of observed over expected cases among them. If indeed one were confident that there was no dose-response relationship at these levels of dose, then that would in-

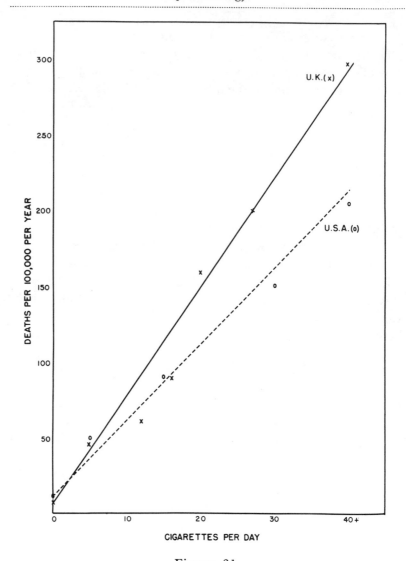

Figure 31

Mortality among males from lung cancer related to cigarette smoking habits. (Data for United Kingdom from Doll and Hill [84]; for United States from Hammond [149].)

deed be an argument against the relationship being causal at low dose levels. In this particular instance, however, it seems more likely that the irregularity of the relationship in the lower exposure categories results from the relatively small numbers of

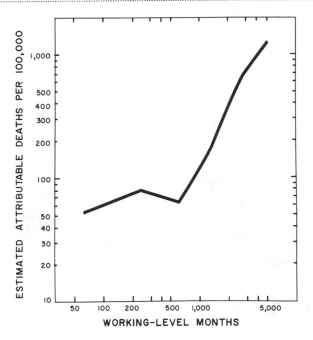

Figure 32

Average annual death rate from lung cancer among U.S. uranium miners estimated as attributable to radon exposure in working-level months. (Estimated from data of Lundin et al. [209].)

men in the individual categories and from uncertainties in the dose estimates at these levels [268].

*Inferences from Different Measures of Risk*

In interpreting the findings of cohort studies, one may find that measures of relative and attributable risk give different impressions as to the importance of a particular exposure. If several factors that are etiologically significant in the same disease are being compared, the same order of importance of the factors will be suggested whether relative or attributable risk is examined. However, when the significance of the same exposure is assessed for several different manifestional entities, this may not be the case. For example, data from Doll and Hill's study (shown in Table 31) indicate that the relative risk from heavy cigarette smoking is far greater for lung cancer and chronic bronchitis than for deaths from other causes, but the attributable death

## Table 31
Relative and attributable risks of death from selected causes associated with heavy cigarette smoking by British male physicians, 1951 to 1961*

| Cause of death | Death rate† among nonsmokers | Death rate† among heavy smokers‡ | Relative risk | Attributable death rate† |
|---|---|---|---|---|
| Lung cancer | 0.07 | 2.27 | 32.4 | 2.20 |
| Other cancers | 1.91 | 2.59 | 1.4 | 0.68 |
| Chronic bronchitis | 0.05 | 1.06 | 21.2 | 1.01 |
| Cardiovascular disease | 7.32 | 9.93 | 1.4 | 2.61 |
| *All causes* | 12.06 | 19.67 | 1.6 | 7.61 |

* From Doll and Hill [84].
† Annual death rates per 1000.
‡ Heavy smokers are defined as smokers of 25 or more cigarettes per day.

rate is greater for cardiovascular disease than for lung cancer. Each of these observations contributes to the evaluation of the findings:

1. The size of the relative risk is a better index than is the attributable risk of the likelihood that a causal relationship exists between the exposure and the disease involved. Thus a difference of 10 per thousand (attributable risk) noted between two exposure categories would be less likely to be an error of measurement if it occurred between rates of 1 and 11 than between rates of 110 and 120. It would take less bias to raise a rate from 110 to 120 than to raise it from 1 to 11, just as it is easier to make an error of 1 inch in measuring a mile than in measuring a foot. Furthermore, the likelihood that an association between two variables results from association of both with a third variable would appear to decrease as relative risk increases, since the higher the relative risk the stronger—and therefore, presumably, more obvious—must be the association between each of the variables and the third variable. Thus, in the present example, on the basis of the evidence in Table 31 alone, one would be inclined to accept the associations with cigarette smoking as evidence of a causal relationship more readily for lung cancer and for chronic bronchitis than for cardiovascular disease.

2. On the other hand, if it is accepted that the observed association is a causal one, then the attributable risk gives a better idea than does the relative risk of the impact that a successful preventive program might have. In the present example, if the associations of cigarette smoking with lung cancer and with cardiovascular disease are both causal in nature, then elimination of cigarette smoking would prevent even more deaths from cardiovascular disease than from lung cancer.

# 12

---

## Case-Control Studies

A case-control study is an inquiry in which groups of individuals are selected in terms of whether they do (the cases) or do not (the controls) have the disease of which the etiology is to be studied, and the groups are then compared with respect to existing or past characteristics judged to be of possible relevance to the etiology of the disease. Such studies might be described more accurately as *case-comparison group* studies, since they do not incorporate the kind of "control" that may be obtainable over compared groups in experimental situations. However, the term *case-control* is in common use and at least has the advantage of brevity, particularly when referring to the individuals constituting the noncase or comparison group, the "controls."

Commonly, in a case-control study, a specific hypothesis is being tested—for example, that a connection exists between lung cancer and prior cigarette smoking habits, or between congenital malformation and maternal rubella during pregnancy. Sometimes, in the absence of a specific hypothesis, this type of study is used to explore the totality of the backgrounds of affected and unaffected persons (to the extent that this can be defined and measured).

### SELECTION OF CASES

In assembling a group of cases for study, consideration must be given to the diagnostic criteria for definition of the disease, to the source of the cases, and to the question of inclusion of incident or prevalent cases.

## Diagnostic Criteria

An important issue in defining manifestational criteria for inclusion and exclusion of potential study cases is whether or not to include cases manifesting criteria currently considered as possible variants of the disease entity under investigation. The criteria must be specific to each investigation and few generalizations are possible. Criteria which provide clear and reproducible applications of definition are obviously desirable, and decisions which tend to provide manifestationally more homogeneous groups of cases are usually preferable. If time and funds are available, establishment of a number of groups of cases based on variously defined criteria is a happy compromise, providing the possibility of separate examination of cases defined by each group of criteria. Depending on whether strong associations with the suspected cause are found, such groupings will assist in judging whether or not certain clinical syndromes should or should not be regarded as part of the disease under investigation.

## Source of Cases

Series of affected individuals in a case-control study commonly include either:

1. All persons with the disease seen at a particular medical care facility or group of facilities in a specified period of time, or,
2. All persons with the disease found in a more general population, such as that of a city or county, at a point or in a period of time.

The first procedure is the more common, since it is relatively easy and inexpensive to carry out. The second procedure, although more laborious because it involves special efforts to locate and obtain the necessary data from all affected individuals in the chosen population, is generally more satisfactory because (a) it avoids the bias arising from the selective factors that guide affected individuals to a particular medical care facility or physician, and (b) it allows computation of rates of the disease in the total population and in subgroups related to the etiologic factors under examination.

In certain situations the advantages of both types of procedure may be obtained. For example, when a defined population is served by a single medical facility or by a group of facilities sharing common record-keeping procedures—such as the population of a prepaid medical care plan—all cases may be readily identifiable and yet still related to the source population of which the size, age, sex, and other demographic characteristics are known. The population need not, of course, be defined in geographic terms. Closed populations, such as those of schools, military establishments, and certain places of work, may offer the same advantages if they are large enough. In the investigation of congenital defects or of disorders of parturition, the related population will then be a certain number of deliveries, and the births occurring in a certain hospital or combination of hospitals may provide all the cases occurring in what, for the purpose of computation of rates, may be regarded as an appropriate population.

## Incident or Prevalent Cases?

Whether the cases have come from selected facilities or from a defined population, it is preferable that they be limited to those who were newly diagnosed within a specified period. Although the inclusion of all cases existent during the period may, in a chronic disease, greatly increase the number of cases available for study, the inclusion of cases at a variety of stages in the disease process and patients undergoing recurrences will complicate the interpretation of the findings. In patients in advanced stages of the disease it may be difficult to differentiate past events causally related to the disease from those consequent to it (as, for example, in a study of the x-ray exposure of patients with chronic leukemia it may be unclear whether x-ray exposures reported by the patient were given for diagnosis of early symptoms of the disease, or even for therapeutic purposes, when the patient himself may have been unaware that he already had the disease). In addition, in studies of prevalent cases, even if the exposures clearly antedated the onset of the present disease, it may not be possible to determine to what extent a particular characteristic noted in excess in the cases has relevance to the duration and course rather than to the etiology of the disease.

## SELECTION OF CONTROLS

Controls are needed in a case-control study to allow evaluation of whether the frequency or level of a characteristic or past exposure among the cases is different from that among comparable persons in the source population who do not have the disease under investigation. The many decisions to be made in the selection of a control group for a particular group of cases involve several kinds of consideration:

1. Assurance that information on study factors can be obtained from the control group in a manner similar to that by which it was obtained from the cases. This includes consideration of the fact that a difference in response rates between cases and controls may raise serious questions about the comparability of the information given by the two groups.

2. Whether or not deliberately to select (match) the controls in such a way as to make them similar to the cases with respect to certain confounding variables. The latter are variables that may introduce differences between cases and controls which do not reflect differences in the variables of primary interest (study variables). For example, cases of breast cancer and controls may be compared with respect to frequency or duration of lactation, to test the hypothesis—suggested by the decrease in risk of breast cancer observed with increase in parity—that lactation protects against the disease. It will obviously be necessary to take account of the low parity of the breast cancer cases—otherwise a low frequency of lactation will be observed in them solely as a consequence of their low parity. To demonstrate that infrequent lactation is the explanation of the low parity of breast cancer cases, it will be necessary to show a difference between cases and controls of the same parity. This may be attempted either in the analysis—by comparing women in the same parity level—or in the selection of controls—by selecting controls who have the same distribution by parity as the cases.

3. The desirability that the controls derive from a population generally similar to that which gave rise to the cases. In addition to the known tangible factors that may introduce spurious differences, as noted in paragraph 2 above, one must also be aware of the possible operation of factors that are intangible or currently unknown. These may be partially dealt with by assuring "general" similarity (with respect, for example, to place of residence, ethnic group, and socioeconomic status) between the cases and controls.

4. Practical and economic considerations. Certain sources of controls are more easily and cheaply accessible than others. In addition, once a particular source has been decided on, the question of how many controls to select from that source, and how they will be selected, must be faced. The greatest amount of information would be obtained if data were obtained for all possible controls in the selected source, but economic considerations usually force compromise between what is desirable and what is feasible.

In discussing the sources and methods of selection of control groups that have been frequently used in the past, reference will be made to these kinds of consideration. We must stress, however, that the weighing of the many separate aspects of these broad questions to arrive at specific decisions in a particular study is one of the most difficult processes in epidemiologic research. The decisions are also usually the ones most critical to the establishment of confidence in the results of case-control studies.

*Sources of Control Groups*

Before selecting individual controls, it is necessary to decide on the general source (in statistical terms, the *sampling frame*) from which they will be selected. An important consideration is whether or not the cases represent all the affected individuals in a defined general population. If they do, then the control group should also be drawn from that population. They either should be representative of the population or the ways in which they are unrepresentative should be known—either because they have been deliberately introduced (for example, by matching) or because they follow from the specific method of selection from the population. If the cases are selected because they attended a particular hospital or physician, then it is preferable to find a source of controls that shares as far as possible those selective processes by which the cases came to attention—for example, persons who, if they had the disease under investigation, would also be likely to attend the same hospitals. Four common sampling frames will be considered.

POPULATION OF AN ADMINISTRATIVE AREA. This is an appropriate source only when the cases represent all, or the great majority of, cases occurring in the same area. When this situation exists, this source is in theory one that can be sampled with assurance that it represents the same source population that gave rise to the patients. However, it also poses certain difficulties. If the information of interest must be obtained from the persons themselves, nonresponse rates are nearly always appreciably higher in randomly selected members of the population than in cases under medical care. In addition, the usual concerns regarding differences in quality of information provided by cases and controls will be reinforced if the circumstances of the interview are different—for example, if cases are interviewed in hospital and controls must be interviewed at home. Further, selection and interview of a sample of the population are generally more expensive and time-consuming than use of other potential sources of control groups.

HOSPITAL PATIENTS. Other patients in or attending the same hospitals as the cases may be used as a source of controls. One rationale behind this choice is that patients with other diseases are subject to the same selective factors that influenced the cases to come to this particular hospital. For example, if the cases in the study are taken from a hospital located in an area inhabited by a particular ethnic group, a control group drawn from other patients attending the same hospital is likely to have the same ethnic distribution as the study group.

On the other hand, this source of controls may be used simply for practical reasons. For example, in a recent collaborative case-control study of breast cancer [224] the cases represented all the identified cases of breast cancer in certain geographically defined areas. However, in several of these areas the population rosters, maps, or other facilities necessary for population sampling were not readily available, and, because of practical and economic restrictions, other hospital patients provided the only source of controls that could be utilized in all the collaborating centers.

Even when all cases in a defined population are to be studied and facilities for population sampling are available, the question whether healthy members of the population are a preferable source of controls to hospital patients is by no means clear-cut. The major disadvantage of hospital controls is, of course, that they are ill, and may therefore be unrepresentative of the population as a whole with respect to factors, such as cigarette smoking or socioeconomic status, that are associated with illness in general. On the other hand, response rates and quality of information will, as noted above, be more comparable if both cases and controls are interviewed in hospital than if they are interviewed under different circumstances. For any particular study these advantages and disadvantages must be weighed in the light of the nature of the cases, their source, and the type of information to be collected. Unfortunately, methodologic studies to provide guidelines for arriving at the most favorable choices are still inadequate.

If a decision to use hospital controls is made, it must be realized that the factors leading a patient to come to a particular hospital are not the same for all diseases. For example, if a hospital has a wide reputation for the treatment of a particular disease, it might be a fruitful source of cases for a case-control study of that disease. But it might be unjustified to compare its patients with this disease with its other patients, since the patients with the specific disease are likely to be drawn from a wider geographic area and perhaps from a generally higher economic group than those with other diseases. Similarly the temptation to use patients who have no known disease but are seen at the hospital—for example, healthy patients attending a screening or cancer detection clinic—should be avoided. Such persons are usually markedly different—in regard to socioeconomic status, ethnic background, and other relevant factors—from patients who come to the same hospital because of illness.

The question will arise whether a control group should be drawn from all patients attending the hospital or only from patients with certain groups of diseases that are believed not to be influenced by the factors being studied. For example, should the smoking habits of a series of patients with lung cancer be compared with those of a sample of all patients in the same hospital or with those of a particular diagnostic group, such as accident cases? The appeal of the second course is that, if there are diseases other than lung cancer that are influenced by smoking, the all-patients-in-the-hospital group will be unrepresentative of the healthy population with respect to smoking, and a difference between lung cancer patients and other patients may reflect the effect of smoking on diseases other than lung cancer. On the other hand, if a diagnostic group can be identified that is known not to be influenced by smoking, then the control group having that diagnosis can be assumed to represent the general population in this respect, and a difference between the lung cancer patients and the group can be presumed to be a true reflection of the influence of smoking on lung cancer. The practical disadvantage of this course is the difficulty of identifying a diagnostic group that is known to be representative of the general population with respect to any particular factor. Consequently, if a difference is found in a situation where the controls were drawn from a single diagnostic category, it is difficult to decide with confidence whether it is the cases or the controls that differ from the general population.

On the whole, a control group drawn from all patients is probably preferable to one drawn from a single diagnostic category. Since the interpretation of differences between cases and controls depends to a large extent on the "reasonableness" of different explanations, it may be desirable to use several control groups, drawn from patients with different diagnoses, and to examine the patterns that appear. For example, patients with cancer of the breast may be compared with patients with cancer of the reproductive system, with patients with cancer of the digestive system, with patients with noncancerous lesions of the breast, with accident victims, and with other patients. If the breast cancer patients differed from *all* the other groups in respect to some study factor, the evidence is strengthened that it is in fact the breast cancer patients whose experience is unusual.

RELATIVES OF THE CASES. Two types of relative are commonly used as sources of controls—spouses and siblings. Both these groups are generally similar in ethnic and social background to the cases. This will usually be an advantage since it will eliminate certain spurious associations. However, if the study factor itself is one in which close relatives are likely to be similar—for example, diet, smoking history, or genetic background—they will not constitute a suitable control group.

The use of spouses is satisfactory only if there are approximately equal numbers of male and female cases available for study, so that comparisons can be made of males with males and females with females. The age range of the cases must also be such that the number of cases with living spouses is adequate.

When siblings are used as the source of controls, it is necessary to select from among the available siblings on a one patient : one-sibling basis. The mistake is occasionally made of comparing a series of patients with all their available siblings. This procedure leads to bias in that the controls will be heavily weighted with the members of large families and will show to an excessive degree (by comparison with the cases) any of the multitude of characteristics that are related to large family size. For the same reason, patients for whom no control sibling is available must be excluded; otherwise the cases, in comparison to controls, will be weighted with one-child families. The feasibility of using sibling controls will depend on the average family size, population mobility, the sources of the information to be assembled, and other factors that will determine whether or not a sibling control will be available for an adequate proportion of the cases.

ASSOCIATES OF THE CASES. Members of the population may be selected on the basis of having shared with the cases attendance at the same school, similar place of employment, or residence in the same neighborhood. This type of control group combines the advantages of comprising healthy individuals for the most part and at the same time providing a large pool from which individuals with specific characteristics can be selected if necessary. A disadvantage of the method is the large amount of field work that may be involved in identification of the controls. In addition, the difficulties relating to differences in rates of nonresponse and quality of information that were referred to earlier (p. 244) also apply here.

## Selection of Individual Controls

Having selected the source from which the controls will be drawn, it is necessary to decide whether the data for the cases will be compared with data on all the individuals who might be available from the chosen source, or whether a sample will be selected. If a sample is decided on, a choice must be made between the various sampling procedures available—the most common of these are random, systematic, and paired sampling. It is said that the selection of the source of a control group is more important than the method of sampling individuals from that source [58]. Although this may be true, it is also true that, however satisfactory its source, the usefulness of a control group can be seriously impaired by unsatisfactory sampling.

TOTAL POPULATION—NO SAMPLING. When the population from which the cases were drawn can be defined and is chosen as the source of a control group, it may be possible to use data on the total population. Clearly this is practical only when data on the frequency of the factors under examination are recorded routinely for the total population.

For example, in studies of diseases of early life—or of diseases of later life in which influences operative in early life may be suspected—it may be possible to obtain, for all the cases in a defined geographic population, information on such variables as birth weight, parity, and age of parents. The information may be compared with data for the same variables routinely published in vital statistics for all births in the same area [226]. Computer storage of information from medical histories—as is now being undertaken on populations in certain prepaid medical care plans—may increase the opportunities for studies of this kind.

However, routine medical histories are not completed with

sufficient consistency, nor, generally speaking, is the information sufficiently accessible, to be used in most kinds of case-control study. Some form of sampling, coupled with special inquiry into historical facts, is usually required when hospital patients form the control group. Similarly, the kinds of detailed historical information usually required in case-control studies is rarely available for general populations.

RANDOM AND SYSTEMATIC SAMPLING. A random sample is one which was drawn in such a way that each member of the total group to be sampled had an equal chance of being represented; for example, each individual may be numbered and the persons for study picked from a table of random numbers. A systematic sample is one in which the group to be sampled is placed in some sort of order and then individuals are selected systematically throughout the series, for example, every second, hundredth, or thousandth individual. Provided the order in which the group is placed prior to systematic sampling is not highly structured with respect to some variable directly or indirectly important to the study, the characteristics of a systematic sample are similar to those of a random sample, and similar tests of statistical significance may be applied. The distinction between these two methods is therefore not of great importance in most situations, and the choice of one or the other method depends primarily on the practicability of each in a given situation.

Random or systematic samples are often used in the selection of controls when a listing of all the potential controls is available. For example, in the instance of the population of births in a maternity hospital, a listing of all births in the hospital may be available. Similarly, population registers may facilitate the drawing of a random sample of the population of a geographic area. However, information on patients in or attending a general hospital is rarely adequate for random or systematic sampling, and paired samples are usually preferred if hospital patients are the source of controls.

To obtain a representative sample, the procedures for random or systematic sampling must be followed explicitly and carefully. No confidence can be placed in a sample that is selected haphazardly. Bias resulting from haphazard selection is frequent and has been discussed by many writers [231, 414]. For example, haphazard selection from lists of names may be influenced by the length of the name (related to ethnicity), its position on the page, or the legibility of the handwriting (possibly related to hospital service and hence to diagnosis). Haphazard selection from files of cards or records may select those which are thicker or more worn and hence of greater medical interest.

PAIRED SAMPLING. To select a random sample, the total population to be sampled must be defined and, at least in theory, enumerated. This is not always possible. For example, if the controls are to be drawn from persons living in the same neighborhoods as the patients, how far do these neighborhoods extend? Similarly, if the sample is to be drawn from other patients attending the same hospital as the cases, it may not be desirable to wait until the total number of such patients is known before beginning to assemble the sample. In these situations, paired sampling is usually undertaken. This involves the selection from the sampling frame of one or more controls for each case. Individuals are selected by virtue of some defined temporal or geographic relationship to the case—for example, the next patient (or next two patients, etc.) admitted after the case, the person living in the nearest residence to that of the case, the student next to the case in an alphabetical class listing, and so on.

Once again it is important that the selection not be haphazard; the rules for selection must be clearly defined and adhered to. For example, in the selection of a neighborhood paired sample it will be necessary to specify whether the interviewer goes to the right or the left of the patient's house, what the procedure is in the case of two-family and apartment houses, and so on. The fact that nobody is at home at the time the interviewer calls is not an adequate reason for rejection of the selected control, since the probability of all members of a family being away from home at any moment is highly correlated with family size and other demographic characteristics. Once an individual has been selected, the use of alternate selectees in place of the individual first selected always raises the question of whether the omission of the difficult-to-locate group biases the sample.

*Matching*

Earlier in this chapter (p. 244) it was noted that one way to eliminate the effects of variables that may confound the analysis of study variables is to select the controls in such a way that the control group has the same distribution as the cases with respect to certain confounding variables. The procedures for doing this are known as matching.

FREQUENCY MATCHING. In frequency matching the group to be sampled is divided into subgroups according to the chosen variables, and different proportions—corresponding to the distribution in the case series—are selected from each subgroup. For example, if the cases contain four times as many males as females, four times as many individuals would be selected from the male subgroups of the control population as from the female. The use of frequency matching (or stratification) in case-control studies has some considerable disadvantages. In the first place, because of lack of the necessary information, it is often very difficult to subdivide the population to be sampled. Secondly, the necessity to know the final composition of the patient series means that the controls cannot be assembled until after the case series is complete. This may mean that all the controls would be interviewed after the cases were interviewed, which could be undesirable. For these reasons, frequency matching is rarely used in case-control studies.

INDIVIDUAL MATCHING. When it is decided to select a control group with some of the characteristics of the patient series, it is usually preferable to use the method of paired sampling as described above, with the additional requirement that the individuals selected from the control population must match the corresponding case with respect to specified criteria. The selected control would then be, for example, not necessarily the next person admitted to the hospital but the next person admitted who satisfied the defined criteria.

In considering whether to use a matched control sample and what variables, if any, should be used in the matching process, it must be borne in mind that, while more often helpful, matching can also be harmful in some circumstances [252]. It should not, therefore, be introduced without a definite reason. The following factors must be considered:

1. Certain confounding variables *must* be taken account of; these are variables that are known to be associated with both the disease under investigation (e.g., breast cancer) and the study variable (e.g., lactation). Such a variable, in this instance, is parity; another would be socioeconomic status. The existence of such variables does not, however, necessitate matching if the decision is to take them into account in the analysis.

2. The more unusual the distribution of cases with respect to a particular confounding variable, the less overlap there will be in unmatched groups, and the less efficient will be the approach of controlling confounding factors only in the analysis. To take an extreme example, there would be rather little overlap in age distribution between a series of stroke cases and an unmatched sample of all hospital patients. The controls under 50 years of age would be wasted, in the sense that there would be no cases to compare them with, and there would be too few controls over 70 years of age for efficient comparison with the many cases in that age group. An unusual distribution of cases with respect to a relevant variable—the most extreme example being perhaps a disease limited to one sex—would therefore argue in favor of matching in control selection.

3. The cost of obtaining the study information must be considered. If this is small, it may be preferable to select multiple controls for each case and take account of differences in confounding variables in the analysis. The selection of more controls than cases helps insure that there will be controls for cases at all relevant levels of the confounding variables, so that adequate comparisons can be made. On the other hand, if the cost of obtaining the study information is high, and an unlimited number of cases is available, the greatest efficiency will be achieved by having equal numbers of cases and controls. In this case, matching will assure comparable distributions with respect to confounding variables.

4. The effects of variables that have been matched obviously cannot be evaluated. Whether or not to match will therefore

depend to some extent on the state of knowledge of the disease. As noted at the beginning of this chapter, case-control studies are sometimes undertaken without specific hypotheses in mind. Even in such studies, the relationship of the disease to such variables as age and sex will usually be known from descriptive data, and these variables have relationships to such a broad spectrum of traits and exposures that it may be wise to match on them. However, more specific matching will generally not be indicated.

If it is decided to match on a particular variable, it is also necessary to specify how close the match must be. For example, must age match within 1 year or 20 years? The decision will be based largely on matters of practicability. If a large sampling frame is available, quite narrow limits may be specified and close similarity with respect to the matched variable may be achieved. However, criteria that are difficult to satisfy lead to added expense and loss of study material, since cases that cannot be matched must be excluded.

Similar considerations relate to the over-all matching plan for a particular study—if too many matching criteria are specified, the assembly of the control series may become inordinately cumbersome, and many unmatched cases may have to be excluded. Three variables that influence the incidence of all diseases and to which a wide variety of events in an individual's background are related are age, sex, and race. If matching is attempted, it should usually include these variables; beyond these, the matching process becomes more difficult with each additional variable, and each one added to the criteria requires justification. It should also be noted that certain selection schemes force a certain amount of indirect matching, even if no attempt is made expressly to match individuals. For example, as noted earlier, the use of other patients in the same hospital may introduce various similarities, depending on the peculiarities of local responsibilities for, and use of, medical care facilities.

One other type of matching should be mentioned. Sometimes, it is necessary to select one control from a limited number of available persons—for example, siblings. The selection of one individual may then be made in terms of an important variable.

For example, if a patient has several siblings, the one nearest in age might be selected, without specification that the patient and the selected sibling must match within so many years of age. While this process tends to reduce dissimilarities between the cases and controls, the groups will not be completely matched, and it may also be necessary to take account of differences in the analysis.

OVERMATCHING. Matching can occasionally be harmful; there are two particular situations in which it is to be avoided if possible. First, variables intermediate in the causal pathway between the study factor and the disease should not be matched. For example, if smoking altered blood cholesterol which in turn was causally associated with cardiovascular disease, smoking would be considered a cause of cardiovascular disease. Yet, in a case-control study, if cases and controls were matched on cholesterol levels, no association of the disease with smoking would emerge. Second, factors should not be matched that are related to the suspected cause but not to the disease. For example, if contraceptive use (the exposure) were related to religion but religion were not related to the disease under study, it would be inappropriate to match on religion. The consequence of matching in this situation would be a loss of statistical efficiency of the study, although the relative risk estimate would not be changed [252]. It is, of course, not always clear whether a factor that is known to be strongly associated with the exposure of interest is also related to the disease. In such a circumstance, the decision to match may be made on the basis that the risk of loss of statistical efficiency (if the factor turns out not to be related to the disease) is more acceptable than the risk of introducing spurious associations (if the factor is indeed related to the disease).

## INFORMATION ON EXPOSURE

### Sources

The most common sources of information on the past experiences and characteristics whose etiologic relevance is examined in case-control studies are interviews with the patient or, in the case of diseases of children, with the parents. Other sources include interviews with relatives, hospital records, birth certificates, employment records, and so on.

Two characteristics of the information on exposure are important—its comparability in cases and controls, and its validity.

*Comparability*

If data are inaccurate or incomplete, spurious differences may be introduced between cases and controls only if the inaccuracy or incompleteness affects the two groups to a different degree. Thus, if only a fraction of the relevant events is reported—for example, if only half the women who took a particular drug in early pregnancy can remember doing so—but this proportion is the same in both the cases and the controls, there will, if there is a true difference, still be a difference between cases and controls in the frequency of women reporting taking the drug. If there is no true difference, no apparent difference will emerge (see p. 263). However, if, say, half the cases and only a quarter of the controls have the recollection of taking the drug, an erroneous conclusion will be reached. If there was no true difference, one will appear, and if there was a difference in favor of the cases, it will be exaggerated. Conceivably, also, a higher frequency of taking the drug among the controls could be hidden. For these reasons, lack of comparability between the accuracy or completeness of information in cases and controls is one of the most serious criticisms that can be levelled against a case-control study.

AVOIDANCE OF BIAS.   While it may be possible to determine that differences in accuracy or completeness of information exist between groups that are to be compared, it is rarely possible to evaluate the extent of such differences and to take account of them adequately in the comparison. Therefore, every effort must be made to achieve comparability during the process of assembling the data. There are two basic considerations:

1. Achieving similarity in the procedures used to obtain information from cases and controls. To the extent possible, staff engaged in abstracting information from records should be una-

ware whether they are dealing with a case or a control. If the information to be obtained is of a medical or personal nature, it is unusual that an interview can be conducted without the interviewer becoming aware of the general state of health of the person being interviewed, but it may sometimes be possible to arrange that the interviewer does not know whether he is interviewing a case or a control. So far as possible, the place and circumstances of the interview should be similar. A given interviewer should interview equal proportions of cases and controls. As much effort should be made to gain cooperation and accurate response from controls as from cases.

2. Use of information recorded prior to the time of diagnosis of the present illness, wherever possible. For example, in a comparison of the birth weights of mentally defective children and controls, birth certificates or hospital records would be superior to the mothers' memories as sources of information on birth weight, not only because of the ordinary deficiencies of human memory, but also because the hospital records were made prior to the identification of the child as mentally defective. While there is no more prolific source of data relative to a person's past experience than his own memory, this source suffers not only from people's propensity to forget or distort past events but, most important in the present context, from the fact that such losses and distortions are affected by subsequent events. For example, the fact that she, or her child, currently has a serious illness may alter a woman's recollection of the events that preceded the illness. In using data from interviews in which the case has a serious illness and the control does not, only factors of a highly objective nature can be compared with confidence. Even if information on the study factors of greatest interest can be obtained only by interview, such information as is recorded should also be assembled and evaluated.

EVIDENCE OF COMPARABILITY. Certain analytic procedures can be undertaken to evaluate to what extent a particular result could be explained by lack of comparability between cases and controls. Although one can never prove that two series are truly comparable, the greater the number and relevancy of the tests that can be applied without revealing lack of comparability, the greater will be the confidence in the belief that it is present in sufficient degree for the current purpose.

First, certain analyses can be conducted to determine whether the procedures planned to assure comparability in the data collection have indeed been carried out. There is no more revealing evidence of lack of comparability between two series than a substantial difference in the proportions of individuals for whom data were not obtained (nonresponse rates). In the case of interview data, times of beginning and ending of interviews can be recorded and the durations compared for evidence of greater interest on the part of the interviewers in one group than in the other. Interviewers, at the end of the interview, can be asked to classify each respondent with respect to level of reliability of his responses; the distributions should usually be similar for cases and controls.

Second, cases and controls can be compared with respect to frequency of reporting (or other ascertainment) of experiences or characteristics that seem unlikely to be relevant to the etiology of the disease under investigation. Such factors are sometimes referred to as dummy variables. It is, of course, difficult to be sure that a particular characteristic does not have etiologic relevance. For example, in the first study in which a high frequency of prenatal exposure to x-rays was observed among children with cancer, a higher rate of maternal x-ray exposure in the cases than in the controls was noted *prior to,* as well as *during,* the relevant pregnancy [384]. If the higher frequency of x-rays reported prior to the pregnancy was used as an index of the extent of bias introduced by more complete reporting on the part of the case mothers, and this index applied to the reports of x-rays during pregnancy, the excess frequency of x-rays reported during the relevant pregnancy was reduced but not eliminated. However, subsequent investigators have also noted a higher frequency of parental x-rays prior to the index pregnancy [133], and it is not at all clear that this finding does not have etiologic relevance. At the same time, cases and controls would not be expected to differ with respect to a large number of such dummy variables—particularly if the difference always appeared in the direction explicable in terms of the anticipated more complete reporting for cases. Similarly, a difference between cases and controls with respect to a single prior experience, and lack of difference with respect to others, will be more readily accepted as evidence of a real difference than if all the ascertained experiences differed.

Lastly, in addition to dummy variables, it may in some circumstances also be possible to examine what might be called a dummy disease—a disease (or group of patients) that would not be expected to share the etiologic background of the true cases although they went through the same study procedures as did the cases. For example, in a study of 1465 patients with lung cancer, Doll and Hill [81] noted that the lung cancer patients differed from their controls in (1) giving a higher percentage of histories of smoking, and in particular of heavy smoking, and (2) reporting a higher frequency of pneumonia and chronic bronchitis in the past. During the course of the same study, 335 patients with chest disease were interviewed in the belief that they had lung cancer. These patients were subsequently found not to have lung cancer and were excluded from the lung cancer series. Nevertheless their histories were compared with those of the lung cancer patients and with those of the controls (patients with diseases other than lung cancer). It was found that, with respect to smoking habits, the incorrectly notified group resembled the controls and not the lung cancer cases, but with respect to history of pneumonia and chronic bronchitis they resembled the lung cancer cases rather than the controls. These comparisons suggested that (1) the difference between the lung cancer cases and the controls in smoking habits was not the result of the patient or the interviewer knowing that the patient had lung cancer, and (2) there was a tendency for patients with diseases of the chest of all forms to report more pneumonia and chronic bronchitis than did patients with other diseases. "Unresolved" pneumonia is, of course, a frequent misdiagnosis in early lung cancer, and its more frequent reporting among lung cancer cases, as among patients with other chest diseases, is readily explicable in nonetiologic terms.

If the disease under investigation is a common one, a comparable situation may exist with respect to the controls—that is, persons may be interviewed as controls but subsequently turn out to be cases. For example, in a study of coronary heart disease in the population of the Health Insurance Plan of Greater New York (HIP), information on exposure variables (smoking history, physical exercise, etc.) was obtained from the patients in a clinical setting after diagnosis of their illness, whereas for the controls—a randomly selected sample of the population—the information was sought by mail questionnaire. It was, therefore, important to assess the comparability of the data obtained on cases and controls—both because there was a nonresponse rate of 17 percent in the control series, and because of the possibility that persons report differently in a clinical interview than in a mail questionnaire. The report [366] contains many examples of the ways in which this comparability may be and was assessed, but, in the present context, the comparison of the two sets of information obtained for 156 persons who both answered the mail questionnaire, having been selected in the random sample, and underwent interview, because of suspicion of cardiovascular disease, is of particular interest. It may indeed be important for the investigator to contrive such dual sets of data—for example, to reinterview at a later date a sample of one or both groups (cases or controls) under the circumstances that prevailed in the other group at the time of the original interview.

*Validity*

Validity refers to the extent to which a situation as observed reflects the "true" situation, or the situation as evaluated by other criteria that are thought to reflect the true situation more accurately. In the present context, the term is used to refer to the extent to which subjects in a case-control study are correctly classified as to the presence or absence, or level, of an exposure of interest.

SENSITIVITY AND SPECIFICITY. The concepts of sensitivity and specificity will be illustrated by reference to the data in Table 32, the hospital record being considered the more accurate source of information on whether or not the patient was x-rayed during pregnancy. *Sensitivity* is the extent to which patients who truly manifest a characteristic are so classified; in the present example the sensitivity of the mother's statement that she had been x-rayed is 24/37, or 65 percent. *Specificity* is the extent

Table 32

Comparison of hospital records and patients' statements as to the presence or absence of prenatal abdominal x-ray*

| Hospital record | Patients' statement | | | |
|---|---|---|---|---|
| | X-rayed | Not x-rayed | Don't know | Total |
| X-rayed | 24 | 10 | 3 | 37 |
| Not x-rayed | 2 | 31 | 5 | 38 |
| *Total* | 26 | 41 | 8 | 75 |

* Source: unpublished data [153].

to which patients who do not manifest a characteristic are correctly classified; in this instance, 31/38, or 82 percent.

PREDICTIVE VALUE. The same information conveyed by the consideration of sensitivity and specificity is provided by computing the predictive values of data from what is considered the less accurate source. The predictive value of the positive statement is the probability that persons who say that they manifest a characteristic truly do—in this case, 24/26, or 92 percent—and the predictive value of the negative statement is the probability that persons who say they do not have the characteristic truly do not—in this instance, 31/41, or 76 percent.

In the context of evaluating screening tests for disease detection in populations, it is preferable to consider validity in terms of sensitivity and specificity than of predictive value [407]. However, in considering the validity of information obtained in case-control studies there is little to choose between the two approaches.

The situation illustrated in Table 32 is not uncommon in case-control studies based on interview information—that is, the predictive value of the positive statement is higher than that of the negative. This results because patients will seldom report the occurrence of a nonexistent event, but they frequently forget to report events that actually occurred. In evaluating the extent of misclassification it is, therefore, important to keep these two kinds of error in mind. Repeating interviews after a lapse of time, checking interview information against records, comparing different records against each other, and other procedures which may reveal the extent of misclassification errors must be aimed at detecting both kinds of error. For example, on the basis of the example in Table 32, checking against hospital records only the patient's positive statements that she had an x-ray would have failed to reveal the major source of misclassification.

EFFECTS OF MISCLASSIFICATION. If misclassification with respect to study variables occurs to a different extent in the cases than in the controls, then the lack of comparability discussed in the previous section (pp. 257 to 261) exists. We are here concerned with the effects of misclassification that exists equally in the compared groups—that is to say, the specificity and sensitivity of the sources of data are the same in cases and controls. In this circumstance, the misclassification, however serious, will not introduce a difference between cases and controls if a true difference does not exist. Thus, if a difference is observed, and one can be confident that misclassification errors applied equally to cases and controls, he can conclude that a true difference exists that is *at least* as great as that observed. However, if such misclassification is substantial, the observed difference may be substantially less than the true difference. Indeed, random misclassification may reduce the difference to a level so low that the particular study is unable to detect it. Thus random misclassification errors may lead to a false negative conclusion, a conclusion that no difference exists when in fact one does.

An example will be taken from the study of Dunn and Buell [98] on the relationship of circumcision of the sexual partner to risk of cancer of the cervix uteri. To evaluate the validity of histories of circumcision, a group of men were asked whether or not they had been circumcised, and were subsequently examined by a physician. The results are shown in Table 33. Of the men who said that they had been circumcised, 52 percent were found to have at least some foreskin; of those who said that they had not been circumcised, 41 percent were found to have less than a complete foreskin. Dunn and Buell computed the effect of this misclassification on studies designed to test various hypotheses. For example, the relative risk of cervical cancer in non-Jewish, compared to Jewish, white women in the United States

## Table 33
Comparisons of patients' statements as to circumcision
status with physician's findings at examination*

| Physician's findings | Patients' statements | | | |
|---|---|---|---|---|
| | Circumcised | | Not circumcised | |
| | Number | Percent | Number | Percent |
| Circumcised | 21 | 47.7 | 8 | 6.6 |
| Partially circumcised | 17 | 38.6⎫ | 42 | 34.4⎫ |
| Not circumcised | 6 | 13.6⎭ 52.2 | 72 | 59.0⎭ 93.4 |
| *Total* | 44 | 99.9 | 122 | 100.0 |

* From Dunn and Buell [98].

is about 5. If this ethnic difference is explained in terms of circumcision of Jewish males, the relative risk associated with lack of circumcision must be at least 5. Suppose that only complete circumcision—as is characteristic of Jewish males—confers protection, and that both partial and complete lack of circumcision are associated with a five-times higher risk of cervix cancer. Then the relative risk of cervix cancer in their sexual partners associated with men's *statements* of not being circumcised can be computed as follows:

$$R = \frac{(5w) + (1x)}{(5y) + (1z)}$$

where $R$ is the apparent relative risk
  $w$ is the proportion of men who say they are not circumcised and indeed are not
  $x$ is the proportion who say they are not circumcised but have complete circumcision
  $y$ is the proportion who say they are circumcised but are not completely circumcised
  $z$ is the proportion who say they are circumcised and indeed have complete circumcision

In the example: $R = \dfrac{(5 \times 93.4) + (1 \times 6.6)}{(5 \times 52.2) + (1 \times 47.7)} = 1.5$

While a difference should still be found between cases and controls, it is much more difficult to demonstrate a difference associated with a relative risk of 1.5 than one associated with a relative risk of 5. Indeed, in a case-control study which had been set up to test the hypothesis of a relative risk of 5, Dunn and Buell found no difference in circumcision status of the husbands of cases and of controls. However, they noted that their numbers were inadequate to reject hypotheses involving relative risks less than 2.5. The error possibly introduced by misclassification was therefore sufficient to invalidate the study as a test of the hypothesized explanation of the low rate of cervix cancer in Jewish women.

Further clarification of the effects of misclassification errors in case-control studies will be found in papers by Rogot [348], Newell [294], and Buell and Dunn [36].

## ANALYSIS

The analysis of a case-control study is basically a comparison between cases and controls with respect to the frequency of factors whose possible etiologic influence is being evaluated. This may be a comparison in a fourfold table, such as Table 34, in which the concern is merely with the presence or absence of the suspect factor, or it may be in the form of two frequency distributions, as in Table 35, where the intensity or duration of exposure is also considered.

In Table 34 it is seen that a higher proportion of the bladder

### Table 34

Number of bladder cancer cases and controls reporting at least 6 months past employment in suspected high-risk industries; males, Boston, 1967 to 1968*

| Employed in suspect industry† | Cases | Controls |
|---|---|---|
| Yes | 118 | 69 |
| No | 257 | 299 |
| *Total* | 375 | 368 |

* From Cole and Hoover [61].
† Shoe, leather, rubber, dye, and chemical industries.

cancer cases than of the controls gave a history of employment in industries suspected of conferring high risk of the disease. Table 35 shows a considerable difference between the lung cancer patients and the control group in the ratio of smokers to nonsmokers; in addition, within the group of smokers there is a difference between the cases and controls in the distribution according to number of cigarettes smoked.

Some study factors can be considered only in terms of two classes (for example, present or absent), but, whenever possible, factors should be considered in multiple classes (as in Table 35). For example, a great deal of information would be lost if the data in Table 35 were considered only in terms of the dichotomy smoker : nonsmoker, or smoker of less than 15 cigarettes: smoker of 15 or more cigarettes. The consideration of a broad range of exposures, as in Table 35, has the advantages of (1)

Table 35

Distribution of 1465 lung cancer patients and a control group according to average number of cigarettes smoked daily over the 10 years preceding onset of the present illness*

| Daily average cigarettes | Males | | Females | |
|---|---|---|---|---|
| | Lung cancer patients | Control group | Lung cancer patients | Control group |
| 0 | 7 | 61 | 40 | 59 |
| 1–4 | 55 | 129 | 16 | 25 |
| 5–14 | 489 | 570 | 24 | 18 |
| 15–24 | 475 | 431 | 14 | 6 |
| 25–49 | 293 | 154 | 14 | 0 |
| 50 + | 38 | 12 | 0 | 0 |
| *Total* | 1357 | 1357 | 108 | 108 |

* From Doll and Hill [81].

being statistically more efficient—that is, more likely to reveal a significant difference if a difference is present, (2) allowing examination of the dose-response relationship, which, as mentioned earlier (pp. 21 and 235), is important in the interpretation of findings, and (3) allowing an estimation of risk in the more extreme exposure categories. With regard to statistical significance, the $\chi^2$ test for linear trend [15, 375] is a powerful test in situations involving several levels of exposure.

When dealing with quantitative variables, a comparison of distributions, such as that in Table 35, gives a clearer picture of the risk associated with the variable than does a comparison in terms of means or other summary statistics. For example, in a case-control study of breast cancer in Japan [432], the mean age at first delivery was found to be 23.8 years for the cases and 22.6 years for the controls. The difference of 1.2 years was statistically significant, but its size does not suggest any more than a tendency of breast cancer patients to have their first delivery at a later age than women without the disease. However, in the same data, comparison of the distributions of cases and controls with respect to age at first delivery showed that women first delivered at age 35 or older had more than four times the breast cancer risk of those first delivered under 20 years of age. The difference between the means of two distributions drawn from cases and controls will, of course, depend not only on the risk associated with being at a given level of the distribution but also on how many individuals there are at the various levels. Thus, in a comparison of means, a high risk associated with a particular level of exposure will be obscured if only a small fraction of the total population receives such exposure. The mean difference between cases and controls in age at first delivery in the study cited appeared fairly small because a relatively small proportion of women had their first deliveries in the categories which showed the greatest discrepancy in breast cancer risk—under 20, and 35 and over.

Apart from the matter of assessing the statistical significance of observed differences—which we consider here only peripherally—there are two important objectives in the further analysis of differences such as those observed in Tables 34 and 35. These are: (1) to estimate the risk associated with the presence or absence or level of exposure, and (2) to determine to what extent the difference observed may be the result of associations of the suspected cause and the disease with some confounding variable. In the actual analysis of a case-control study, attempts to resolve the second question would usually precede the estimates of risk, since there is little profit in estimating apparent risks if the associations are subsequently shown to be spurious. However, the matter of risk estimation will be described here first, since a knowledge of the methods involved in analyzing a simple table, such as Table 34 or 35, is necessary to an understanding of the more complex procedures that are involved when the influence of confounding variables is taken into account.

## Estimates of Risk

The concepts of relative and attributable risk were introduced in Chapter 11. As described there, these estimates of risk were computed directly from estimates of disease rates among persons exposed, and among persons not exposed, to the study factor. Such rates are obtained directly in cohort studies. Disease rates are not obtained directly in case-control studies, the orientation of such studies being toward the computation of *exposure* rates among diseased and not-diseased individuals. Nevertheless, under certain conditions in case-control studies, estimates can be made of disease risk associated with reported exposures or other study factors.

STUDIES OF CASES REFERABLE TO A POPULATION. When the cases represent all cases of the disorder in a defined population or are a sample of such cases selected in a known way, and the control group is representative of the same population, it will be possible to estimate rates of the disease in exposed and nonexposed persons and to derive relative and attributable risks from these estimates.

For example, the cases of bladder cancer shown in Table 34 were a representative sample of the 547 bladder cancer cases in males that were diagnosed in the population of the Boston metropolitan area during an 18-month period. All cases were identified, but, for reasons of economy, a sample was selected for interview. The controls were randomly selected from the population of the same geographic area, in age and sex groups corresponding to those of the cases. The assumptions may be made that, with respect to frequency of industrial exposure, the 375 interviewed cases were representative of the total of 547 cases, and that the controls were representative of the population of the same age and sex as the cases. The male population of the area aged 20 or over was approximately 850,000. Since 18.8 percent of the controls gave a history of the occupations of interest, the population may be supposed to consist of approximately 850,000 × (18.8/100), or 159,800, men who were exposed and 690,200 who were not. Similarly, from the data shown in Table 34, the 547 total cases can be estimated as including 172 who were exposed and 375 who were not. Applying these numerators to the estimated populations, incidence rates in the exposed and not-exposed population during the 18-month period can be derived; division by 1.5 yields the average annual incidence rates.

Average annual incidence rate in the exposed

$$= \frac{172}{159,800 \times 1.5} \times 10^5 = 72 \text{ per } 100,000$$

Average annual incidence rate in the not-exposed

$$= \frac{375}{690,200 \times 1.5} \times 10^5 = 36 \text{ per } 100,000$$

From these rates, the relative risk can be estimated as 2.0, and the attributable risk among exposed persons as 36 per 100,000 per year.

Note that in this particular example the controls were not representative of the total population, in that they were matched to the age distribution of the cases. If the exposure under consideration were one that varied in frequency with age the procedure outlined above would not be appropriate. In such circumstances rates should be estimated within individual age groups and total rates in exposed and not-exposed individuals derived by standardization.

OTHER STUDIES: ESTIMATES OF RELATIVE RISK. The data in Table 35 cannot be related to a defined population. The lung cancer patients were patients attending selected hospitals and no attempt was made to limit the group according to place of residence or to determine what proportion these represented of the total lung cancer patients in the areas served by the hospitals. Similarly, the control group was selected from patients with other diseases in the same hospitals, and although it was therefore believed to be a sample of the same population from which the lung cancer patients were drawn, it was not known what proportion of that population the sample represented. Since the populations at risk are not known, it is impossible to derive estimates of rates in the exposed and the nonexposed populations. However, it is possible to derive an estimate of the relative risk.

It was noted in Chapter 3 that a population can be divided among the cells of a fourfold table as follows:

| Suspected cause | Disease | | Total |
|---|---|---|---|
| | Present | Absent | |
| Present | $a$ | $b$ | $a + b$ |
| Absent | $c$ | $d$ | $c + d$ |
| *Total* | $a + c$ | $b + d$ | 1 |

In this table, $a$, $b$, $c$, and $d$ represent the frequencies of individuals in the various cells. In a case-control study, only derivatives of such frequencies are available. A case-control study may be represented by the following table, $a'$, $b'$, $c'$, and $d'$ being the numbers of individuals in each cell:

| Suspected cause | Cases | Controls |
|---|---|---|
| Present | $a'$ | $b'$ |
| Absent | $c'$ | $d'$ |
| *Total* | $a' + c'$ | $b' + d'$ |

The right-hand column has been omitted since, as already noted, in the type of study under discussion the cases and controls represent unknown, and nearly always different, fractions of the affected and unaffected individuals in the population; the values $(a' + b')$ and $(c' + d')$ therefore have no meaning.

From the first diagram, showing the distribution of the total population, the relative risk would be:

$$\frac{\text{Rate in exposed persons}}{\text{Rate in nonexposed persons}} = \frac{a}{a + b} \div \frac{c}{c + d} = \frac{a(c + d)}{c(a + b)}$$

When the number of persons affected by the disease is small compared to the number unaffected (the usual situation in disease studies), $d$ is approximately equal to $(c + d)$ and $b$ is approximately equal to $(a + b)$. The formula then reduces to:

$$\frac{ad}{cb}$$

When the cases represent only a sample of all cases in the population, and the control group is a sample of the population, then $a' = as_1$, $c' = cs_1$, $b' = bs_2$, and $d' = ds_2$, where $s_1$ is the sampling fraction used in selecting the cases and $s_2$ is the sampling fraction used in selecting the controls. The formula becomes:

$$\text{Relative risk} = \frac{a's_1d's_2}{c's_1b's_2} = \frac{a'd'}{c'b'}$$

It is clear therefore that for the derivation of relative risk it is not necessary to know the values $s_1$ and $s_2$.

For example, from the data in Table 34 one can estimate the relative risk of bladder cancer in exposed males as:

$$\frac{118 \times 299}{257 \times 69} = 2.0$$

This figure is consistent with that estimated earlier (p. 269) by direct comparison of estimated rates.

From the data in Table 35, in which the values $s_1$ and $s_2$ are not known,* the relative risk for male smokers (any number of cigarettes) compared to nonsmokers is $\dfrac{1350 \times 61}{7 \times 1296} = 9.1$. Further, the formula can be used to compare any two exposure categories. For example, the relative risk for male smokers of 50 or more cigarettes per day, relative to the risk for nonsmokers, is:

$$\frac{38 \times 61}{12 \times 7} = 27.6$$

Table 36 shows a series of relative risks computed from the data in Table 35. In column (a), the risk in each exposure

---

* Note that since the sampling fractions are irrelevant, the formula can be applied equally well to either the actual numbers or the percentages of cases and controls in the exposure categories.

## Table 36

Relative risks as derived from the data for males in
Table 35

| Daily average cigarettes | Lung cancer patients | Control group | Relative risk (a)* | (b)† |
|---|---|---|---|---|
| 0 | 7 | 61 | — | 1.0 |
| 1–4 | 55 | 129 | 3.7 | 3.7 |
| 5–14 | 489 | 570 | 2.0 | 7.4 |
| 15–24 | 475 | 431 | 1.3 | 9.6 |
| 25–49 | 293 | 154 | 1.7 | 16.3 |
| 50 + | 38 | 12 | 1.7 | 27.7 |

\* Relative to persons in the adjacent lower category of smoking.
† Relative to nonsmokers.

category is expressed relative to that in the adjacent lower category; for example, 3.7 is the relative risk for smokers of 1 to 4 cigarettes compared to the risk for nonsmokers. That the relative risk is greater than 1 in each comparison of a higher with a lower exposure category indicates the existence of a clear dose-response relationship. This is also evident in column (b), which expresses the risk for each exposure category relative to that of nonsmokers. The values in this column can be computed either by direct comparison with nonsmokers—as illustrated above for the smokers of 50 cigarettes or more—or by cumulative multiplication of the individual relative risks. Thus, since smokers of 1 to 4 cigarettes have 3.7 times the risk of nonsmokers, and smokers of 5 to 14 cigarettes have 2.0 times the risk of smokers of 1 to 4 cigarettes, it follows that smokers in the 5 to 14 cigarette category have $2.0 \times 3.7 = 7.4$ times the risk of nonsmokers.

The use of this formula for computation of relative risk involves two assumptions: (1) that the disease under study is relatively infrequent in both exposed and unexposed persons, and (2) that neither cases nor controls are selected in favor of either exposed or nonexposed individuals—that is, that the fraction $s_1$ applies equally to exposed and nonexposed cases and the fraction $s_2$ equally to exposed and nonexposed controls.

The first of these assumptions is of little practical importance. Whether or not the disease is infrequent, the ratio $ad/bc$ is still a good measure of difference in disease risk between groups.

When dealing with diseases or defects in which more than, say, 20 percent (but not more than 80 percent) of either exposed or unexposed persons are affected, it may be preferable to give the ratio its more correct name, the *relative odds*—that is, the ratio of affected to unaffected individuals in one group divided by the same ratio in another group. Under such circumstances the ratio is still a useful index of association. With disease frequencies below 20 percent of both exposed and unexposed persons, the relative odds so closely approximates the relative risk that it is common to use the two terms interchangeably.

The second assumption may cause greater difficulty. For example, the relative risk of lung cancer in relation to smoking has been found to be generally smaller in studies in which hospital patients formed the controls than in cohort studies in which the comparison group derived from the general population. It has been pointed out [246] that the reported proportion of non-smokers among hospital patients is smaller than among the population at large, presumably because a number of diseases other than lung cancer are positively associated with smoking. Thus, in case-control studies in which hospital patients are used as controls, the proportion sampled from the general population may be higher for those exposed (smokers) than for those not exposed (nonsmokers). In this instance the error is in favor of understatement. The relationship to smoking is so much stronger for lung cancer than for other diseases that the understatement was not large enough to obscure the relationship. In other instances, bias of this type could readily operate in the direction of overstatement.

OTHER STUDIES: ESTIMATES OF ATTRIBUTABLE RISK. Sometimes estimates of the incidence or mortality rate of a disease are available from other sources, even though they cannot be derived from the study being analyzed. Thus the data in Table 35 do not supply estimates of lung cancer incidence, but such estimates are available for many populations and the disease is such that the even more numerous mortality data could be used to provide reasonable estimates of incidence among males in London in the time period of this study. An approximate figure would be 480 per million per year [79]. Given this information and an estimate of the relative risk as derived above, estimates of the disease incidence in the various exposure categories can be derived on the following basis.

The over-all incidence of a disease in a population is the average of the incidence in the various exposure classes, the individual averages being weighted according to the proportion of the population in each exposure class. Thus, in the simple situation where there are only two classes, exposed and not-exposed, the over-all incidence ($I$) is:

$$I = I_e P_e + I_o P_o$$

where $I_e$ is the incidence and $P_e$ the proportion of the population in the exposed category, and $I_o$ and $P_o$ are corresponding values for the nonexposed. The formula has equal validity whether incidence is expressed in terms of numbers of cases or rates.

Since $I_e = R \times I_o$, where $R$ is the relative risk, the formula can be written:

$$I = R I_o P_e + I_o P_o$$

or, in terms of $I_o$:

$$I_o = \frac{I}{R P_e + P_o}$$

If $I$ is known, and $R$ has been estimated, and the assumption can be made that the distribution of the controls in the study approximates the distribution of the population with respect to exposure categories, then $I_o$ can be estimated.

For example, in the data for males in Table 35, $I$ can be taken from other sources as 480 per million per year [79], $R$ for smokers vis-à-vis nonsmokers was estimated as 9.1 (p. 271), and the proportions of smokers and nonsmokers in the control group are 0.955 and 0.045, respectively. Therefore:

$$I_o = \frac{480/10^6/\text{yr}}{(9.1 \times 0.955) + 0.045} = 54.9/10^6/\text{year}$$

$$I_e = 9.1 \times 54.9/10^6/\text{yr} = 500.0/10^6/\text{year}$$

Given a rate of 55 per million per year for nonsmokers, estimates of incidence for each of the exposure classes can be computed by applying the relative risks shown in column (b) of Table 36. From these estimates of rates, estimates of attributable risk can be computed.

Even if $I$ is unknown, an estimate of the attributable risk can be obtained in terms of percentage of the total risk in the exposed group. In the example already used:

$$I_o = \frac{I}{(9.1 \times 0.955) + 0.045} = 0.1145I$$

$$I_e = 9.1 \times 0.1145I = 1.0420I$$

Attributable risk for smokers (%) is estimated as:

$$\frac{1.0420I - 0.1145I}{1.0420I} \times 100 = 89 \text{ percent}$$

Thus, even if the actual disease rate in smokers is unknown, it can be estimated that 89 percent of their rate is attributable to smoking.

Caution is needed in applying these procedures in situations in which the frequency of exposure varies with age or other variables that may be used as the basis of estimation of standardized rates. The basic formula $I = I_e P_e + I_o P_o$ applies only when crude unstandardized rates are being considered.

### Adjustment for Confounding Variables

The fact that association of disease and study factor with a third variable may introduce spurious differences between cases and controls has been mentioned earlier (p. 244). It was also pointed out (p. 244) that consideration of such confounding variables may be taken either in the selection of controls—by matching the controls to the cases with respect to relevant variables—or in the analysis—by comparing cases and controls with similar characteristics.

ANALYSIS OF PAIRED SAMPLES. When paired matched controls have been drawn, more correct estimates of both risk and statistical significance are obtained when the analysis maintains the pairing—that is to say, each case is compared with the specific control that was paired with it. The basic difference introduced by matched-pair analysis is that pairs in which case and control are similar with respect to the study factor are not considered, and estimates are based solely on pairs in which one member has, and the other does not have, the factor under study. Thus the following arrangement represents the distribution of all the pairs in a paired-sample study. (Note that presence or absence of the factor may be defined in terms of specified levels of the factor, as well as simple presence or absence.)

|  | Case | |
|---|---|---|
| Control | Factor present | Factor absent |
| Factor present | $r$ | $s$ |
| Factor absent | $t$ | $u$ |

In this table, $r$, $s$, $t$, and $u$ are the number of pairs—that is, their sum is half the number of individuals in the study. The most appropriate test of statistical significance in such a situation is the McNemar or marginal $\chi^2$ test, where

$$\chi^2 = \frac{(s - t)^2}{(s + t)}. \text{ The relative risk is estimated as } \frac{t}{s}.$$

These procedures will be illustrated by reference to a case-control study of thromboembolism in females, in which prior use of oral contraceptives was the study factor of primary interest [352]. The data are shown in Table 37. The 10 pairs in which both case and control used the contraceptives and the 95

Table 37

Distribution of 175 case-control pairs according to whether or not oral contraceptives were used within 1 month before admission for thromboembolism; women aged 15 to 44, five American cities, 1964 to 1968*

| Oral agent used by control? | Oral agent used by case? | | Total pairs |
|---|---|---|---|
|  | Yes | No |  |
| Yes | 10 | 13 | 23 |
| No | 57 | 95 | 152 |
| *Total pairs* | 67 | 108 | 175 |

* From Sartwell et al. [352].

pairs in which neither used them provide no information on the association between pill use and thromboembolism. Such information comes only from the discordant pairs:

Relative risk is estimated as $\dfrac{57}{13} = 4.4$, and

$$x^2 = \frac{(57 - 13)^2}{57 + 13} = 27.7 \ \text{(degrees of freedom} = 1, P < 0.001)$$

In this particular instance the values for $x^2$ and for relative risk do not differ appreciably from those which could be calculated from the usual formulas applied to unmatched data: 28.9 and 4.1, respectively. This is a reflection of the fact that, in spite of the comprehensive matching plan used in this study, little similarity between pair members was introduced. Given the frequencies of contraceptive use by cases and controls shown in Table 37, one can compute that if the pairing had been random there would have been 8.8 pairs in which both members used the agents and 93.8 pairs in which neither used them. Thus the matching plan introduced only 2 similar pairs in excess of the 103 expected by chance. The error introduced by analyzing paired data as if they were not paired is a function of the strength of the association between the study factor and the matching factor. When pairing has been used primarily for convenience or when the influence of matching factors is small, so that appreciable similarity within pairs with respect to study factors has not been introduced, the pairing may be ignored in the analysis. However, there is no advantage to be gained by ignoring the pairing if all the confounding variables to be considered entered into the matching process. If confounding variables are to be analyzed that were not considered, or were inadequately dealt with in the matching process, it may be reasonable to treat the series as if they had not been matched.

The use and analysis of matched samples in epidemiologic studies, under different conditions, have been discussed by Worcester [420]. Miettinen has considered the problems of power, sample size, and efficiency [250] and relative risk estimation [253], and the question of significance testing when there are multiple matched controls [251].

STRATIFICATION IN ANALYSIS. Even when cases and controls have been matched with respect to certain relevant variables, other relevant, and possibly confounding, differences may be identified in the analysis. For example, in the study of thrombo-embolism just referred to, controls and cases were matched on marital status, parity, race, city of residence, year of discharge from hospital, hospital pay status, and age. Nevertheless, differences between cases and controls were found in regard to family income, religion, weight, education, proportion employed, and proportion working at a medically related job [352]. Obviously, some of these differences could confound a comparison of oral contraceptive use in the two series.

The first problem is to identify such possible confounding variables. This involves a systematic search of the data on cases and controls to ascertain the ways in which they differ. For each factor in which a significant or substantial difference between cases and controls is found, the question must be asked as to whether that factor is also related to the study variable under analysis. For example, if the cases and controls differ with respect to family income, does use of oral contraceptives differ among family income groups? Only those confounding factors that *both* differ between cases and controls *and* are related to the study variable need be considered further.

Having identified the confounding variables that must be considered, a procedure for evaluating their effects must be decided upon. Sometimes, exclusion of certain cases and controls will suffice. In the oral contraceptive study, the excess of cases employed in medically related occupations was in part due to the inclusion of 26 pairs in which the case was a student nurse. Analyses were therefore run after exclusion of these pairs, with no appreciable change in the results. Such a procedure, however, is economical only when the subgroup responsible for the difference is relatively small, or when there is *no* comparable subgroup among one or the other of the groups being compared. For example, if there are no student nurses among the controls, and being a student nurse is considered a variable that must be accounted for, then the only way to attain comparability is the procedure that was followed.

A more usual procedure is to stratify the cases and controls

*278*

according to various levels of the confounding factor or factors, and to compare the groups within these levels. An example is shown in Table 38, taken from a study comparing smoking

### Table 38

Percentage of smokers of 20 or more cigarettes a day
among patients with tuberculosis and a control group,
in age and sex groups*

| Age (years) | Number of patients | | | | Percentage smoking 20 or more cigarettes a day | | | |
|---|---|---|---|---|---|---|---|---|
| | Males | | Females | | Males | | Females | |
| | Tuber-culous | Other | Tuber-culous | Other | Tuber-culous | Other | Tuber-culous | Other |
| 30–39 | 211 | 126 | 130 | 113 | 48.3 | 46.0 | 9.2 | 2.7 |
| 40–49 | 164 | 141 | 36 | 94 | 51.8 | 44.6 | 19.4 | 3.2 |
| 50–59 | 104 | 103 ⎫ | 19 | 42 | 51.0 | 41.8 ⎫ | 10.5 | 0.0 |
| 60 + | 41 | 49 ⎭ | | | 51.2 | 36.8 ⎭ | | |
| 30 + | 520 | 419 | 185 | 249 | 50.1 | 43.4 | 11.4 | 2.4 |
| 30 +† | — | — | — | — | 50.3 | 43.7 | 12.4 | 2.5 |

\* From Lowe [208].
† Standardized to the age distribution of the combined cases and control group.

habits of tuberculosis patients with those of accident and general surgical patients, unmatched with respect to age or sex [208]. Since smoking and tuberculosis are both markedly associated with both age and sex, it was necessary to determine whether a difference noted between the smoking habits of the patients with tuberculosis and those of the patients in the control group was due to differences in age or sex distribution of the groups. For simplicity, only the percentages of smokers of 20 or more cigarettes a day are shown in the table, although total distributions according to amount smoked could also be compared in each age and sex category. The table shows that for each sex, in each 10-year age category examined, the percentage of heavy smokers was higher among the tuberculous than among the control patients. The difference between the tuberculous patients and the control group in smoking habits cannot, therefore, be explained by differences in their age or sex composition.

In conducting analyses such as these, the range of measurements covered in the subgroups is important. It is desirable for

the subgroups to contain a sufficient number of cases for separate examination, but the range must not be so inclusive that
the desired similarity between compared series is not obtained.
For example, if a disease is markedly related to age, the use of 20-
year age groups may not eliminate the effect of age, since within
20-year age groups there may be sufficient difference between
cases and controls to produce appreciable differences in study
variables. It may be difficult to decide whether the adopted
grouping has been sufficiently fine to equalize the compared
series effectively. If an apparent difference between compared
groups is eliminated by holding a confounding variable constant, it may usually be assumed that the grouping was satisfactory. However, if the difference is reduced but not eliminated,
the effect of finer grouping should be ascertained. If finer grouping is impractical because of inadequate numbers, it may be possible to estimate by indirect methods the maximum possible
influence of variation within the chosen groups by making assumptions about the maximum extent of variation possible
within the adopted grouping and the maximum change in incidence that might be associated with it. Some general idea about
the possible effect of finer grouping may also be obtained by
noting the change in the summary risk estimates, as discussed in
the next paragraph, that results from consideration of the subgroups that can be examined.

In addition to visual inspection of the differences between the
case and control groups in each subdivision of the data, it is usually desirable to obtain some kind of summary statement as to
the statistical significance of the difference and of the estimated
risk in all the subgroups considered together. For example, in
the data for males shown in Table 38, the relative risks for
smokers of 20 or more cigarettes a day are 1.10, 1.33, 1.45, and
1.80, respectively, in the four age groups shown. The problem
then is to derive an over-all relative risk which is a summary of
the relative risks within each of the subclassifications. One procedure is to apply the formula to the total distribution after
standardization. For example, using the standardized
data for males in the table, the relative risk would be
$\dfrac{50.3 \times 56.3}{43.7 \times 49.7} = 1.30$. In this particular case, the effect of stand-

ardization is small, the relative risk being practically identical with that which might be calculated from the total crude data for males, that is, 1.31. However, the summary relative risk estimated in this way is unreliable—it may even give a result that is outside the range of the component values. A more satisfactory method, described by Mantel and Haenszel [239], is one in which the summary relative risk is an average of the relative risks in the individual subcategories, weighted according to the precision of the individual estimates.

Mantel and Haenszel [239] also present a modification and generalization of a summary $\chi^2$ test, earlier described by Cochran [59], that tests the statistical significance of the deviation of the observed relative risk from 1. The procedure has been further extended by Mantel [237] to derive a summary $\chi^2$ test for linear trend, when the individual tables in subcategories of the confounding variables involve several ordered levels of exposure.

## INTERPRETATION

The two basic questions likely to be asked in interpreting the results of a study are the same in a case-control as in a cohort study: (1) Do the findings reflect the true situation with respect to the presence or absence of association between the disease and the study factor? (2) If an association is observed, is it a causal one?

In attempting to answer the first question, consideration should be given to matters of comparability and representativeness of cases, controls, and sources of information, and to the thoroughness of the analysis. These matters have been touched on throughout this chapter. In addition, the findings of the study must be considered as a whole, with a review of all the items on which the cases and controls differ. When the data for cases and controls are generally similar, but sharp differences are found with respect to one or two items, such differences are more likely to be accepted as real than if a great number of apparent associations emerges. Thus, Table 39 shows, for the study of oral contraceptives already referred to, the distribution of cases and controls by method of contraception used within 2

## Table 39

Methods of contraception reported as used during 2
years preceding hospitalization for thromboembolism
(same study as Table 37)*

| Contraceptive used | Cases | Controls |
|---|---|---|
| Oral contraceptive | 67 | 30 |
| Condom | 41 | 42 |
| Diaphragm | 40 | 34 |
| Rhythm | 21 | 14 |
| Jelly, cream | 19 | 9 |
| Douche | 11 | 11 |
| Withdrawal | 8 | 8 |
| Other | 18 | 15 |
| *Total number using*  *one or more methods†* | 114 | 101 |

\* From Sartwell et al. [352].

† Many women had used several methods; therefore the numbers are not additive.

years prior to admission. The general similarity in the frequency of reporting of different methods except for oral agents (the difference in the use of jellies and creams is not statistically significant) strongly supports the view that the difference with respect to oral agents is a real one and not explicable by differences in selecting, or obtaining information from, the cases and controls.

In judging whether or not the associations observed are causal, the results of the particular study must be viewed in light of other knowledge of the disease and the exposures involved. Relevant considerations have been described in Chapter 2 and in the final section of Chapter 11 (pp. 235 to 239).

# 13

Intervention Studies

The types of studies described so far in this book have aimed at the accumulation of sufficient knowledge about the etiology of a disease to permit the design of a practical program for its prevention. When this objective has been attained, there remains the necessity of determining whether or not the program that has been devised is effective. To the extent that this determination requires the measurement of disease frequencies in populations, epidemiologic skills may be required in the process.

Not infrequently in the past, programs aimed at disease prevention have been initiated on a large scale without adequate field studies of their value under the actual circumstances in which they are to be carried out. Some programs, soundly based on theory, experimental work, or even observations on man, have proved impractical or ineffective under real-life conditions; well-known examples include the amendment to the U.S. Constitution that sought to prohibit consumption of liquor containing more than 2.5 percent alcohol, and the failure of gamma globulin to stop the spread of poliomyelitis under epidemic conditions [68]. Perhaps more frequent are untested programs which are able to be operated and which achieve acceptance by the public and by those responsible because of intuitive feelings as to the "reasonableness" of the program—assisted often by the selective recollection of favorable rather than unfavorable outcomes. In such circumstances, harm may stem from the fact that questions as to the efficacy of intervention programs inevitably arise sooner or later—even if they are not raised initially—and there are great practical and ethical problems in evaluating programs that have already achieved acceptance, whether on a sound or unsound basis. The field of cancer therapy is replete with examples of new modalities that were taken up with enthusiasm and proved worthless only after they had resulted in many years of futile cost and suffering.

Occasionally the benefits of a program of therapy or prevention appear so obvious—either in terms of health directly (penicillin, for example) or because there are obvious other benefits, whether or not health is affected (provision of clean air and water, for example)—that formal evaluation studies seem unnecessary, and perhaps even undesirable. However, such programs represent only a small fraction of the total medical and public health effort, and much more commonly the value of a program is not so great that it can be adequately assessed without properly designed studies. There is increasing recognition that, in addition to asking whether it is ethical in the light of current knowledge to plan a randomized trial in which some people will not be offered the new measure, it is also necessary to ask whether it is ethical *not* to plan a randomized trial, since failure to do so may subject the population as a whole to the perpetuation of an ineffective program [160]. Ethical questions that are in most situations more significant than the question of whether or not to undertake a therapeutic or preventive trial revolve around the procedures that must be incorporated to protect the rights and safety of individuals who agree to participate in such experiments [72].

The intervention studies described in this chapter are those that have been designed and carried out specifically as studies of procedures or programs considered to have possibilities for disease prevention. Not described are attempts to evaluate the effects of programs that have been set up as programs, rather than as studies. The programs-as-programs fall more into the category of the observational kinds of research described elsewhere in the book—the program to be evaluated corresponding to the "exposure" or cause, of which the relevance to changes in disease risk is to be ascertained. Special problems of this kind of evaluative study in the field of preventive medicine, as well as of the type of study to be described here, have been discussed by Hutchison [173]. Campbell [44] gives many interesting examples of nonexperimental types of evaluation in other fields of social action.

The defining characteristic of the type of intervention study considered in this chapter is that the investigators determine the presence or absence of the program or programs to be evaluated in accordance with an experimental design of adequate rigor.

## STUDY AND CONTROL GROUPS

The group of individuals offered the particular measure to be evaluated is commonly referred to as the *study group,* and the individuals not offered this measure the *control group.* As noted below, some form of intervention may be offered to both groups. In adopting this terminology, we should stress that the implication that one group is studied and the other not is to be avoided. The steps in the formation of study and control groups in an experimental study are outlined in Figure 33.

### Reference and Experimental Populations

The *reference population* is the population that the investigator has in mind as the one to which the results of the study are expected to be generally applicable. Even though this population may be defined in very broad terms, it is important to be clear as to what the terms are, so that steps can be taken to insure that the *experimental population*—the actual population in which the study is to be undertaken—does not differ from the reference population in such a way that generalization to the latter is not possible.

The reference population may be as broad as all mankind, if the benefits of a particular procedure are felt to be universally applicable. On the other hand, it may be geographically restricted if the intervention program—a mental health consultation service, for example—has particular applicability to a certain culture or region. The reference population may be limited with respect to age, sex, socioeconomic status, marital status, and

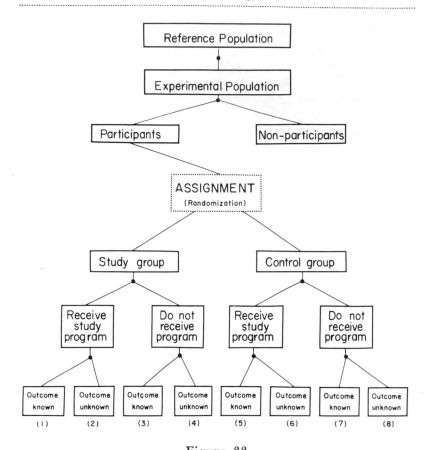

Figure 33

Steps in the selection of participants in a controlled intervention study.
(Adapted from Hutchison [173].)

so on, if such variables influence the frequency of either the disease to be prevented or the causal factors against which the program is directed.

Considerations in selecting the experimental population include the following:

1. Similarity of its demographic characteristics to those of the reference population.

2. Matters of convenience and accessibility. These include not only geographic accessibility but such aspects as the availability of medical resources, compactness of the population, and

so on. Features that are introduced for reasons of convenience must be evaluated to determine whether they limit generalization of the findings to the reference population originally considered. For example, suppose a dietary supplement is to be evaluated for its effect on intellectual development. The reference population might then be children. It would probably be easier to supplement the diet of children in school than those of a younger age. In this instance, however, one would be reluctant to accept from a negative finding in a study of schoolchildren the generalization that this dietary supplement is ineffective at any age of childhood. On the other hand, a beneficial finding might not affect willingness to generalize the results to a broader age range. The willingness to generalize will depend in part on the outcome of the study and in part on the nature of the program being evaluated, as well as on the characteristics of the specific population being used.

3. Incidence of the disease to be prevented. Generally speaking, it will be beneficial to select a population that has—or is expected to have in the near future—a high incidence of the disease. The higher the incidence, the smaller the groups necessary to demonstrate a difference in disease rates. Thus a study of the efficacy of a vaccine against meningococcal meningitis was carried out in military recruits because of the known high incidence of the disease in this population [18]. At the same time, the investigator must be aware that the factors responsible for the high incidence of disease in the selected population may be peculiar to the population and the ability to generalize from the study may be jeopardized. A population of American Indians might well be selected for a trial of a program to prevent congenital dislocation of the hip because of the extraordinarily high frequency of this condition in Indian populations. However, the causes of the defect may be different in Indian and other populations, and a program effective in one group may not be so in others.

4. Size of the population required. The expected incidence of disease, together with estimates as to the differences that might be expected between the compared groups, is the basis for deciding the size of the groups that will be required for the demonstration of statistically significant differences. Since predictions

both of incidence and of differences between groups must of necessity be crude (otherwise the trial would not be required), it is usual to include considerably more persons in the study than statistical tests indicate to be the minimum required for confidence in the significance of predicted differences. Often, reasonable estimates cannot be made ahead of time as to how effective a measure is going to be. In these circumstances, a certain size of difference between study and control groups may be selected for use in sample size estimates on the grounds that this is the smallest difference that, in the light of the expense and other practical considerations involved in implementing the program, would make it a worthwhile public health measure.

## Selection and Assignment of Participating Individuals

When an experimental population has been defined, its members must be invited to participate. While it is sometimes thought that volunteers make unsuitable subjects for experimental studies, as Bradford Hill remarked [161]: "There is (fortunately) no other way of setting up a trial." Current practice requires that when individuals are offered the opportunity to participate in an experimental study, they must be fully informed as to its purposes, procedures, and possible dangers. This includes telling potential participants that they may be allocated to a control group (if this is the case), and having reasonable assurance that this information and its implications are understood by the participants. Thus, while the investigator may select an experimental population, the selection of individuals from that population to participate in the study is in great part beyond his control.

It must be recognized that persons who agree to participate in a study are likely to differ from those who do not in many ways that may affect the outcome under investigation. This was demonstrated in several early studies in which those who volunteered to participate were considered as the study group and those who did not as the controls. Volunteering is likely to be associated with socioeconomic status, education, age, family size, and other less tangible variables. Therefore the separation into study and control groups must be made *after* the individuals have agreed to participate. As noted, this agreement must include agreement to serve as either study or control group member and, in some instances, to not being informed as to the group to which they have been assigned, even after the assignment has taken place.

RANDOMIZATION OF INDIVIDUALS. When the preventive measure being evaluated is one that can be applied to individuals, random assignment to study and control groups is the procedure that will give the greatest confidence that the groups are comparable. Random assignment must be distinguished from haphazard and systematic allocation. The dangers of haphazard assignment are obvious, and have been referred to in the discussion of selection of controls in case-control studies (p. 251). Systematic selection (for example, the assignment of alternate individuals to study and control groups, or allocation on the basis of whether the date of birth is odd or even) was employed in many early studies. Although this procedure is often satisfactory in case-control studies, since the systematic nature of the selection does not usually bias the group (p. 251), it is not recommended in experimental designs. Its major disadvantages are two. First, if the system becomes known it may be manipulated —either by the participants themselves or by the study staff—for purposes which seem worthy but which may destroy the similarity of the groups. Second, even if the system is not manipulated, knowledge of the assignment procedure reveals whether an individual is a member of the study group or a control, and therefore complicates procedures that are necessary to insure that the later ascertainment of outcome is equally complete in all the groups to be compared (see p. 295).

Since the individuals to be included in an intervention study are usually not all available at one time—and cannot therefore be randomly assigned by the usual processes of random selection (e.g., giving each individual a number and then drawing numbers from a table of random numbers)—it is common to assign an individual by entering his or her name on the first empty line on a roster of eligible participants. The lines have been previously designated, in random order, as indicating assignment to study or control groups. The individual's eligibility (for either study or control group) must be determined before the name is entered on the roster, and it is preferable that the assignment determined by a particular line not be apparent until after the name is entered—for example, sealed envelopes bearing the line number may be opened to reveal the assignment allotted to a particular line only after the name is entered on the line.

In studies where a placebo is being used, it may be possible to randomize the measure, rather than the individuals who receive it. For example, vials of vaccine and placebo may be assembled in random order and given to individuals in order as they appear.

BLIND ASSIGNMENT. The so-called double-blind procedure is designed to insure that ascertainment of outcome is not biased by knowledge of the group to which an individual was assigned. It involves two safeguards—blind assignment to study and control groups, and blind assessment of outcome. The blind assignment component implies that neither the study staff nor the participants know to which group an individual was assigned, until after the study is completed. For example, vials of vaccine and placebo may be identified only by number. The number of the vial used for each individual is recorded but, except in instances involving the immediate welfare of an individual participant, the master list indicating whether that number identified a vial of vaccine or placebo is not consulted until the outcome has been determined and the results are to be analyzed. Such a procedure was followed by the Medical Research Council [243] in a study of whooping cough vaccine and by Hammon et al. [148] in evaluating gamma globulin in the prophylaxis of paralytic poliomyelitis. These investigations have become classic examples of this particular form of intervention study.

Clearly the blind assignment procedure depends on having study and placebo programs that are indistinguishable. How far to go towards this end requires difficult judgments. The scientific advantages must be weighed against the added complexity and inconveniences to persons assigned to the control group. In addition to inconveniences and discomforts, more serious consequences of attempts to make placebos similar to study procedures have been reported [32, 258]. Mechanisms must be available for ready access to the code in the event that unexpected reactions occur or that persons responsible for the care of the participants find it necessary to know the allocation of any individual in order to deal with his particular clinical situation.

The need for a placebo—and for blind assignment to study and placebo groups—is highly related to the subjectivity of the measure of outcome. For example, dead is dead and no amount of knowledge of the history of the corpse will bias a reasonable observer's evaluation of the situation. The blind assignment procedure is not always necessary for objective evaluation of outcome and should not be introduced into a study design merely as a scientific tour de force.

When blind assignment has been used and the procedure has proved effective, it will be necessary to inform the members of the control group that they were controls, since they may be under the impression that they have received the protection conferred by a new procedure (e.g., a vaccine) when they have not.

STRATIFICATION OF GROUPS. If the disease to be prevented varies appreciably in frequency between age, sex, or other demographic subgroups of the experimental population, it will usually be desirable to attempt to obtain study and control groups that are equally distributed with respect to such variables. This may be accomplished by randomization within specified age, sex, or other subgroups, separate rosters being kept for each of the subgroups considered important. The randomization within each subgroup may be restricted (prior to the assignment of individuals) so as to equalize the numbers of study and control individuals. This procedure is known as *blocking,* in the terminology of experimental design. In addition to assuring closer comparability of the study and control groups, blocking increases the efficiency of the statistical analysis.

*Selection of Participating Groups or Communities*

Some preventive measures can be applied only to groups, or on a community-wide basis, even though the individuals constituting the community are the target of the measure. Fluoridation of public water supplies and changing the milieu in mental hospitals are examples. In such situations, individuals cannot be randomized to study and control groups. In the case of measures such as fluoridation, which can be practically applied only to large communities, two communities as similar as possible—particularly with respect to frequency and characteristics of the disease to be prevented—may be selected. One of them is then arbitrarily or randomly chosen to provide the study group and the other the control. Even though each community consists of many individuals, and subsequent difference in rates of outcome may be statistically highly significant on this account, such a study is in one sense a study of only two individuals—a single case and a control. Even though the two individuals (communities) were very similar at the beginning of the study, something might readily happen by chance in one but not in the other—unknown to the investigator—and confound the results of the experiment. Confidence that such an extraneous change did not occur may be high if the outcome is one, like dental caries, that does not usually vary in frequency over short periods of time. Even so, the results of several such trials, or a great deal of collateral supporting evidence, will usually be required before the evaluation is considered conclusive. When the disease to be prevented is one that does fluctuate in frequency from time to time and place to place, this design is to be avoided if at all possible.

There are some examples of trials in which a number of relatively small communities have been randomly assigned to study and control groups. For example, in a comparison of three different regimens for poliomyelitis vaccination, the 74 administrative subdivisions of the Swiss canton of Basel-land were allocated at random into three groups [355]. In such a procedure it is essential to evaluate similarities and dissimilarities between the populations assigned to the groups to be compared. In this instance it was ascertained that the administrative subdivisions allocated to each of the three groups were distributed throughout the canton, that they contained similar proportions of large and small communities and of urban and rural areas, and that the persons immunized included similar proportions with poliomyelitis antibodies prior to the immunization. Such comparisons of study and control groups are, of course, a necessary safeguard in all experimental studies, whatever the process of randomization, but one is particularly concerned that significant differences may be present if the number of units randomized was small.

For a more detailed account of methods of selection and assignment of individuals to study and control groups—as well as many other aspects of intervention studies—the reader is referred to a useful manual prepared under the auspices of the World Health Organization [327].

## STUDY AND CONTROL PROGRAMS

### The Study Program

In an experiment on a human population, the total program *offered* to the individuals randomized to the study group is what is evaluated. A specific preventive measure, even if it is the sole component of the program, is tested only indirectly. Suppose, for example, that it is desired to evaluate the effect of regular physical exercise in the prevention of coronary vascular disease. A program of exercise may be offered to the individuals selected for the study group but not to the controls. If no difference is found in coronary disease rates between the study and control groups, it can be concluded that the offering of a program of physical exercise in the manner in which this was done in the study is not protective against coronary disease. It cannot be concluded that physical exercise does not protect against coronary disease, since it may be that nobody in the study group followed the offered regimen. On the other hand, if a majority of the study group followed the prescribed program and the group experienced a lower disease rate than the control group, it is a reasonable implication that the reduced disease rate is a consequence of the physical exercise.

Even though individuals' agreements to participate in an experiment are obtained prior to their allocation to study or control groups, it will almost invariably happen that certain members of the study group do not undergo the procedure under test. Individuals may leave the population prior to initiation of the program, they may dislike the program when they try it, or they may simply change their minds. The effects of such losses are similar to those of misclassification in case-control studies (p. 263): they will not introduce spurious differences between study and control groups, but they may conceal a real effect of the specific measure under test. If extent of conformity to the offered program can be measured, estimates can be made of the extent to which real differences between those receiving and not receiving the measure will be reflected in differences between the study and control groups (see p. 263).

*The Control Program*

The program offered to the individuals selected for the control group cannot be *no* program. At least, the controls must have free access to the facilities normally available to the community in which they reside. This means that, just as certain members of the study group may not receive a vaccine or other test procedure, some members of the control group may receive it through channels other than the study program. The effects of this on the study results are similar to those of lack of involvement in the study program by members of the study group, as described in the preceding section. Both problems are in fact problems of misclassification, as discussed in Chapter 12. The extent of misclassification in an experimental study will be highly related to the length of time that study group members and controls are expected to adhere to the program, as well as to what is expected of them. Even if the duration of the study has been explained at the beginning, an increasing proportion of study group members can be expected to drop out as time passes, and an increasing proportion of the controls will receive the study program through other mechanisms. Even when participation involves only three administrations of vaccine separated by monthly intervals, a substantial number of dropouts may occur [243, 355]. The duration of adherence to the program that would be necessary is a major difficulty in the implementation of such intervention studies in the field of coronary artery disease as can be devised on the basis of present knowledge [285].

Preferably the program offered to the control group will offer benefits beyond those available in the community generally. This may be another vaccine or dietary supplement, for example, or free medical supervision. The first Medical Research Council trial of pertussis vaccine, already referred to, was followed by a study in which participants were randomized to receive vaccine from different manufacturers, there being no unvaccinated group. The trial showed significant differences in attack rates among children receiving different vaccines [244]. In addition to removing a burden from the investigator's conscience, the possibility that benefit can be offered to both study and control groups will encourage continued participation of individuals, and hence facilitate follow-up.

## ASCERTAINMENT OF OUTCOME

Ascertainment of outcome in study and control groups may require relatively short follow-up—as with the determination of disease incidence in the few months following administration of a vaccine—or it may require many years of follow-up with physical examination of the participants—as with attempts to lower rates of coronary artery disease by diet manipulation. Naturally the difficulties increase considerably as the necessary length of follow-up increases. The problems of follow-up are similar to those discussed in connection with cohort studies (pp. 214 to 221).

Even more important than measures taken to achieve as complete a follow-up as possible are those designed to insure that bias is not introduced by more complete or more accurate ascertainment of outcome in one or the other of the groups to be compared. This is most convincingly achieved by having those responsible for the ascertainment of outcome remain unaware of whether they are dealing with a member of the study group or a control—so-called *blind assessment* (see p. 290). When the ascertainment involves contact with the participants—physical examination of them, for example—blind assessment will usually be possible only when the participants themselves are also unaware as to the group to which they have been assigned—that is, when the assignment has also been blind. Other procedures used to prevent bias in ascertainment of outcome include the use of material such as x-ray photographs and sera, which can be examined by different examiners without knowledge of their source.

## Selection of Outcome

Even in the relatively simple situation in which a vaccine against a specific disease is being tested, there is usually more than one outcome that can be assessed. Thus one may be concerned not only with the frequency of occurrence of the specific disease in the compared groups but also with its severity and frequency of complications or death. Since a change in any one of these outcomes may have public health significance, it is not necessary to single out any one of them as *the* criterion of success or failure of the preventive measure.

However, it is always necessary to consider whether the particular outcome assessed does reflect the real preventive significance of the program. For example, a difference between two groups or communities in rates of utilization of mental hospital inpatient facilities may or may not reflect a difference in frequency of mental illness; an intervention program could conceivably change the patterns of use of facilities without changing the disease frequency, and one must ask whether the change in use of facilities (if this is the outcome being assessed) is in itself an adequate measure of the utility of the program.

Programs aimed at the prevention of morbidity and mortality from cancer by means of early detection and treatment offer special difficulties in this regard. If one group of persons is receiving periodic screening examinations and another is not, it will be extremely difficult to interpret differences between them in rates of incidence of new cases. The fact that survival rates for treated cases in the screened population are better than those in cases in the unscreened population does not indicate that the program is reducing morbidity and mortality—it may merely reflect the fact that cases are diagnosed earlier in the course of the disease in the screened population and that the average interval from diagnosis to death is therefore longer. Some of the problems involved in assessing the extent to which earlier cases may be being detected, and what implications this may have to the cancer frequency rates observed in an early-detection program, are discussed by Hutchison and Shapiro [175]. The definitive measure of effectiveness of such a program is, of course, a difference between the study and control populations in the mortality rates from the particular cancer.


## Sequential Designs

In most preventive intervention studies, a predetermined number of individuals is assigned to study and control groups and then outcomes are compared, usually after all the individuals to be included in the trial have been assigned to one or the other group. In a situation in which individuals are assigned to groups over an extended period of time, and the outcome for those assigned early in the study becomes known while other individuals are still being assigned, the design poses the dilemma that, although significant beneficial results may be obtained before all the individuals have been assigned, the double-blind design continues to conceal the significant result. Controls may therefore be unnecessarily jeopardized by being denied an effective measure. Conversely, if the measure under test is harmful rather than beneficial, this may not be revealed until unnecessary damage has been done.

To overcome these difficulties, the method of sequential design has been developed. In this design the data are continuously analyzed as the outcomes become known, and the trial is interrupted as soon as statistical significance is obtained in one direction or the other. There is no predetermined group size. This does not necessarily conflict with the use of double-blind procedures, because the decision to stop the trial can be made by an investigator who is not participating in the clinical work but makes his decision on the basis of results submitted to him sequentially.

The particular circumstances that make sequential methods appropriate (that is, that knowledge of outcome is obtained concurrently as new participants are admitted to the trial) have so far been found more often in trials of therapeutic than of preventive procedures.

The methods of sequential experimentation are described in some detail by Armitage [16].

## ANALYSIS

The considerations that enter into the analysis of intervention studies are in many ways similar to those discussed in connection with the analysis of cohort studies (pp. 226 to 235), and these should be kept in mind in the present context.

Referring to Figure 33, one might, in the analysis of results, be tempted to compare individuals in box (1) with those in box (5)—that is, persons who received the study program with those who received the control program, and for whom the outcome is known. However, these individuals represent only a part of the total population that was assigned to study and control groups, and it is the groups assigned by randomization that are truly comparable—that is, the sum of boxes (1) through (4) and of (5) through (8).

There may be no choice with respect to omission from the analysis of individuals for whom outcome is unknown, but a careful comparison of individuals in boxes (2) and (4) with those in (6) and (8) is necessary. Differences between study and control populations in the proportions of individuals with unknown outcome, or in the characteristics of such individuals, may seriously reflect on the comparability of those for whom outcome is known.

There is a choice, however, with regard to deciding between comparison of (1) with (5), or (1) + (3) with (5) + (7). The latter is the more correct comparison, in that the groups compared approach more closely the total groups selected by randomization. The problem of dilution of the effect of the preventive measure by misclassification of the participants has been referred to (pp. 293 and 294). If it is quite certain that the likelihood of, and the reasons for, controls not receiving the control program are the same as those for the study group—as it may be, for example, under the conditions of a blind-assignment vaccine trial—then a more accurate estimate of the size of the beneficial effect of the preventive measure *may* be obtained by comparison of (1) with (5). Such conditions are unusual, however, and under all circumstances the comparison most essential to the demonstration of a difference with potential for a program of prevention is of (1) + (3) with.(5) + (7).

The problem described in the last paragraph is particularly evident when there is an opportunity for one group (usually the study group) to refuse the program and not for the other. For example, to evaluate the effectiveness of screening for breast cancer, two stratified random samples of 30,000 women were selected from among the enrollees of the Health Insurance Plan of Greater New York [363, 364]. One sample, the study group, was offered a special program of repeated screening examinations. The other sample, the control group, received the normal medical care available to all enrollees in the insurance plan. Some of the women selected for the study group refused to participate, and others will drop out of the program as time passes. Nevertheless, in evaluating the effectiveness of the program it will be necessary to compare the control group with *all* the women selected for the study group, whether or not they participated in the program.

# 14

Genetics and Epidemiology

Human genetics and epidemiology have much in common. Genes, being a major determinant of disease frequency and distribution, must be considered in the development of any hypothesis proposed to explain epidemiologic observations. There is, in addition, overlap in methodology of the two sciences, in that both depend on the collection of data dealing with the frequency of disease in man and both draw heavily on the application of statistics and mathematics to the analysis of patterns of disease distribution. Lastly, there are certain kinds of study (for example, twin studies) and certain variables (for example, birth order) that are of interest to workers in both disciplines. Indeed, since one usually does not know, at the beginning of the investigation of a disease, whether its determinants will turn out to be heritable, one frequently cannot decide a priori whether a disease would be more appropriately investigated by epidemiologists or geneticists.

In this chapter we will describe some of the ways in which genetic and environmental disease determinants interact and some of the kinds of study that are commonly undertaken to elucidate their relative roles.

## GENE AND ENVIRONMENT

At first sight the dichotomy between gene and environment seems simple and unequivocal: genes are factors transmitted in the chromosomes received from one's parents; the environment consists of the things to which one is exposed after conception. With the growth of knowledge, however, this dichotomy becomes less and less clear.

## Interaction of Genes and Environment

No disease is determined solely by either gene or environment —any more than any disease is determined by a single cause.

In 1933 Hogben [167] illustrated a simple instance of gene-environment interaction by reference to yellow shanks—a characteristic occurring in certain strains of fowl when fed yellow corn. He noted that a farmer using only yellow corn as feed and owning several strains of fowl would observe the trait only in certain strains; he would therefore regard it as genetically determined. Another farmer owning only a genetically susceptible strain of fowl, and feeding some of them on yellow and some on white corn, would note that the trait appeared only in those fed yellow corn; he would conclude that the condition was environmentally determined. Thus this trait cannot accurately be described as either genetic or environmental; within a certain range of genetic background environmental factors determine its occurrence, and within a certain range of environmental conditions the trait is genetically determined.

Phenylketonuria and the consequences of certain other metabolic errors dependent on single major genes now provide quite comparable models in man. Within our present environment, in which phenylalanine is a universal component of the diet, phenylketonuria behaves as a purely genetic trait, dependent on a single autosomal recessive gene. However, in a population homozygous for the recessive allele and having a diet in which phenylalanine might or might not be present, the occurrence of phenylketonuria would be determined by the environment— the level of phenylalanine in the diet. Indeed, this is how phenylketonuria is treated—by provision of an *environment* (phenylalanine-free diet) that does not allow the expression of the genetic potential of susceptible individuals. Thus the characterization of phenylketonuria as a genetic trait holds only within the particular limits of our environment. While environmental limits have not been identified for most of the human diseases that we now regard as genetic, this does not mean that they do not exist. Twenty years ago there was nothing to distinguish phenylketonuria from hundreds of other genetic diseases in this respect. The issue is not whether environmental factors are involved, but whether they have been identified and whether they are alterable. Similarly, genetic factors—so far largely unidentified—are without doubt involved as etiologic factors in infections and other diseases now regarded as environmental. Rather than ask whether a disease is determined by genes or environment, one should inquire as to the limits and characteristics of the disease-producing factors of each kind.

While both gene and environment enter into the determination of the disease as a whole, particular features—familial incidence or seasonal variation of a disease, for example—are often explained in terms of one or the other type of factor. And so one can ask to what extent particular *patterns* of disease frequency are attributable to environmental or genetic factors. Yellow shanks is determined by both genetic and environmental factors, but the fact that it occurs only in fowl fed yellow corn is explained in environmental terms alone. Analogously, certain diseases tend to occur in several members of a family; the question that follows from this observation is not whether or not the disease may be genetic, but rather to what extent the familial recurrence is due to the repetition of specific gene combinations in families, and to what extent to shared environmental factors.

Very complex gene-environment interactions have been uncovered in experimental research on cancer. The effects of carcinogenic viruses, chemicals, and physical agents are specific for species, strain, and sometimes sex. Viruses that cause mild diseases in one species produce cancer in others. In species in which specific tumors usually occur in almost all animals, the disease can be almost eliminated by environmental manipulation. These environmental modifications are also strain-specific—for example, removal of the thymus will protect certain strains of mice against radiation-induced leukemia, but will not protect other strains. As perhaps the ultimate in intimacy of gene-environment relations, there are examples of tumors resulting from the incorporation of virus particles into the host genetic structure in a relationship so intimate that what was formerly environment can no longer be distinguished from what is now gene.

## *Time of Action of Genetic and Environmental Agents*

The distinction between genetic and environmental agents is basically one of the time at which the agent exerted its effect, for the individual's genotype is itself the end result of his ancestors' accumulated environments—those which induced mutations, as well as those which selectively determined which mutants would survive. Again, as knowledge accumulates, the dichotomy becomes less clear. For example, those cases of Down's syndrome due to trisomy involving group G chromosomes (numbers 21 and 22) are clearly due to a defect with a genetic basis. Yet manifest genetic damage may not occur until the final stages of the meiotic divisions of the oocyte, around the time of ovulation and fertilization, or perhaps even during one of the earliest divisions of the fertilized ovum that subsequently developed into the affected child. If an environmental factor is responsible, as is suggested by the association of this disease with maternal age, it may be a factor active around the time of ovulation and fertilization, or it may be something to which the mother was exposed earlier in her life but which did not exert its effect until this time. Whichever the case, it is clear that the environment at the time of ovulation and fertilization may have an important influence on the genotype of the conceptus. Thus there is the possibility of environmental determination of an individual's genotype in the days immediately prior to his conception, or even after his conception.

The occurrence of genetic mosaicism and of a variety of chromosomally aberrant cells in adults shows that genetic change takes place throughout the life of an individual. Those mutations which become incorporated into the individual's own germ cells are called genetic, and those which do not are called somatic. The distinction is, of course, crucial from the point of view of the individual's descendants. From the point of view of the individual himself, however, a somatic mutation occurring in, say, a stem cell in his bone marrow may also have significant health implications.

## Mechanisms of Action of Genetic and Environmental Agents

In the previous section the point of view was presented that environmental agents (mutagens) may produce their effects through genetic mechanisms (transmission of mutant genes). Some examples of the reverse process are now being identified in man. Thus pregnancies have been reported in women with unrecognized phenylketonuria. Phenylalanine crosses the placenta, and high maternal blood levels produce mental retardation in the child, regardless of its genotype. Here, then, is a defect which is determined by the environment of the child but is highly dependent on the genotype of another person who is providing that environment. Similarly Rh incompatibility is a condition affecting the fetus but highly dependent on the genotype of the mother. While the genotype of the fetus is also a factor in this condition, the "susceptible" genotype is so common that the variation in frequency of the disease is much more dependent on the genotype of the mother than on that of the fetus. Similar possibilities—in the area of behavioral rather than chemical or immunologic factors—seem worthy of investigation in the field of mental illness [222].

## Implications

The foregoing discussion pointing to the complexity of the relations between gene and environment is not intended to discourage attempts to distinguish genetic from environmental causes of disease. It may indeed be important to determine whether a particular disease pattern results from genetic or environmental factors. For example, it will usually be very helpful to the epidemiologist to know whether the familial occurrence of a particular disease is likely to have a genetic or an environmental explanation. If the former, then he may choose to disregard the familial pattern in forming his own hypotheses, regarding it as evidence of variation in genetic susceptibility to whatever environmental factors are involved in the etiology of the disease. If, on the other hand, the familial pattern seems likely to have an environmental explanation, the tendency to recur or persist in families might be a characteristic to be considered in developing hypotheses as to what specific environmental factors may be involved.

Recognition of the existence of the types of gene-environment relationship illustrated by phenylketonuria is important also for the reason that it may forestall the pessimism that might otherwise lead to abandonment of the search for environmental causes of diseases that appear on the surface to be determined solely by genetic factors.


## FAMILIAL DISEASE

Diseases that are most commonly investigated by both geneticists and epidemiologists include those that exhibit a tendency to familial recurrence but in which the pattern does not fit clearly into any specific genetic model. Most of the common congenital malformations and many other diseases of early infancy are in this category, and many diseases of adult life show similar patterns. As already noted, the question of interest deals with the extent to which the familial occurrence may be explained by genetic susceptibility and the extent to which it may be due to some environmental factor that persists or recurs in particular families.

The question is approached both by investigating the characteristics of the familial pattern itself and by searching for other evidence of genetic or environmental determination. Other evidence of the existence of etiologic factors of one type or the other does not necessarily imply that the familial pattern results from those factors, but the nature of the identified factors may suggest whether or not it is likely that they could produce familial recurrence.

### Familial Patterns

The investigation of familial disease patterns may be technically quite complex, and its consideration makes up much of the material in textbooks of genetic methodology [290, 382]. In general, if the familial pattern of a disease is found to conform to the pattern expected for a single major gene, this may be taken as strong evidence that it is in fact genetically determined. Failure to identify a simple genetic hypothesis compatible with the familial pattern does not rule out its genetic determination, but does suggest that environmental explanations may be sought with profit. Similarly a high familial recurrence rate need not be attributed to genetic factors unless accompanied by other evidence of genetic etiology—for example, high concordance rates in monozygous twins.

In general, in investigating family histories the epidemiologist will be interested in kinds of observation similar to those that concern the geneticist—comparisons of persons in various levels of relationship to the proband (index case), of rates in maternal and paternal relatives, of rates by sex in relation to sex of the proband, and so on. However, there is one relation that may be of particular interest to the epidemiologist, especially in investigating diseases of early life. This is the incidence of a disease in half-siblings of affected individuals, and, in particular, in half-siblings who have their mother in common with the proband. A high frequency in this group of the same disease manifested by the proband is of special interest because the mother is such an important component of the fetal and infant environment. The finding of an incidence in half-siblings as high, or almost as high, as that in full siblings is compatible with genetic explanations, but the kind of genetic hypotheses that must be invoked to explain such an observation—specifically, those calling on single dominant genes—are such that they can usually be readily either supported or ruled out on the basis of other kinds of evidence.

## Time Clustering Within Families

In examining the possibility of environmental explanations of a familial pattern, it is useful to determine whether there is any clustering in time of the familial cases. The most obvious instances of this are of course in the childhood infectious diseases. The explanation of the high familial incidence of these diseases is made obvious by the close temporal relationship between primary and secondary cases. However, the examination of time relationships may also be useful in other contexts. For example, Table 40 shows the incidence of congenital neural tube defects in siblings according to the interval since the birth of the first affected child in the family. The risk decreases as the

Table 40

Prevalence of neural tube defects in siblings of affected
infants according to interval since birth of the first
affected, Rhode Island, 1936 to 1967*

| Interval (months) | Number of siblings | Number of siblings affected | Percent of siblings affected |
|---|---|---|---|
| <18 | 210 | 13 | 6.2 |
| 18–35 | 307 | 14 | 4.6 |
| 36–59 | 296 | 16 | 5.4 |
| 60–119 | 327 | 12 | 3.7 |
| 120 + | 121 | 3 | 2.5 |
| *Total* | 1261 | 58 | 4.6 |

* From Yen and MacMahon [430].
$\chi^2$ for linear trend = 2.7, degrees of freedom = 1, $P \sim 0.1$.

interval becomes longer. The trend is not statistically significant in these data, but if such a trend were confirmed by additional observations it would suggest environmental rather than genetic determination of the familial risk, since the genetic risk should remain constant for all offspring of the same parents whereas an environmental factor might well vary over time.

Similarly it may be possible to discriminate whether familial concentration results from genetic or environmental similarities by comparing cases within families according to their age at, and the chronologic time of, onset. In a genetic disease with a tendency for onset at a particular age, one would expect affected siblings to develop the disease at similar ages (after allowing for chance fluctuations), and one would not expect the chronologic time of onset to be similar except insofar as siblings tend to reach similar ages within a few years of each other. On the other hand, an environmental factor producing familial concentration, particularly an infectious agent, might produce onsets at similar times regardless of the ages of the siblings. Thus greater similarity in time of onset than in age at onset suggests an environmental interpretation. Lack of similarity in time of onset does not rule out environmental interpretation but it implies that if there is a responsible environment it must be one that is not limited to a short time period. This method of analysis has been applied in attempts to clarify the familial nature of Hodgkin's disease [221] and of multiple sclerosis [354].

When a disease shows other characteristics in addition to familial recurrence, it is useful to examine the familial incidence in relation to those characteristics. For example, in the same study referred to in Table 40, rates of familial recurrence were examined in different time periods, because it had been observed that incidence of neural tube defects as a whole had decreased markedly during the study period (Table 41). The fact

Table 41

Prevalence of neural tube defects in siblings of affected infants and in the general population, according to year of birth, Rhode Island, 1936 to 1967*

| Year of birth | Number of siblings | Number of siblings affected | Percent of siblings affected | Percent of general population affected |
|---|---|---|---|---|
| 1936–45 | 186 | 16 | 8.6 | 0.53 |
| 1946–50 | 291 | 17 | 5.8 | 0.41 |
| 1951–55 | 281 | 9 | 3.2 | 0.29 |
| 1956–60 | 246 | 8 | 3.3 | 0.19 |
| 1961–67 | 253 | 8 | 3.3 | 0.19 |

* From Yen and MacMahon [430].
$\chi^2$ for linear trend in siblings $= 8.4$, degrees of freedom $= 1$, $P < 0.01$.

that the risk of familial recurrence declined over the period to an extent quite comparable to the trend in the population as a whole implies that the familial risk is environmentally determined. Alternative explanations are possible—for example, that the trend in familial cases may be due to a change in the frequency of factors necessary for the expression of a genetic potential, the latter having remained constant—but the decline in familial risk indicates at least that the environmental factors responsible for the general decline also have relevance to the occurrence of familial cases.

## TWIN STUDIES

### Comparisons of Monozygotic and Dizygotic Twins

Twin studies provide the single most powerful method of detecting genetic etiology in human disease. The basic premise of classical twin studies is that monozygotic twins, being formed by the division of a single fertilized ovum, carry identical genes, while dizygotic twins, being formed by the fertilization of two ova by two different spermatozoa, are genetically no more similar than two siblings born after separate pregnancies. More frequent similarity with respect to the presence (or absence) of a disease or trait (called *concordance*) between the members of monozygotic pairs than between the members of dizygotic pairs is therefore evidence of the existence of a genetic component in the etiology of the trait.

PROBLEMS IN METHODOLOGY. Before coming to the conclusion that monozygotic sets are concordant for a particular disease more frequently than dizygotic sets, the possibility of biases in studies which suggest such a difference must be considered. Two biases are most common:

1. Errors in the ascertainment of zygosity. Most early twin studies, and many recent ones, have used less than adequate criteria of zygosity. The ascertainment of zygosity is not easy; accounts of the different methods and of their reliability are given by Neel and Schull [290] and Stern [382]. At the present time, blood groups and dermatoglyphics provide the most reliable information. Of particular interest—since it suggests the possibility of assembling far larger series of twins than have been customary in the past—are recent studies [50, 179] indicating that reasonably reliable information on zygosity can be obtained by mail questionnaire to the twins themselves.

It is important to realize that, in general, inaccurate ascertainment of zygosity tends to bias in the direction of concordant twins being considered as monozygotic and discordant pairs as dizygotic. First, the trait itself—for example, a physical or mental characteristic—if present in both twins may tend to make the twins, their relatives, or the investigator think of them as "similar," and therefore monozygotic. Second, if the concordance is due to similar environments rather than similar genes, the environmental similarity of concordant pairs may also tend to produce concordance with respect to characteristics that are being used to determine zygosity.

2. Bias in assembly of the study series. Inferences about the frequency of concordance in monozygotic and dizygotic sets are sometimes made from "series" of twins assembled from case reports published in the medical literature. In such reviews the fact that zygosity and concordance both influence the likelihood of publication of a twin set must be considered. Thus, up to 1953 there had been reported in the literature 47 sets of twins in which at least one member had pyloric stenosis of infancy; 12 of the 18 monozygotic sets were reported as concordant, in contrast to only 1 of the 29 dizygotic sets [248]. These data would suggest that the concordance rate of monozygotic sets is quite high, and certainly higher than that of dizygotic sets. However, in a study in 1955 [225] of 3982 consecutive cases of pyloric stenosis, there were 87 patients who were twins, and only 6 concordant pairs. Analysis of this series suggested that the concordance rate was quite low for both kinds of twin, and that the rate for monozygotic sets was little, if any, higher than that for dizygotic. It thus seemed clear that affected monozygotic twins were much more likely to be reported in the literature if they were concordant than if they were discordant. Similar biases in ascertainment may exist within a single series if the series does not include all affected sets in a defined population.

PROBLEMS IN INTERPRETATION. Even if there is a real difference in the concordance rates between monozygotic and dizygotic sets, one can not conclude that it necessarily reflects the existence of genetic etiology. Besides greater similarity of genes, members of monozygotic twin pairs may share more similar environments than do members of dizygotic pairs. In fetal life, closer placental relations and frequent anastomoses of placental vessels may lead to greater similarity in exposures to substances that must traverse the placenta to affect the fetus. Such close relations, however, may also lead to a competitive intrauterine situation. For example, monochorial monozygotic pairs (whose placental arrangement is such that vascular communication between the two members of the pair is commonly, if not invariably, present) have larger intrapair relative birth weight differences than dichorial pairs as early as the 24th week of gestation [267]. In this connection it is important to recall that about two-thirds of all monozygotic pairs are monochorial [26], whereas all dizygotic pairs are dichorial. A detailed consideration of the bias that may arise in twin studies as a result of these differences has been given by Price [330].

Postnatally, if the twins are of the same sex and look alike, the parents may make a ritual of dressing, feeding, and in other ways treating them similarly, while the dissimilarity of dizygotic twins may be the feature that is noted and developed, consciously or subconsciously. On the other hand, if the twins are markedly different in birth weight—as would happen more frequently in monozygotic sets—preferential, or different, treatment might be given to the lighter twin. Monozygotic twins themselves may also tend to choose more similar diets and other environmental experiences than do dizygotic sets.

For conditions that may produce death in fetal life—for example, serious malformations—the possibility that concordant sets may be aborted more frequently than discordant sets and that this may affect monozygotic more frequently than dizygotic sets must be evaluated. This particular set of circumstances would tend to reduce the concordance rate for monozygotic sets.

### Statistical Assessment of Zygosity

The determination of the zygosity of each set of twins in a study series may be impractical. For example, if the disease is one of high fatality the series must be assembled prospectively, since information rarely is available in routine records that would allow diagnosis of the zygosity of a twin set in which one member is deceased.

In such circumstances, however, inferences can be made from the sexes of the twin sets as to the frequency of the two types of twins in a series, even if the zygosity of the individual pairs is unknown. This method depends on the fact that, since sex is genetically determined, all monozygotic pairs must be of like sex, and the recognition that the proportion of like-sex sets observed in unselected series of human twins is in excess of that which would be expected if all the like-sex sets were dizygotic. If $p$ is the frequency of a male and $q$ the frequency of a female and both values are taken as 0.5 in an unselected population of births, the relative frequencies of dizygotic MM, MF, and FF pairs would be expected to be $p^2$, $2pq$, and $q^2$, which gives a ratio of 1:2:1. In other words, there should be equal numbers of like-sex and unlike-sex pairs if all the pairs are dizygotic. The excess in the number of like-sex pairs over the number of unlike-sex pairs can, then, be used as an estimate of the number of monozygotic pairs. It is an easy arithmetic maneuver, therefore, to estimate the number of monozygotic sets in a series of twins simply by subtracting the number of unlike-sex pairs from the total number of like-sex pairs and to estimate the total number of dizygotic sets by multiplying the number of unlike-sex sets by two. This method is attributed to Weinberg [412].

Take, for example, the series of twins shown in Table 42.

### Table 42
Distribution of 261 sets of twins in which at least one
member had anencephaly or spina bifida*

| Sex | Number affected | | Total |
| | One | Both | |
| --- | --- | --- | --- |
| Like | 164 | 10 | 174 |
| Unlike | 84 | 3 | 87 |
| *Total* | 248 | 13 | 261 |

* Sources: Gittelsohn and Milham [128], Horowitz and McDonald [169], Stevenson et al. [383], and Yen and MacMahon [430].

This was assembled from published reports of consecutive series of infants with congenital neural tube defects. Isolated reports of single twin sets were excluded to reduce the reporting bias referred to earlier. No information on zygosity was available for any of these sets. However, 87 of the 261 sets were reported as being of unlike sex and 174 as of like sex. If the unlike-sex sets constitute half the dizygotic sets, then the series contains about 174 dizygotic sets, of which at least 3 (the MF pairs), and more likely 6 (2 × 3), were concordant. The number of monozygotic sets is estimated as 87 (174 — 87), of which at most 10, and more probably 7 (10 — 3), were concordant. The estimates of concordance rates are then 7 of 87 monozygotic sets and 6 of 174 dizygotic sets. Thus the concordance rate of monozygotic sets appears to be relatively low, particularly in the light of a significant occurrence of concordance in dizygotic sets. This observation should lead to suspicion of the existence of important environmental etiologic factors.

In such calculations $p$ and $q$ refer to the frequencies of males and females in the population of births, and are therefore, to all intents and purposes, always 0.5. The fact that a disease affects predominantly one sex or other will change the ratio of MM to FF sets and the frequency with which the male or female is affected in MF sets. However, except in the most extreme circumstances, the ratio of like-sex to unlike-sex pairs among all affected sets will be changed only slightly. For example, in a disease that affects one sex four times as frequently as the other, the unlike-sex pairs will constitute 53 percent, rather than 50 percent, of the total affected dizygotic sets. On the other hand, among concordant sets the ratio will be changed more markedly. For example, in the same disease, concordant unlike-sex sets would comprise only 32 percent of the concordant dizygotic sets. Estimates of the effect of such sex differences in disease incidence can be made by considering the rates for the two sexes in the disease under investigation and computing the likelihood of no, one, or both members of twin pairs of each sex distribution being affected. For neural tube defects—the disease considered in Table 42—a rate for females twice as high as that for males would be the maximum difference in sex ratio that is likely to pertain. Such a difference would give 51 percent of all affected dizygotic sets, and 44 percent of concordant dizygotic sets, being of unlike sex. In light of the numbers of sets available, 50 percent is a reasonable figure for all practical purposes in both instances.

In applying this method to diseases that do not become manifest until some time after birth, account must be taken of the fact that in some sets both twins may not have been at risk for similar lengths of time because of earlier death of one twin, or for other reasons. Sets in which both members did not survive the period of risk for reasons other than the disease under investigation would normally be excluded.

## Studies of Discordant Monozygotic Sets

Since the members of a monozygotic pair are genetically identical, any manifestational differences between them must be due to differences in environmental experiences. Comparison of the environments of the individuals in discordant sets might, therefore, identify factors of etiologic significance. There are two possible approaches. One is to select monozygotic twins that are discordant with respect to a trait or disease of unknown etiology and search for dissimilarities of environment. This approach (comparable to a case-control study) has been followed by a number of investigators in studying instances of twins discordant for mental illness. In one study of 11 monozygotic pairs discordant for schizophrenia [326], it was found that the schizophrenic twin had the lower birth weight in all the sets and a number of other features of the life course were consistently different between the schizophrenic and the nonschizophrenic twin.

The other approach (comparable to a cohort study) is to select monozygotic twins that are discordant with respect to some environmental factor and then determine whether there are differences in the diseases they manifest. Examples of this approach are the studies by Newman et al. [297] and Shields [368] of monozygotic twins reared apart. Opportunities for studying twins reared apart are of course relatively few. Interesting recent examples of the general approach are the studies of Swedish [51] and American [49] twins in which symptoms of coronary and pulmonary disease have been studied in monozygotic sets in which one member had a high and the other a low tobacco-smoking exposure (Table 43).

## Characteristics of Twins

The studies described above exploit the genetic similarity of monozygotic twins. Other studies of twins are based on the fact that being a twin is itself an experience that may have its own effects. In most studies differences have not been found between disease rates in twins and those in persons born of single pregnancy, except for diseases consequent to prematurity or the spe-

Table 43

Prevalence of certain symptoms in monozygotic twins
discordant for smoking habits*

| Symptom | Percent of low-exposure twins affected | Percent of high-exposure twins affected |
|---|---|---|
| Bronchitis | 3.2 | 7.7 |
| Prolonged cough | 4.3 | 9.5 |
| Cough | 6.1 | 15.0 |
| Angina pectoris | 4.6 | 4.9 |
| Severe chest pain | 3.9 | 4.9 |

* From Cederlöf et al. [49].

cial dangers of delivery. Nevertheless there is no doubt that the environment of twins is unusual in many respects (Fig. 34).

The method of determining whether twins experience an abnormally high frequency of a particular disease has usually been to assemble a large series of cases of the disease, note how many of the affected were twins, and compare the observed number of twins with an expected number. The frequency of twin confinements among white births in the United States is approximately 1 percent; among newborn white infants the proportion of twins is therefore approximately 2 percent, since each twin confinement yields two infants. In such estimates the substantial ethnic and geographic variation in rates of twinning—affecting dizygotic twins predominantly—must be considered. Adjustment for birth order and maternal age may also be necessary, since the frequency of twins is influenced by these variables. The prenatal and early infant mortality of twins is higher than that of single births, and adjustment may be required for the mortality likely to have occurred prior to the age at which the disease under study makes its appearance.

*Twin Registries*

The variety and uniqueness of the contributions that studies of twins can make to epidemiologic and genetic knowledge has led to the establishment of registries of twins in several countries. The role of these registries and the potential value of in-

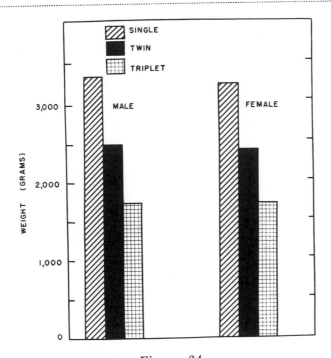

### Figure 34

Median birth weight of livebirths from single, twin, and triplet pregnancies, by sex; United States, white births, 1967. (From *Vital Statistics of the United States* [278].)

ternational collaboration to overcome the practical problems, such as the infrequency of twins with particular diseases, has been described by a study group assembled by the World Health Organization [425].

## BIRTH ORDER

In theory, parental genes are distributed to their offspring independently of the order of birth in the sibship. Association of a disease with order of birth should therefore be clear evidence at least of the existence of an environmental component to its etiology, even if the explanation of the association is not readily apparent.

There are two general methods of examining for birth order associations. One is the usual case-control approach, in which order of birth is the "exposure" being investigated (see Chap. 12). Care must be taken, in the selection of controls and in the analysis, to allow for the close association of birth order with such variables as socioeconomic status, age of mother, and year of birth. While association with any of these variables may equally be regarded as evidence of environmental determination, they must nevertheless be taken into account if an effect intrinsic to birth order is being sought. The case-control method is the method of choice for studies of illnesses of infancy or childhood that are undertaken within a short time of the events being studied, because the alternative approach (the Greenwood-Yule method) requires that the sibships containing affected individuals be completed.

## Method of Greenwood and Yule

The method of Greenwood and Yule [136] is to compare the observed distribution of affected individuals by birth order with the distribution that would be expected if an affected individual had an equal probability of being born in each of the birth orders represented in his sibship. The expected distribution will, of course, depend on the number of birth orders in the sibship—that is, on the size of the sibship. The information required, therefore, is the total eventual size of the sibships into which the patients were born, and the patients' own birth orders.

For example, the data shown in Table 44 are taken from a study by Norton [300] of 2500 patients with neurosis. The information necessary for the calculation of the expected distribution is the distribution by size of sibship, shown in the right-hand column of the table. The calculation, in which the data for each sibship size are considered separately, is shown in Table 45. The 226 affected individuals who had no siblings are obviously all first births. In a condition randomly distributed by birth order, the 358 affected individuals who came from sibships of size two would be expected to be half (179) first births and half (179) second births. Similarly the 374 affected individuals in sibships of size three would be expected to be represented equally in the first, second, and third birth orders. Thus the expected distribution by birth order is calculated for each sibship

## Table 44

### Distribution of 2500 patients with neurosis according to birth order and size of sibship*

| Size of sibship | Birth order of patient | | | | | | | | | | | | | | | | | Total |
|---|---|---|---|---|---|---|---|---|---|---|---|---|---|---|---|---|---|---|
| | 1 | 2 | 3 | 4 | 5 | 6 | 7 | 8 | 9 | 10 | 11 | 12 | 13 | 14 | 15 | 16 | 17 | |
| 1 | 226 | | | | | | | | | | | | | | | | | 226 |
| 2 | 172 | 186 | | | | | | | | | | | | | | | | 358 |
| 3 | 124 | 128 | 122 | | | | | | | | | | | | | | | 374 |
| 4 | 89 | 90½† | 77½ | 91 | | | | | | | | | | | | | | 348 |
| 5 | 41 | 59 | 72½ | 73½ | 89 | | | | | | | | | | | | | 335 |
| 6 | 36 | 32 | 39 | 37 | 40 | 41 | | | | | | | | | | | | 225 |
| 7 | 24 | 26 | 16 | 21 | 24 | 32 | 35 | | | | | | | | | | | 178 |
| 8 | 11 | 11 | 18 | 20 | 17 | 19 | 22 | 21 | | | | | | | | | | 139 |
| 9 | 11 | 10 | 11 | 7 | 19 | 12 | 16 | 14 | 18 | | | | | | | | | 118 |
| 10 | 6 | 4 | 4 | 8 | 13 | 9 | 10 | 6 | 7 | 17 | | | | | | | | 84 |
| 11 | 5 | 1 | 4 | 4 | 3 | 0 | 2 | 3 | 3 | 3 | 5 | | | | | | | 33 |
| 12 | 0 | 2 | 2 | 1 | 0 | 5 | 1 | 3 | 3 | 3 | 8 | 2 | | | | | | 30 |
| 13 | 2 | 4 | 1 | 1 | 2 | 0 | 1 | 2 | 3 | 1 | 0 | 2 | 6 | | | | | 25 |
| 14 | 2 | 0 | 1 | 0 | 0 | 1 | 0 | 1 | 0 | 0 | 2 | 1 | 0 | 1 | | | | 9 |
| 15 | 1 | 0 | 1 | 0 | 0 | 1 | 0 | 1 | 0 | 0 | 0 | 0 | 0 | 1 | 4 | | | 9 |
| 16 | 0 | 0 | 0 | 1 | 0 | 0 | 0 | 0 | 0 | 0 | 0 | 0 | 0 | 0 | 0 | 1 | | 2 |
| 17 | 1 | 0 | 0 | 0 | 0 | 0 | 0 | 0 | 0 | 0 | 0 | 0 | 0 | 0 | 0 | 1 | 1 | 3 |
| 18 | 0 | 0 | 0 | 2 | 0 | 0 | 0 | 1 | 0 | 0 | 0 | 0 | 0 | 0 | 0 | 0 | 0 | 3 |
| 19 | 0 | 0 | 0 | 0 | 0 | 0 | 0 | 0 | 0 | 0 | 0 | 0 | 0 | 0 | 0 | 0 | 1 | 1 |
| *Total* | 751 | 553½ | 369 | 266½ | 207 | 121 | 87 | 52 | 34 | 24 | 15 | 5 | 6 | 2 | 4 | 1 | 2 | 2500 |

* From Norton [300].

† The halves are due to the treatment of twin pairs, which were assigned as ½ to each of two consecutive birth orders, both members of the twin pair being counted in the calculation of sibship size.

## Table 45

Expected distribution by birth order derived from observed distribution by sibship size*

| Size of sibship | Observed number of affected | Expected numbers of affected individuals occurring at each birth order | | | | | | | | | | | | | | | | | | |
|---|---|---|---|---|---|---|---|---|---|---|---|---|---|---|---|---|---|---|---|---|
| | | 1 | 2 | 3 | 4 | 5 | 6 | 7 | 8 | 9 | 10 | 11 | 12 | 13 | 14 | 15 | 16. | 17 | 18 | 19 |
| 1 | 226 | 226.0 | | | | | | | | | | | | | | | | | | |
| 2 | 358 | 179.0 | 179.0 | | | | | | | | | | | | | | | | | |
| 3 | 374 | 124.7 | 124.7 | 124.7 | | | | | | | | | | | | | | | | |
| 4 | 348 | 87.0 | 87.0 | 87.0 | 87.0 | | | | | | | | | | | | | | | |
| 5 | 335 | 67.0 | 67.0 | 67.0 | 67.0 | 67.0 | | | | | | | | | | | | | | |
| 6 | 225 | 37.5 | 37.5 | 37.5 | 37.5 | 37.5 | 37.5 | | | | | | | | | | | | | |
| 7 | 178 | 25.4 | 25.4 | 25.4 | 25.4 | 25.4 | 25.4 | 25.4 | | | | | | | | | | | | |
| 8 | 139 | 17.4 | 17.4 | 17.4 | 17.4 | 17.4 | 17.4 | 17.4 | 17.4 | | | | | | | | | | | |
| 9 | 118 | 13.1 | 13.1 | 13.1 | 13.1 | 13.1 | 13.1 | 13.1 | 13.1 | 13.1 | | | | | | | | | | |
| 10 | 84 | 8.4 | 8.4 | 8.4 | 8.4 | 8.4 | 8.4 | 8.4 | 8.4 | 8.4 | 8.4 | | | | | | | | | |
| 11 | 33 | 3.0 | 3.0 | 3.0 | 3.0 | 3.0 | 3.0 | 3.0 | 3.0 | 3.0 | 3.0 | 3.0 | | | | | | | | |
| 12 | 30 | 2.5 | 2.5 | 2.5 | 2.5 | 2.5 | 2.5 | 2.5 | 2.5 | 2.5 | 2.5 | 2.5 | 2.5 | | | | | | | |
| 13 | 25 | 1.9 | 1.9 | 1.9 | 1.9 | 1.9 | 1.9 | 1.9 | 1.9 | 1.9 | 1.9 | 1.9 | 1.9 | 1.9 | | | | | | |
| 14 | 9 | 0.6 | 0.6 | 0.6 | 0.6 | 0.6 | 0.6 | 0.6 | 0.6 | 0.6 | 0.6 | 0.6 | 0.6 | 0.6 | 0.6 | | | | | |
| 15 | 9 | 0.6 | 0.6 | 0.6 | 0.6 | 0.6 | 0.6 | 0.6 | 0.6 | 0.6 | 0.6 | 0.6 | 0.6 | 0.6 | 0.6 | 0.6 | | | | |
| 16 | 2 | 0.1 | 0.1 | 0.1 | 0.1 | 0.1 | 0.1 | 0.1 | 0.1 | 0.1 | 0.1 | 0.1 | 0.1 | 0.1 | 0.1 | 0.1 | 0.1 | | | |
| 17 | 3 | 0.2 | 0.2 | 0.2 | 0.2 | 0.2 | 0.2 | 0.2 | 0.2 | 0.2 | 0.2 | 0.2 | 0.2 | 0.2 | 0.2 | 0.2 | 0.2 | 0.2 | | |
| 18 | 3 | 0.2 | 0.2 | 0.2 | 0.2 | 0.2 | 0.2 | 0.2 | 0.2 | 0.2 | 0.2 | 0.2 | 0.2 | 0.2 | 0.2 | 0.2 | 0.2 | 0.2 | 0.2 | |
| 19 | 1 | 0.1 | 0.1 | 0.1 | 0.1 | 0.1 | 0.1 | 0.1 | 0.1 | 0.1 | 0.1 | 0.1 | 0.1 | 0.1 | 0.1 | 0.1 | 0.1 | 0.1 | 0.1 | 0.1 |
| Total | 2500 | 794.7 | 568.7 | 389.7 | 265.0 | 178.0 | 111.0 | 73.5 | 48.1 | 30.7 | 17.6 | 9.2 | 6.2 | 3.7 | 1.8 | 1.2 | 0.6 | 0.5 | 0.3 | 0.1 |

* Data from Table 44.

size, and the total expected distribution is derived by summation (bottom row of Table 45).

When the expected distribution by birth order has been obtained, it may be compared with the observed distribution, as in Table 46. Note that, while birth orders may be grouped for the

### Table 46

Comparison of total observed and expected distributions by birth order of 2500 patients with neurosis*

| Birth order | Observed distribution | Expected distribution | Observed/ Expected |
|---|---|---|---|
| 1 | 751 | 794.7 | 0.95 |
| 2 | 553.5 | 568.7 | 0.97 |
| 3 | 369 | 389.7 | 0.95 |
| 4 | 266.5 | 265.0 | 1.01 |
| 5 | 207 | 178.0 | 1.16 |
| 6 + | 353 | 304.5 | 1.16 |
| *Total* | 2500 | 2500.6 | — |

* Data from Tables 44 and 45.

purpose of comparison of observed and expected distributions (as in this example into "6 +"), they cannot be so grouped during the derivation of the expected values, since the calculation requires use of exact family size. In this example there was a higher than expected frequency of patients with neurosis in birth orders higher than 4, and a lower than expected frequency in birth orders 1, 2, and 3.

Another test for birth order effect, based on similar premises to that of Greenwood and Yule, has been proposed by Haldane and Smith [147].

The Greenwood-Yule method has an advantage over the case-control method in that the analysis of birth order occurs *within* sibships and is therefore not liable to biases resulting from association of disease risk with size of sibship. The analysis is therefore less likely to be influenced by socioeconomic and certain other demographic differentials.

On the other hand, the method has the serious limitation of requiring that the sibships examined be complete. Use of the method on a series of incomplete sibships would result in over-representation of affected individuals in the higher birth orders. For example, in the extreme situation in which all sibships were included immediately after the birth of the affected individual, all the last-born children—that is, the later birth orders—would be affected. The shorter the interval between birth of the affected individual and the time of the study, the greater will be the bias from this source.

The extent and types of this error have been considered by McKeown and Record [216], who list a number of studies in which erroneous conclusions have resulted. These authors also suggest a modification of the method for use when sibships are incomplete. The method is suitable for use when cases have been assembled during a limited period and all siblings born within that same period (either before or after the patients) are known. In this method the expected distribution by birth order is derived in the same way as in the Greenwood-Yule method, except that siblings born outside the period during which the patients were assembled are excluded.

In the use of the Greenwood-Yule method, the question of inclusion or exclusion of deceased siblings in the calculation of sibship size is of some importance. Neonatal and infant deaths occur more frequently in certain birth orders—particularly the first and the late orders. Therefore, if the characteristic under consideration is one which is not manifest in early life, there will appear to be a proportionately lower risk of being af-fected in these birth orders. Consequently, in the calculation of sibship size, only those individuals who lived long enough to have been at risk of exhibiting the characteristic should be included.

In a series of sibships, those persons occupying the early birth orders will be on the average older than those in the later ranks. The possibility that this difference accounts for apparent differences in disease incidence should be considered.

EFFECT OF VARIATION IN FERTILITY. Variation in parental fertility may suggest birth order associations that do not stand up under close examination. In particular, the following possibilities should be considered:

1. Is the disease dependent on sibship size rather than on position within the sibship? In a case-control study, a disease with a tendency to occur in small sibships may give the appearance of being more common in lower birth orders since the higher birth orders are not represented in such sibships. In such a situation the Greenwood-Yule method—carried out on completed sibships—would not suggest an artificial association with birth order but neither would it indicate that there was an association between the disease and small sibship size.

2. Did the birth of the affected individual affect the subsequent fertility of the parents? For example, voluntary limitation of further reproduction might follow the birth of children with certain congenital malformations or the birth of twins. Involuntary limitation might result from such conditions as ectopic pregnancy. The effect of either type of limitation of reproduction on the assessment of birth order association by the Greenwood-Yule method would be the same as the effect that would result from including sibships of incomplete size—an artificial excess in the ratio of observed to expected affected individuals in the later birth orders. Data collected in the course of a case-control study, however, can cast some light on whether limitation of reproduction had or had not occurred. Cases and controls can be compared with respect to the number of children born during the interval between the time of birth of the affected child and the time that data collection for the study was undertaken.

### Interpretation of Birth Order Associations

As already noted, if the frequency of a condition is related to birth order, it can be assumed that some environmental influence is involved in its etiology, since genetic recombination is independent of order of birth. Birth order associations may be found in conditions in which genetic factors are known to be important, but then the existence of environmental factors modifying expression of the genetic potential must be presumed. The acquisition of such evidence is alone enough to justify studies of birth order.

Unfortunately birth order associations have so far not been

particularly fruitful in suggesting hypotheses as to what the specific environmental influences involved might be—perhaps because of the great variety of environmental circumstances that can be envisioned to change with order of birth.

DEMOGRAPHIC CHARACTERISTICS. It is, of course, necessary first to establish that the association with birth order is not the result of more direct associations with sibship size, parental age, socioeconomic status, or other variables. The effect of sibship size was discussed above; the interrelation between birth order and parental age will be considered in the discussion of parental age.

In many cultures low socioeconomic status is associated with large family size, so that observed birth order associations may be more a reflection of association with socioeconomic circumstance than with birth order itself. In addition, socioeconomic status may change over time within a family so that a late child may be born into either more or less affluent circumstances than was the first. Other demographic characteristics that may reflect associations with disease through associations with birth order include race, religion, and nativity. The complex, U-shaped association between fetal death rates and birth order is shown in Figure 35. A similar association exists for early infant deaths. These associations are no doubt due largely to socioeconomic and other demographic factors, as well as to phenomena more intrinsic to birth order itself.

PRENATAL ENVIRONMENT. That the prenatal environment varies with birth order is convincingly illustrated by the increase in mean birth weight with increase in birth order. This association presumably has its origin in less adequate mechanisms for fetal nutrition in the early birth orders, particularly towards the end of pregnancy. The effect of previous pregnancies, through changes in the maternal antibody system, is seen in the increase in frequency and severity of erythroblastosis with increasing birth order. Local abnormalities of the uterus, which may be more frequent in the later pregnancies, have been postulated as causes of congenital malformations, although there is little evidence to

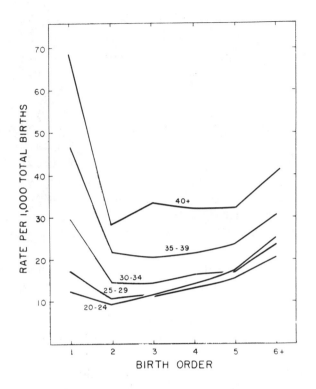

Figure 35

Fetal death rate by birth order in selected maternal age groups; United States, 1963. (Data from McCarthy [212].)

support this possibility. The greater concern that may be felt over first than over later pregnancies may lead to birth order differences in fetal exposure to drugs, nutritional supplements, and other experiences.

PERINATAL EXPERIENCES. The more prolonged and difficult labor characteristic of first pregnancies may lead to higher rates of abnormalities resulting from anoxia, trauma, prolonged anesthesia, and other factors connected with the confinement. An intriguing suggestion in this connection is that the relatively high frequency of patent ductus arteriosus in first births may be due in part to such factors acting at a time when the physiologic stimulus for closure should occur [336].

POSTNATAL ENVIRONMENT. Differences in postnatal environment associated with birth order seem even more numerous and varied than those in the prenatal environment. Psychosocial differences are obvious and stem from changes in parental psychology with increasing family size, as well as from dependence of interpersonal relations on the number, sex, and age of the siblings. There is a need for more comprehensive and definitive investigations than have so far been reported of the relation of personality traits to order of birth, with cognizance being taken of sex and spacing of siblings. Child-rearing practices are also unlikely to remain static within a sibship, even in the absence of major psychologic changes in the parents. Nutrition, patterns of exercise and recreation, and strength of parental prodding with respect to scholastic achievement are all likely to change with birth order. Being born into a sibship already containing children is also an important determinant of the frequency and timing of exposure to infectious agents.

One of the strongest associations of disease with birth order is that of hypertrophic pyloric stenosis, a disease with onset usually within 6 weeks of birth (Fig. 36). First births experience a rate three times as high as that of births after the third. While either prenatal or postnatal factors could be involved, the fact that the birth order association is absent among cases with onset within 2 weeks of delivery (Fig. 37) suggests that the influence is proba-

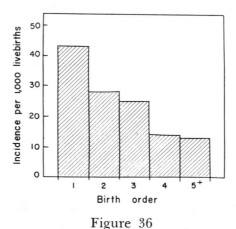

Figure 36

Cases of pyloric stenosis of infancy per 1000 livebirths by birth order; Birmingham, 1940 to 1949. (From McKeown et al. [214].)

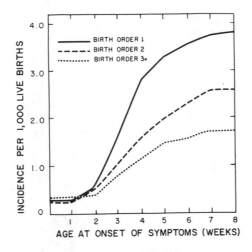

Figure 37

Cumulative incidence of pyloric stenosis by age, in three birth order groups;
Birmingham, 1942 to 1949. (From McKeown et al. [215].)

bly postnatal for the most part. That onset of the disease is about
1 week later among infants born in hospital than among those
born at home suggests that some aspect of maternal care may be
involved [215]. The association is, however, still unexplained.


PARENTAL AGE

A variable that is closely related to order of birth is the age of
the parents at the time of an individual's conception and birth.
The most striking association of this variable with disease frequency so far observed is that between age of mother and prevalence of Down's syndrome. As shown in Figure 38, the prevalence of Down's syndrome is less than one per 1000 in infants
born to mothers under 30 years of age but more than one per
100 in infants of mothers over 40. Another striking association
of maternal age is with the frequency of dizygotic twinning,
which is about six times higher for the maternal age group 35 to
39 years than for the age group 15 to 19. Associations with age
of father seem less frequent—perhaps in part because they
have been less often sought. However, the frequency of achondroplasia [313] and the secondary sex ratio [301] have been
found to be related to paternal age.

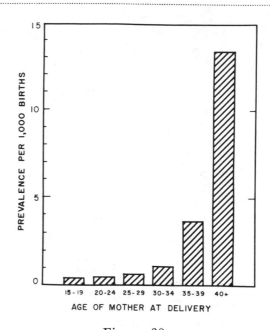

Figure 38

Prevalence of Down's syndrome per 1000 births, by age of mother; Massachusetts, 1954 to 1965. (From Fabia [111].)

## Study Methods

The methods of detecting associations with parental age are comparable to those described in the discussion of birth order. If the distribution of the related population of births is known, rates can be computed directly, as for the data in Figure 38. If not, the case-control or the Greenwood-Yule method can be utilized.

In applying the Greenwood-Yule method to the analysis of maternal or paternal age, the null hypothesis is that in a disease unassociated with parental age the affected individual will have an equal probability of being born at any of the maternal ages represented in his sibship. In addition to sibship size, information on maternal age at birth of all the members of the sibship is therefore required. The computation is similar to that described for birth order, as are the limitations of the method.

The ages of parents are, of course, highly correlated, and parental age is also highly correlated with birth order. It is therefore necessary to separate the effects of these variables if hypotheses are to be related specifically to any one of them. Although other statistical methods are available for such analyses [375], the most direct and most satisfactory procedure—if adequate numbers are available—is simply to examine disease rates in a cross-tabulation of two variables.

For example, prevalence rates of Down's syndrome by age of mother and birth order are shown in Table 47. The rates in-

Table 47

Prevalence of Down's syndrome at birth, by age of
mother and birth order, lower Michigan, 1950 to 1964*

| Maternal age | Number per 1000 livebirths affected in birth order | | | | | Total | |
| | 1 | 2 | 3 | 4 | 5 + | Crude | Adjusted |
|---|---|---|---|---|---|---|---|
| <20 | 0.5 | 0.4 | — | — | — | 0.4 | 0.3 |
| 20–24 | 0.4 | 0.5 | 0.4 | 0.4 | 0.2 | 0.4 | 0.4 |
| 25–29 | 0.5 | 0.5 | 0.5 | 0.5 | 0.5 | 0.5 | 0.5 |
| 30–34 | 1.0 | 1.0 | 0.8 | 0.9 | 0.8 | 0.9 | 0.9 |
| 35–39 | 2.7 | 3.0 | 2.4 | 3.0 | 2.5 | 2.6 | 2.7 |
| 40 + | 8.5 | 7.5 | 8.6 | 9.4 | 8.5 | 8.6 | 8.4 |
| *Total:* | | | | | | | |
| crude | 0.6 | 0.7 | 0.8 | 1.1 | 1.7 | 0.9 | — |
| adjusted | 0.9 | 0.9 | 0.8 | 0.9 | 0.7 | — | — |

* From Stark and Mantel [380].

crease from 0.4 per 1000 for mothers under 20 to 8.6 per 1000 in infants of mothers aged 40 or more.* There is also a distinct trend with birth order—from 0.6 in first births to 1.7 per 1000 in fifth and later births—when birth order is considered without respect to maternal age. The two trends can be examined independently by considering the body of the table. Reading along the rows—that is, within each maternal age group—there is no consistent trend with birth order: it must therefore be concluded that the over-all association with birth order is a conse-

* The differences between the over-all rates by maternal age seen in this table and those illustrated in Figure 38 are probably due to differences between the two surveys in ascertainment of cases.

quence of the association between birth order and maternal age. On reading down the columns, one sees that the trend with maternal age is present within each birth order. In these data the association with maternal age is therefore the more direct association and the one to be explained in biologic terms.

Also illustrated in Table 47 is a method of summarizing the separate effects of the two variables. The adjusted total rates by maternal age are rates that are standardized to allow for differences in birth order distribution between maternal age categories, and the adjusted total rates for each birth order are standardized to allow for variation in maternal age distribution between birth orders. The results reflect the impression derived from inspecting the individual rates—the trend with maternal age is virtually unaffected by the adjustment for birth order, but the trend with birth order is eliminated by the adjustment for maternal age.

Separation of the effects of maternal and paternal age will usually not be possible by this method unless very large numbers are available, because of the very high correlation between these two variables. More complex statistical methods, such as partial correlation, may also be applied.

Penrose has described a modification of the Greenwood-Yule method to separate the effects of parental age and birth order, but, apart from its initial utilization by Penrose on mongolism [311], the method has rarely been used.

### Interpretation

The factors responsible for associations with parental age are no better understood than those responsible for birth order effects. The variables discussed in connection with the interpretation of birth order effects are pertinent in assessing associations with parental age. In addition, the association between maternal age and frequency of Down's syndrome shows that strong parental age effects may be seen in conditions for which genetic mechanisms have been identified. In spite of knowledge of the chromosomal mechanism of Down's syndrome, the way in which maternal age contributes to the production of the genetic defect is still not known.

In considering associations with age of the mother, it must be remembered that a woman's full complement of oocytes has already been produced by the time of her own birth. The oocytes then remain in a late resting phase of meiosis until within a few weeks of ovulation. It is conceivable that events occurring during a woman's life, such as exposure to ionizing radiation [369], the cumulative risk of which would increase with age, may produce changes that will interfere with chromosomal separation just prior to ovulation. Alternatively, there may be circumstances whose frequency increases with age which, if present at the time of the final stages of meiosis, increase the probability of nondisjunction.

Selective death of oocytes during life, or selective ovulation of "healthier" ova first, may also lead to changes in the "quality" of ova discharged at different maternal ages, although there is no evidence on this point.

It is of interest that, so far, no maternal age association has been identified that is in the direction of higher rates of abnormality in children of young mothers, other than associations resulting indirectly from higher rates of abnormality in early birth orders.

With respect to paternal age, the above considerations are also pertinent. The increasing frequency of various exposures with age may be more relevant here because the germ cells in the male are being formed continuously throughout life. Such exposures might include dietary factors, alcohol, cigarette smoke, therapeutic drugs, medical procedures, and all the other causes and consequences of the deterioration of the male organism with age.

It has been suggested [124] that the maternal age effect in Down's syndrome may result from the decreasing frequency of coitus with age, leading to a greater likelihood that the fertilized ovum will be one that was discharged several days before fertilization. Experimentally, abnormalities have been produced by delay in fertilization of ova, but there is little to support this hypothesis as it applies specifically to Down's syndrome in man [111, 314]. Nevertheless the hypothesis is a reminder that a great many biologic and social variables that change with parental age surround the final stages of meiosis, fertilization, and the prenatal and postnatal development of the fertilized ovum. When the relation of some of these to specific illnesses has been elucidated, analogies to conditions in which parental age effects are still unexplained may become more apparent.

# References

1. Abou-Daoud, K. T.   Epidemiology of carcinoma of the cervix uteri in Lebanese Christians and Moslems. *Cancer* 20: 1706–1714, 1967.
2. Acheson, E. D.   *Medical Record Linkage.* Oxford University Press, London, 1967.
3. Acheson, E. D. (Ed.).   *Record Linkage in Medicine.* Williams & Wilkins, Baltimore, 1968.
4. Acheson, R. M. (Ed.).   *Comparability in International Epidemiology.* Milbank Memorial Fund, New York, 1965.
5. Ad Hoc Committee on the Implications of Record Linkage for Health-Related Research.   *Health Research Uses of Record Linkage in Canada.* Medical Research Council of Canada, Ottawa, Ont., 1968.
6. Ahmed, P.   *Disability Days, United States, July 1965–June 1966.* Public Health Service Publ. No. 1000, Series 10, No. 47. U.S. Govt. Printing Office, Washington, D.C., 1968.
7. Aird, I., Bentall, H. H., Mehigan, J. A., and Roberts, J. A. F.   The blood groups in relation to peptic ulceration and carcinoma of colon, rectum, breast, and bronchus. *Brit. Med. J.* 2: 315–321, 1954.
8. Alderson, M. R., and Meade, T. W.   Accuracy of diagnosis on death certificates compared with that in hospital records. *Brit. J. Prev. Soc. Med.* 21:22-29, 1967.
9. Allison, A. C.   The distribution of the sickle-cell trait in East Africa and elsewhere, and its apparent relationship to the incidence of subtertian malaria. *Trans. Roy. Soc. Trop. Med. Hyg.* 48:312–318, 1954.

10. Alter, M., Halpern, L., Kurland, L. T., Bornstein, B., Leibowitz, U., and Silberstein, J.  Multiple sclerosis in Israel. Prevalence among immigrants and native inhabitants. *Arch Neurol.* 7:253–263, 1962.

11. Alter, M., Leibowitz, U., and Speer, J.  Risk of multiple sclerosis related to age at immigration to Israel. *Arch. Neurol.* 15: 234–237, 1966.

12. American Psychiatric Association.  *Diagnostic and Statistical Manual of Mental Disorders* (2nd ed., DSM-II). American Psychiatric Association, Washington, D.C., 1968.

13. American Public Health Association.  *The Control of Communicable Diseases in Man* (10th ed.). American Public Health Association, New York, 1965.

14. Andvord, K. F.  What can we learn by studying tuberculosis by generations? *Norsk Mag. Laegevidensk.* 91:642–660, 1930.

15. Armitage, P.  Tests for linear trends in proportions and frequencies. *Biometrics* 11:375–386, 1955.

16. Armitage, P.  *Sequential Medical Trials.* Thomas, Springfield, Ill., 1960.

17. Arnold, F. A., Jr., Likins, R. C., Russell, A. L., and Scott, D. B.  Fifteenth year of the Grand Rapids fluoridation study. *J. Amer. Dent. Ass.* 65:780–785, 1962.

18. Artenstein, M. S., Gold, R., Zimmerly, J. G., Wyle, F. A., Schneider, H., and Harkins, C.  Prevention of meningococcal disease by group C polysaccharide vaccine. *New Eng. J. Med.* 282:417–420, 1970.

19. Ast, D. B., Smith, D. J., Wachs, B., and Cantwell, K. T.  Newburgh-Kingston caries-fluorine study. XIV. Combined clinical and roentgenographic dental findings after ten years of fluoride experience. *J. Amer. Dent. Ass.* 52:314–325, 1956.

20. Aycock, W. L., and Luther, E. H.  The occurrence of poliomyelitis following tonsillectomy. *New Eng. J. Med.* 200: 164–167, 1929.

21. Bahn, A. K., Gardner, E. A., Alltop, L., Knatterud, G. L., and Solomon, M.  Admission and prevalence rates for psychiatric facilities in four register areas. *Amer. J. Public Health* 56:2033–2051, 1966.

22. Bailar, J. C., III.  The Third National Cancer Survey. *CA* 19: 228–231, 1969.

23. Beebe, G. W.  Lung cancer in World War I veterans: possible relation to mustard-gas injury and 1918 influenza epidemic. *J. Nat. Cancer Inst.* 25:1231–1252, 1960.

24. Beebe, G. W., Ishida, M., and Jablon, S.  Studies of the mortality of A-bomb survivors. 1. Plan of study and mortality in the medical subsample (Selection 1), 1950–1958. *Radiation Res.* 16:253–280, 1962.

25. Beebe, G. W., and Simon, A. H.  Ascertainment of mortality

in the U.S. veteran population. *Amer. J. Epidem.* 89:636–643, 1969.

26. Benirschke, K.   Accurate recording of twin placentation: a plea to the obstetrician. *Obstet. Gynec.* 18:334–347, 1961.

27. Berkson, J.   The statistical study of association between smoking and lung cancer. *Proc. Staff Meetings Mayo Clinic* 30:319–348, 1955.

28. Berkson, J.   The statistical investigation of smoking and cancer of the lung. *Proc. Staff Meetings Mayo Clinic* 34:206–244, 1959.

29. Berman, C.   Primary carcinoma of the liver in the Bantu races of South Africa. *S. Afr. J. Med. Sci.* 5:54–72, 1940.

30. Bizzozero, O. J., Jr., Johnson, K. G., and Ciocco, A.   Radiation-related leukemia in Hiroshima and Nagasaki, 1946–1964. I. Distribution, incidence and appearance time. *New Eng. J. Med.* 274:1095–1101, 1966.

31. Blayney, J. R., and Hill, I. N.   Fluorine and dental caries. *J. Amer. Dent. Ass.* 74:225–302, 1967.

32. Bodian, D.   Viremia in experimental poliomyelitis. II. Viremia and the mechanism of the "provoking" effect of injections or trauma. *Amer. J. Hyg.* 60:358–370, 1954.

33. Brill, N. Q., and Beebe, G. W.   *A Follow-up Study of War Neuroses.* VA Medical Monograph. U.S. Govt. Printing Office, Washington, D.C., 1956.

34. Brown, J., Bourke, G. J., Gearty, G. F., et al.   Nutritional and epidemiologic factors related to heart disease. *World Rev. Nutr. Diet.* 12: in press, 1970.

35. Budd, W.   *Typhoid Fever. Its Nature, Mode of Spreading, and Prevention.* London, 1874. Reprinted by Delta Omega Society, American Public Health Association, New York, 1931.

36. Buell, P., and Dunn, J. E., Jr.   The dilution effect of misclassification. *Amer. J. Public Health* 54:598–602, 1964.

37. Bureau of the Census.   *Historical Statistics of the United States, 1789–1945.* U.S. Govt. Printing Office, Washington, D.C., 1949.

38. Bureau of the Census.   *United States Census of the Population: 1950. State of Birth.* Special Report P–E, No. 4A, U.S. Govt. Printing Office, Washington, D.C., 1953.

39. Bureau of the Census.   *United States Census of the Population: 1960. Subject Reports. Lifetime and Recent Migration.* Final Report PC(2)–2D. U.S. Govt. Printing Office, Washington, D.C., 1963.

40. Bureau of the Census.   *Estimates of the Population of the United States, by Single Years of Age, Color and Sex, 1900 to 1959.* Current Population Reports, Series P–25, No. 311. U.S. Govt. Printing Office, Washington, D.C., 1965.

41. Bureau of the Census.   *Evaluation and Research Program of*

*the U.S. Censuses of Population and Housing, 1960.* Series ER 60. U.S. Govt. Printing Office, Washington, D.C., Periodic.

42. Bureau of the Census. *Current Population Reports. Population Estimates.* Series P–25. U.S. Govt. Printing Office, Washington, D.C., Periodic.

43. Cairns, M., and Stewart, A. Pulmonary tuberculosis mortality in the printing and shoemaking trades. Historical survey, 1881–1931. *Brit. J. Soc. Med.* 5:73–82, 1951.

44. Campbell, D. T. Reforms as experiments. *Amer. Psychol.* 24: 409–429, 1969.

45. Case, R. A. M., Hosker, M. E., McDonald, D. B., and Pearson, J. T. Tumours of the urinary bladder in workmen engaged in the manufacture and use of certain dyestuff intermediates in the British chemical industry. *Brit. J. Industr. Med.* 11:75–104, 1954.

46. Case, R. A. M., and Lea, A. J. Mustard gas poisoning, chronic bronchitis, and lung cancer. *Brit. J. Prev. Soc. Med.* 9:62–72, 1955.

47. Case, R. A. M., and Pearson, J. T. *Cancer Death Rates by Site, Age and Sex; England and Wales, 1911–55. Supplement, 1956–65.* Institute of Cancer Research, Royal Cancer Hospital, London (Mimeographed), 1956, 1968.

48. Caverly, C. S. Preliminary report of an epidemic of paralytic disease, occurring in Vermont, in the summer of 1894. *Yale Med. J.* 1:1–5, 1894.

49. Cederlöf, R., Friberg, L., and Hrubec, Z. Cardiovascular and respiratory symptoms in relation to tobacco smoking. A study of American twins. *Arch. Environ. Health* 18:934–940, 1969.

50. Cederlöf, R., Friberg, L., Jonsson, E., and Kaij, L. Studies on similarity diagnosis in twins with the aid of mailed questionnaires. *Acta Genet.* 11:338–362, 1961.

51. Cederlöf, R., Friberg, L., Jonsson, E., and Kaij, L. Respiratory symptoms and "angina pectoris" in twins with reference to smoking habits. *Arch. Environ. Health* 13:726–737, 1966.

52. Chen, K. P., and Wu, H. Y. Epidemiologic studies on blackfoot disease. 2. A study of source of drinking water in relation to the disease. *J. Formosan Med. Ass.* 61:611–618, 1962.

53. Chen, K. P., and Wu, H. Y. Epidemiologic studies on blackfoot disease in Taiwan, China. 6. Effect of the piped water supply on occurrence and disease progress of blackfoot disease. *J. Formosan Med. Ass.* 68:291–296, 1969.

54. Ciocco, A. On the mortality in husbands and wives. *Hum. Biol.* 12:508–531, 1940.

55. Clark, D. W., and MacMahon, B. (Eds.). *Preventive Medicine.* Little, Brown, Boston, 1966.

56. Clemmesen, J. *Statistical Studies in Malignant Neoplasms.*

*II. Basic Tables, Denmark 1943–52.* Munksgaard, Copenhagen, 1964.

57. Clemmesen, J., and Nielsen, A.   Comparison of age-adjusted cancer incidence rates in Denmark and the United States. *J. Nat. Cancer Inst.* 19:989–998, 1957.

58. Cochran, W. G.   Modern methods in the sampling of human populations. General principles in the selection of a sample. *Am. J. Public Health* 41:647–653, 1951.

59. Cochran, W. G.   Some methods for strengthening the common $\chi^2$ tests. *Biometrics* 10:417–451, 1954.

60. Cohen, J., and Steinitz, R.   Underlying and contributory causes of death of adult males in two districts. *J. Chronic Dis.* 22:17–24, 1969.

61. Cole, P., and Hoover, R. N.   Bladder cancer risk and occupation. In preparation, 1970.

62. Cole, P., MacMahon, B., and Aisenberg, A.   Mortality from Hodgkin's disease in the United States. Evidence for the multiple-aetiology hypothesis. *Lancet* 2:1371–1376, 1968.

63. College of General Practitioners.   A diabetes survey. Report of a working party. *Brit. Med. J.* 1:1497–1503, 1962.

64. Collins, S. D.   Causes of illness in 9,000 families based on nation-wide periodic canvasses, 1928–1931. *Public Health Rep.* 48:283–308, 1933.

65. Commission on Chronic Illness.   *Chronic Illness in the United States. Vol. IV. Chronic Illness in a Large City: The Baltimore Study.* Harvard University Press, Cambridge, Mass., 1957.

66. Commission on Chronic Illness.   *Chronic Illness in the United States. Vol. III. Chronic Illness in a Rural Area: The Hunterdon Study.* Harvard University Press, Cambridge, Mass., 1959.

67. Commonwealth of Massachusetts, Division of Vital Statistics. *Annual Report on the Vital Statistics of Massachusetts.* Secretary of the Commonwealth, Boston, Annual.

68. Communicable Disease Center, National Advisory Committee for Evaluation of Gamma Globulin.   Evaluation of gamma globulin in prophylaxis of paralytic poliomyelitis in 1953. *J.A.M.A.* 154:1086–1090, 1954.

69. Court Brown, W. M., and Doll, R.   *Leukaemia and Aplastic Anaemia in Patients Irradiated for Ankylosing Spondylitis.* Medical Research Council Special Report Series No. 295. Her Majesty's Stationery Office, London, 1957.

70. Court Brown, W. M., and Doll, R.   Mortality from cancer and other causes after radiotherapy for ankylosing spondylitis. *Brit. Med. J.* 2:1327–1332, 1965.

71. Cullen, W.   *Synopsis Nosologicae Medicae* (1785). Quoted by Hosack, D., *A System of Practical Nosology* (2d ed.). O. S. Van Winkle, New York, 1821.

72. Curran, W. J. Governmental regulation of the use of human subjects in medical research: the approach of two Federal agencies. *Daedalus* 98:542–595, 1969.

73. David, F. N., and Barton, D. E. Two space-time interaction tests for epidemicity. *Brit. J. Prev. Soc. Med.* 20:44–48, 1966.

74. Dawber, T. R., Kannel, W. B., and Lyell, L. P. An approach to longitudinal studies in a community: the Framingham study. *Ann. N.Y. Acad. Sci.* 107:539–556, 1963.

75. Dawber, T. R., Meadors, G. F., and Moore, F. E., Jr. Epidemiological approaches to heart disease. The Framingham Study. *Amer. J. Public Health* 41:279–286, 1951.

76. Dayton, N. A. *New Facts on Mental Disorders.* Thomas, Springfield, Ill., 1940.

77. Dean, H. T. Some general epidemiological considerations. In Moulton, F. R. (Ed.), *Dental Caries and Fluorine.* American Association for the Advancement of Science, Washington, D.C., 1946.

78. DeBakey, M. E., and Beebe, G. W. Medical follow-up studies on veterans. *J.A.M.A.* 182:1103–1109, 1962.

79. Doll, R. Bronchial carcinoma: incidence and aetiology. *Brit. Med. J.* 2:521–527, 585–590, 1953.

80. Doll, R. *Prevention of Cancer. Pointers from Epidemiology.* The Nuffield Provincial Hospitals Trust, 1967.

81. Doll, R., and Hill, A. B. A study of the aetiology of carcinoma of the lung. *Brit. Med. J.* 2:1271–1286, 1952.

82. Doll, R., and Hill, A. B. The mortality of doctors in relation to their smoking habits. A preliminary report. *Brit. Med. J.* 1:1451–1455, 1954.

83. Doll, R., and Hill, A. B. Lung cancer and other causes of death in relation to smoking. A second report on the mortality of British doctors. *Brit. Med. J.* 2:1071–1081, 1956.

84. Doll, R., and Hill, A. B. Mortality in relation to smoking: ten years' observations of British doctors. *Brit. Med. J.* 1:1399–1410, 1460–1467, 1964.

85. Doll, R., Payne, P., and Waterhouse, J. *Cancer Incidence in Five Continents.* International Union Against Cancer, Springer-Verlag, New York, 1966.

86. Dorn, H. F. Methods of analysis for follow-up studies. *Hum. Biol.* 22:238–248, 1950.

87. Dorn, H. F. Tobacco consumption and mortality from cancer and other diseases. *Public Health Rep.* 74:581–593, 1959.

88. Dorn, H. F. Some considerations in the revision of the International Statistical Classification. *Public Health Rep.* 79:175–179, 1964.

89. Dorn, H. F. Underlying and contributory causes of death. In

Haenszel, W. (Ed.), *Epidemiological Approaches to the Study of Cancer and Other Chronic Diseases.* Nat. Cancer Inst. Monogr. 19. U.S. Govt. Printing Office, Washington, D.C., 1966.

90. Dorn, H. F., and Cutler, S. J. *Morbidity from Cancer in the United States.* Public Health Monogr. No. 56. U.S. Govt. Printing Office, Washington, D.C., 1959.

91. Downes, J. Chronic disease among spouses. *Milbank Mem. Fund Quart.* 25:334–358, 1947.

92. Downes, J., and Collins, S. D. A study of illness among families in the Eastern Health District of Baltimore. *Milbank Mem. Fund Quart.* 18:5–26, 1940.

93. Doyle, J. T., Heslin, A. S., Hilleboe, H. E., Formel, P. F., and Korns, R. F. A prospective study of degenerative cardiovascular disease in Albany: report of three years' experience. 1. Ischemic heart disease. *Amer. J. Public Health,* Suppl. Apr. 1957, 25–32, 1957.

94. Duffy, E. A., and Carroll, R. E. *United States Metropolitan Mortality 1959–1961.* Public Health Service Publ. No. 999–AP–39, U.S. Public Health Service, National Center for Air Pollution Control, 1967.

95. Dunn, H. L., and Shackley, W. Comparison of cause-of-death assignments by the 1929 and 1938 revisions of the International List: deaths in the United States, 1940. *Vital Statistics Special Reports* 19, No. 14:153–277, 1944.

96. Dunn, J. E., Jr. Preliminary findings of the Memphis-Shelby County uterine cancer study and their interpretation. *Amer. J. Public Health* 48:861–873, 1958.

97. Dunn, J. E., Jr. The presymptomatic diagnosis of cancer with special reference to cervical cancer. *Proc. Roy. Soc. Med.* 59: 1198–1204, 1966.

98. Dunn, J. E., Jr., and Buell, P. Association of cervical cancer with circumcision of sexual partner. *J. Nat. Cancer Inst.* 22: 749–764, 1959.

99. Dunn, J. E., Jr., and Martin, P. L. Morphogenesis of cervical cancer. Findings from San Diego County cytology registry. *Cancer* 20:1899–1906, 1967.

100. Dunning, J. M. The influence of latitude and distance from seacoast on dental disease. *J. Dent. Res.* 32:811–829, 1953.

101. Eaton, J. W., and Weil, R. J. *Culture and Mental Disorders.* Free Press, Glencoe, Ill., 1955.

102. Ederer, F., Myers, M. H., and Mantel, N. A statistical problem in space and time: Do leukemia cases come in clusters? *Biometrics* 20:626–628, 1966.

103. Edwards, J. H. Congenital malformations of the central nervous system in Scotland. *Brit. J. Prev. Soc. Med.* 12:115–130, 1958.

104. Edwards, J. H. The recognition and estimation of cyclic trends. *Ann. Hum. Genet.* 25:83–87, 1961.
105. Edwards, J. H. Seasonal incidence of congenital disease in Birmingham. *Ann. Hum. Genet.* 25:89–93, 1961.
106. Ehrlich, P. R., and Holm, R. W. Patterns and populations. *Science* 137:652–657, 1962.
107. Eisenberg, H., Campbell, P. C., and Flannery, J. T. *Cancer in Connecticut. Incidence Characteristics 1935–62.* Connecticut State Department of Health, Hartford, 1967.
108. Enterline, P. E. Mortality among asbestos products workers in the United States. *Ann. N.Y. Acad. Sci.* 132:156–165, 1965.
109. Erhardt, C. L., and Nelson, F. G. Reported congenital malformations in New York City, 1958–1959. *Amer. J. Public Health* 54:1489–1506, 1964.
110. Erhardt, C. L., and Weiner, L. Changes in mortality statistics through the use of the new International Statistical Classification. *Amer. J. Public Health* 40:6–16, 1950.
111. Fabia, J. Illegitimacy and Down's syndrome. *Nature* 221:1157–1158, 1969.
112. Feinleib, M. Breast cancer and artificial menopause: a cohort study. *J. Nat. Cancer Inst.* 41:315–329, 1968.
113. Feinleib, M., and Garrison, R. J. Interpretation of the vital statistics of breast cancer. *Cancer* 24:1109–1116, 1969.
114. Ferris, B. G., Jr., Anderson, D. O., and Burgess, W. A. Prevalence of respiratory disease in a flax mill in the United States. *Brit. J. Industr. Med.* 19:180–185, 1962.
115. Finlay, C. Yellow fever: its transmission by means of the Culex mosquito. *Amer. J. Med. Sci.* 92:395–409, 1886.
116. Fletcher, W. Rice and beri-beri: preliminary report of an experiment conducted at the Kuala Lumpur Lunatic Asylum. *Lancet* 1:1776–1779, 1907.
117. Florey, C. du V., and Acheson, R. M. *Blood Pressure as It Relates to Physique, Blood Glucose, and Serum Cholesterol.* Public Health Service Publ. No. 1000, Series 11, No. 34. U.S. Govt. Printing Office, Washington, D.C., 1969.
118. Fox, J. P., Hall, C. E., and Elveback, L. R. *Epidemiology. Man and Disease.* Macmillan, London, 1970.
119. Francis, T., Jr., and Epstein, F. H. Survey methods in general populations. I. Studies of a total community. Tecumseh, Michigan. In Acheson, R. M. (Ed.), *Comparability in International Epidemiology.* Milbank Memorial Fund, New York, 1965.
120. Friedman, M., Rosenman, R. H., and Carroll, V. Changes in the serum cholesterol and blood clotting time in men subjected to cyclic variation of occupational stress. *Circulation* 17:852–861, 1958.

121. Frost, W. H.   The age selection of mortality from tuberculosis in successive decades. *Amer. J. Hyg., Sect. A* 30:91–96, 1939.

122. Gaon, J. A.   Endemic nephropathy in Yugoslavia. In Pemberton, J. (Ed.), *Epidemiology. Reports on Research and Teaching, 1962.* Oxford University Press, London, 1963.

123. Gentry, J. T., Nitowsky, H. M., and Michael, M., Jr.   Studies on the epidemiology of sarcoidosis in the United States: the relationship to soil areas and to urban-rural residence. *J. Clin. Invest.* 34:1839–1856, 1955.

124. German, J.   Mongolism, delayed fertilization and human sexual behaviour. *Nature* 217:516–518, 1968.

125. Gilliam, A. G.   A note on evidence relating to the incidence of primary liver cancer among the Bantu. *J. Nat. Cancer Inst.* 15:195–199, 1954.

126. Gilliam, A. G.   Trends of mortality attributed to carcinoma of the lung: possible effects of faulty certification of deaths to other respiratory diseases. *Cancer* 8:1130–1136, 1955.

127. Gilliam, A. G.   Geographic distribution and trends of leukaemia in the United States. *Acta Unio Int. Contra Cancr.* 16: 1623–1628, 1960.

128. Gittelsohn, A. M., and Milham, S., Jr.   Vital record incidence of congenital malformations in New York State. In Neel, J. V., Shaw, M. W., and Schull, W. J. (Eds.), *Genetics and the Epidemiology of Chronic Diseases.* Public Health Service Publ. No. 1163. U.S. Govt. Printing Office, Washington, D.C., 1965.

129. Glazebrook, P. R., Smith, A., and Witts, L. J.   Symposium on confidentiality of medical records and related problems. In Acheson, E. D. (Ed.), *Record Linkage in Medicine.* Williams & Wilkins, Baltimore, 1968.

130. Goldberger, J.   The etiology of pellagra. The significance of certain epidemiological observations with respect thereto. *Public Health Rep.* 29:1683–1686, 1914. Reprinted in Terris, M. (Ed.), *Goldberger on Pellagra.* Louisiana State University Press, Baton Rouge, La., 1964.

131. Goldberger, J., and Wheeler, G. A.   The experimental production of pellagra in human subjects by means of diet. *Hyg. Lab. Bull.* 120:7–116, 1920. Reprinted in Terris, M. (Ed.), *Goldberger on Pellagra.* Louisiana State University Press, Baton Rouge, La., 1964.

132. Gove, P. B. (Ed.).   *Webster's Third New International Dictionary of the English Language.* G. & C. Merriam, Springfield, Mass., 1963.

133. Graham, S., Levin, M. L., Lilienfeld, A. M., Schuman, L. M., Gibson, R., Dowd, J. E., and Hempelmann, L.   Preconception, intrauterine and postnatal irradiation as related to leukemia. In Haenszel, W. (Ed.), *Epidemiological Approaches to the*

*Study of Cancer and Other Chronic Diseases.* Nat. Cancer Inst. Monogr. 19. U.S. Govt. Printing Office, Washington, D.C., 1966.

134. Graunt, J. *Natural and Political Observations made upon the Bills of Mortality.* London, 1662. Republished by The Johns Hopkins Press, Baltimore, 1939.

135. Greenwood, M. *Epidemics and Crowd-Diseases. An Introduction to the Study of Epidemiology.* Macmillan, New York, 1935.

136. Greenwood, M., Jr., and Yule, G. U. On the determination of size of family and of the distribution of characters in order of birth from samples taken through members of the sibships. *J. Roy. Statist. Soc.* 77:179–197, 1914.

137. Grove, R. D. *The 1968 Revision of the Standard Certificates.* Public Health Service Publ. No. 1000, Series 4, No. 8. U.S. Govt. Printing Office, Washington, D.C., 1968.

138. Grove, R. D., and Hetzel, A. M. *Vital Statistics Rates in the United States, 1940–1960.* Public Health Service Publ. No. 1677. U.S. Govt. Printing Office, Washington, D.C., 1968.

139. Guralnick, L. Mortality by occupation level and cause of death among men 20 to 64 years of age, United States, 1950. *Vital Statistics Special Reports* 53, No. 5:439–612, 1963.

140. Guralnick, L. Some problems in the use of multiple causes of death. *J. Chronic Dis.* 19:979–990, 1966.

141. Haddow, A. J. An improved map for the study of Burkitt's lymphoma syndrome in Africa. *E. Afr. Med. J.* 40:429–432, 1963.

142. Haddow, A. J. Age incidence in Burkitt's lymphoma syndrome. *E. Afr. Med. J.* 41: 1–6, 1964.

143. Hadley, J. N. Health conditions among Navajo Indians. *Public Health Rep.* 70:831–836, 1955.

144. Haenszel, W. (Ed.). *Epidemiological Approaches to the Study of Cancer and Other Chronic Diseases.* Nat. Cancer Inst. Monogr. 19. U.S. Govt. Printing Office, Washington, D.C., 1966.

145. Haenszel, W., and Kurihara, M. Studies of Japanese migrants. I. Mortality from cancer and other diseases among Japanese in the United States. *J. Nat. Cancer Inst.* 40:43–68, 1968.

146. Haenszel, W., Marcus, S. C., and Zimmerer, E. G. *Cancer Morbidity in Urban and Rural Iowa.* Public Health Monogr. No. 37, Public Health Service Publ. No. 462. U.S. Govt. Printing Office, Washington, D.C., 1956.

147. Haldane, J. B. S., and Smith, C. A. B. A simple exact test for birth-order effect. *Ann. Eugenics* 14:117–124, 1947.

148. Hammon, W. McD., Coriell, L. L., and Stokes, J., Jr., Evaluation of Red Cross gamma globulin as a prophylactic agent for poliomyelitis. *J.A.M.A.* 150:739–760, 1952.

149. Hammond, E. C.  Smoking in relation to mortality and morbidity. Findings in first thirty-four months of follow-up in a prospective study started in 1959. *J. Nat. Cancer Inst.* 32:1161–1188, 1964.

150. Hammond, E. C.  Life expectancy of American men in relation to their smoking habits. *J. Nat. Cancer Inst.* 43:951–962, 1969.

151. Hammond, E. C., and Horn, D.  Smoking and death rates—report on forty-four months of follow-up of 187,783 men. *J.A.M.A.* 166:1159–1172, 1294–1308, 1958.

152. Hanhart, E.  Zur geographischen Verbreitung der Erbkrankheiten (Mutationen) mit besonderer Berücksichtigung der Schweiz. *Schweiz. Med. Wschr.* 22:861–864, 1941.

153. Harvard School of Public Health, Department of Epidemiology.  Unpublished data.

154. Heasman, M. A.  Accuracy of death certification. *Proc. Roy. Soc. Med.* 55:733–736, 1962.

155. Heath, C. W., Jr., and Hasterlik, R. J.  Leukemia among children in a suburban community. *Amer. J. Med.* 34:796–812, 1963.

156. Hempel, C. G.  Introduction to problems of taxonomy. In Zubin, J. (Ed.), *Field Studies in the Mental Disorders.* Grune & Stratton, New York, 1961.

157. Henderson, D. A.  Chronic nephritis in Queensland. *Aust. Ann. Med.* 4:163–177, 1955.

158. Henderson, D. A.  The aetiology of chronic nephritis in Queensland. *Med. J. Australia* 1:377–386, 1958.

159. Hewitt, D.  Regional variations in the incidence of spina bifida. In Neel, J. V., Shaw, M. W., and Schull, W. J. (Eds.), *Genetics and the Epidemiology of Chronic Diseases.* Public Health Service Publ. No. 1163. U.S. Govt. Printing Office, Washington, D.C., 1965.

160. Hill, A. B.  The clinical trial. *New Eng. J. Med.* 247:113–119, 1952.

161. Hill, A. B.  Observation and experiment. *New Eng. J. Med.* 248:995–1001, 1953.

162. Hill, A. B.  *Principles of Medical Statistics* (8th ed.). Oxford University Press, New York, 1966.

163. Hippocrates.  *On Airs, Waters, and Places.* Translated and republished in *Medical Classics* 3:19–42, 1938.

164. Hirohata, T.  Mortality from gastric cancer and other causes after medical or surgical treatment for gastric ulcer. *J. Nat. Cancer Inst.* 41:895–908, 1968.

165. Hirohata, T., and Kuratsune, M.  The geographical comparison of mortality from cancer of the stomach and ulcer of the stomach in Japan. *Brit. J. Cancer* 23:465–479, 1969.

166. Hirsch, A. *Handbook of Geographical and Historical Pathology. Vols. I–III.* Translated from the Second German Edition by Creighton, C. The New Sydenham Society, London, 1883–1886.
167. Hogben, L. *Nature and Nurture.* Williams and Norgate, London, 1933.
168. Hollingshead, A. B., and Redlich, F. C. *Social Class and Mental Illness. A Community Study.* Wiley, New York, 1958.
169. Horowitz, I., and McDonald, A. D. Anencephaly and spina bifida in the Province of Quebec. *Canad. Med. Ass. J.* 100:748–755, 1969.
170. Hueper, W. C. Age aspects of environmental and occupational cancers. *Public Health Rep.* 67:773–779, 1952.
171. Hume, D. *Treatise of Human Nature* (1739). Selby-Bigge (Ed.). Oxford, Clarendon, 1896.
172. Humphreys, N. A. (Ed.). *Vital Statistics: A Memorial Volume of Selections from the Reports and Writings of William Farr, 1807–1883.* The Sanitary Institute of Great Britain, London, 1885.
173. Hutchison, G. B. Evaluation of preventive measures. In Clark, D. W., and MacMahon, B. (Eds.), *Preventive Medicine.* Little, Brown, Boston, 1966.
174. Hutchison, G. B. Leukemia in patients with cancer of the cervix uteri treated with radiation. A report covering the first 5 years of an international study. *J. Nat. Cancer Inst.* 40:951–982, 1968.
175. Hutchison, G. B., and Shapiro, S. Lead time gained by diagnostic screening for breast cancer. *J. Nat. Cancer Inst.* 41:665–681, 1968.
176. Huxley, J. Genetics, evolution and human destiny. In Dunn, L. C. (Ed.), *Genetics in the 20th Century.* Macmillan, New York, 1951.
177. Ipsen, J., Jr. Prevalence and incidence of multiple sclerosis in Boston, 1939–1948. *Arch. Neurol. Psychiat.* 64:631–640, 1950.
178. Jablon, S., Angevine, D. M., Matsumoto, Y. S., and Ishida, M. On the significance of cause of death as recorded on death certificates in Hiroshima and Nagasaki, Japan. In Haenszel, W. (Ed.), *Epidemiological Approaches to the Study of Cancer and Other Chronic Diseases.* Nat. Cancer Inst. Monogr. 19. U.S. Govt. Printing Office, Washington, D.C., 1966.
179. Jablon, S., Neel, J. V., Gershowitz, H., and Atkinson, G. F. The NAS-NRC twin panel: methods of construction of the panel, zygosity diagnosis, and proposed use. *Amer. J. Hum. Genet.* 19:133–161, 1967.
180. Jaco, E. G. *The Social Epidemiology of Mental Disorders—A Psychiatric Survey of Texas.* Russell Sage Foundation, New York, 1960.

181. Jaffe, A. J. *Handbook of Statistical Methods for Demographers.* Preliminary Edition—Third Printing. U.S. Bureau of the Census. U.S. Govt. Printing Office, Washington, D.C., 1960.

182. James, G., Patton, R. E., and Heslin, A. S. Accuracy of cause-of-death statements on death certificates. *Public Health Rep.* 70:39–51, 1955.

183. Jenner, E. *An Inquiry into the Causes and Effects of the Variolae Vaccinae.* Law, London, 1798.

184. Kahn, H. A. The Dorn study of smoking and mortality among U.S. veterans: report on eight and one-half years of observation. In Haenszel, W. (Ed.), *Epidemiological Approaches to the Study of Cancer and Other Chronic Diseases.* Nat. Cancer Inst. Monogr. 19. U.S. Govt. Printing Office, Washington, D.C., 1966.

185. Källén, B., and Winberg, J. A Swedish register of congenital malformations. *Pediatrics* 41:765–776, 1968.

186. Kashgarian, M. The concepts of prevalence and incidence as applied to the study of development and duration of disease. *Meth. Inform. Med.* 7:111–117, 1968.

187. Keys, A. Atherosclerosis: A problem in newer public health. *J. Mt. Sinai Hosp. N. Y.* 20:118–139, 1953.

188. Knobloch, H., and Pasamanick, B. Seasonal variation in the births of the mentally deficient. *Amer. J. Public Health* 48: 1201–1208, 1958.

189. Knox, G. Detection of low intensity epidemicity. Application to cleft lip and palate. *Brit. J. Prev. Soc. Med.* 17:121–127, 1963.

190. Knox, G. Epidemiology of childhood leukaemia in Northumberland and Durham. *Brit. J. Prev. Soc. Med.* 18:17–24, 1964.

191. Koch, R. The aetiology of tuberculosis. *Berlin. Klin. Wschr.* 19:221, 1882. Translated and reprinted in *The Aetiology of Tuberculosis.* Pinner, M. (Transl.). National Tuberculosis Association, New York, 1932.

192. Kraepelin, E. *General Paresis.* Authorized English Translation by Moore, J. W. Nervous and Mental Disease Monograph Series, No. 14. Journal of Nervous and Mental Disease Publishing Co., New York, 1913.

193. Krueger, D. E. New numerators for old denominators—multiple causes of death. In Haenszel, W. (Ed.), *Epidemiological Approaches to the Study of Cancer and Other Chronic Diseases.* Nat. Cancer Inst. Monogr. 19. U.S. Govt. Printing Office, Washington, D.C., 1966.

194. Kurtzke, J. F., Beebe, G. W., Nagler, B., Nefzger, M. D., Auth, T. L., and Kurland, L. T. Studies on the natural history of multiple sclerosis. 5. Long-term survival in young males. *Arch. Neurol.* 22:215–225, 1970.

195. Lancaster, H. O. Deafness as an epidemic disease in Australia. *Brit. Med. J.* 2:1429–1432, 1951.

196. Leck, I. Incidence and epidemicity of Down's syndrome. *Lancet* 2:457–460, 1966.
197. Leck, I., and Rogers, S. C. Changes in the incidence of anencephalus. *Brit. J. Prev. Soc. Med.* 21:177–180, 1967.
198. Leighton, D. C., Harding, J. S., Macklin, D. B., Macmillan, A. M., and Leighton, A. H. *The Stirling County Study of Psychiatric Disorder and Sociocultural Environment. Vol. III.* Basic Books, New York, 1963.
199. Lenz, W. Thalidomide and congenital abnormalities (Letter to the Editor). *Lancet* 1:45, 1962.
200. Leren, P. *The Effect of Plasma Cholesterol Lowering Diet in Male Survivors of Myocardial Infarction.* Universitelsforlaget, Oslo, 1966.
201. Lewis, E. B. Leukemia, multiple myeloma, and aplastic anemia in American radiologists. *Science* 142:1492–1494, 1963.
202. Lilienfeld, A. M., Pedersen, E., and Dowd, J. E. *Cancer Epidemiology: Methods of Study.* Johns Hopkins Press, Baltimore, 1967.
203. Lind, J. *A Treatise of the Scurvy.* Kincaird & Donaldson, Edinburgh, 1753. Reprinted in Steward, C. P., and Guthrie, D. (Eds.), *Lind's Treatise on Scurvy.* University Press, Edinburgh, 1953.
204. Linder, F. E. National Health Survey. *Science* 127:1275–1280, 1958.
205. Linder, F. E., and Grove, R. D. *Vital Statistics Rates in the United States, 1900–1940.* U.S. Govt. Printing Office, Washington, D.C., 1943.
206. Livingstone, F. B. Anthropological implications of sickle cell gene distribution in West Africa. *Amer. Anthrop.* 60:533–562, 1958.
207. Lombard, H. C. Observations suggested by a comparison of the post mortem appearances produced by typhous fever in Dublin, Paris and Geneva. *Dublin J. Med. Sci.* 10:17–24, 101–104, 1836.
208. Lowe, C. R. An association between smoking and respiratory tuberculosis. *Brit. Med. J.* 2:1081–1086, 1956.
209. Lundin, F. E., Jr., Lloyd, J. W., Smith, E. M., Archer, V. E., and Holaday, D. A. Mortality of uranium miners in relation to radiation exposure, hard-rock mining and cigarette smoking —1950 through September 1967. *Health Phys.* 16:571–578, 1969.
210. McBride, W. G. Thalidomide and congenital abnormalities (Letter to the Editor). *Lancet* 2:1358, 1961.
211. McCarroll, J., and Bradley, W. Excess mortality as an indicator of health effects of air pollution. *Amer. J. Public Health* 56:1933–1942, 1966.

212. McCarthy, M. A. *Infant, Fetal, and Maternal Mortality. United States, 1963*. Public Health Service Publ. No. 1000, Series 20, No. 3. U.S. Govt. Printing Office, Washington, D.C., 1966.

213. McKay, F. S., and Black, G. V. An investigation of mottled teeth: an endemic developmental imperfection of the enamel of the teeth, heretofore unknown in the literature of dentistry. *Dental Cosmos* 58:627–644, 1916.

214. McKeown, T., MacMahon, B., and Record, R. G. The incidence of congenital pyloric stenosis related to birth rank and maternal age. *Ann. Eugenics* 16:249–259, 1951.

215. McKeown, T., MacMahon, B., and Record, R. G. Evidence of postnatal environmental influence in the aetiology of infantile pyloric stenosis. *Arch. Dis. Child.* 27:386–390, 1955.

216. McKeown, T., and Record, R. G. Maternal age and birth order as indices of environmental influence. *Amer. J. Hum. Genet.* 8:8–23, 1956.

217. MacKenzie, A., Court Brown, W. M., Doll, R., and Sissons, H. A. Mortality from primary tumours of bone in England and Wales. *Brit. Med. J.* 1:1782–1790, 1961.

218. MacKenzie, I. Breast cancer following multiple fluoroscopies. *Brit. J. Cancer* 19:1–8, 1965.

219. MacMahon, B. Epidemiological evidence on the nature of Hodgkin's disease. *Cancer* 10:1045–1054, 1957.

220. MacMahon, B. Cohort fertility and increasing breast cancer incidence. *Cancer* 11:250–254, 1958.

221. MacMahon, B. Epidemiology of Hodgkin's disease. *Cancer Res.* 26:1189–1200, 1966.

222. MacMahon, B. Gene-environment interaction in human disease. *J. Psychiat. Res.* 6 (Suppl. 1):393–402, 1968.

223. MacMahon, B., and Clark, D. Incidence of the common forms of human leukemia. *Blood* 11:871–881, 1956.

224. MacMahon, B., Lin, T. M., Lowe, C. R., Mirra, A. P., Ravnihar, B., Salber, E. J., Trichopoulos, D., Valaoras, V. G., and Yuasa, S. Lactation and cancer of the breast. Summary of an international study. *Bull. WHO* 42:185–194, 1970.

225. MacMahon, B., and McKeown, T. Infantile hypertrophic pyloric stenosis: data on 81 pairs of twins. *Acta Genet. Med. (Roma)* 4:320–329, 1955.

226. MacMahon, B., and Newill, V. A. Birth characteristics of children dying of malignant neoplasms. *J. Nat. Cancer Inst.* 28:231–244, 1962.

227. MacMahon, B., and Pugh, T. F. Suicide in the widowed. *Amer. J. Epidem.* 81:23–31, 1965.

228. MacMahon, B., Pugh, T. F., and Ingalls, T. H. Anencephalus, spina bifida, and hydrocephalus. Incidence related to sex, race,

and season of birth, and incidence in siblings. *Brit. J. Prev. Soc. Med.* 7:211–219, 1953.

229. MacMahon, B., Pugh, T. F., and Ipsen, J. *Epidemiologic Methods.* Little, Brown, Boston, 1960.

230. MacMahon, B., Record, R. G., and McKeown, T.   Congenital pyloric stenosis. An investigation of 578 cases. *Brit. J. Soc. Med.* 5:185–192, 1951.

231. Mainland, D.   Chance and random sampling. *Meth. Med. Res.* 6:127–137, 1954.

232. Malzberg, B.   *Social and Biological Aspects of Mental Disease.* State Hospitals Press, Utica, N.Y., 1940.

233. Malzberg, B.   *Cohort Studies of Mental Disease in New York State, 1943–1949.* National Association for Mental Health, New York, 1958.

234. Malzberg, B., and Lee, E. S.   *Migration and Mental Disease; A Study of First Admissions to Hospitals for Mental Disease, New York, 1939–41.* Social Science Research Council, New York, 1956.

235. Mancuso, T. F., and Coulter, E. J.   Methods of studying the relation of employment and long term illness—cohort analysis. *Amer. J. Public Health* 49:1525–1536, 1959.

236. Manos, N. E.   *Comparative Mortality Among Metropolitan Areas of the United States, 1949–51; 102 Causes of Death.* Public Health Service Publ. No. 562. U.S. Govt. Printing Office, Washington, D.C., 1957.

237. Mantel, N.   Chi-square tests with one degree of freedom; extensions of the Mantel-Haenszel procedure. *J. Amer. Statist. Ass.* 58:690–700, 1963.

238. Mantel, N.   The detection of disease clustering and a generalized regression approach. *Cancer Res.* 27:209–220, 1967.

239. Mantel, N., and Haenszel, W.   Statistical aspects of the analysis of data from retrospective studies of disease. *J. Nat. Cancer Inst.* 22:719–748, 1959.

240. Markush, R. E.   National chronic respiratory disease mortality study. 1. Prevalence and severity at death of chronic respiratory diseases in the United States, 1963. *J. Chronic Dis.* 21:129–141, 1968.

241. Martin, W. J.   Vital statistics of the County of London in the years 1901 to 1951. *Brit. J. Prev. Soc. Med.* 9:126–134, 1955.

242. Mathews, J. D., Glasse, R., and Lindenbaum, S.   Kuru and cannibalism. *Lancet* 2:449–452, 1968.

243. Medical Research Council.   The prevention of whooping cough by vaccination. *Brit. Med. J.* 1:1463–1471, 1951.

244. Medical Research Council.   Vaccination against whooping cough. *Brit. Med. J.* 2:454–462, 1956.

245. Medical Research Council, Research Committee.   Controlled

trial of soya-bean oil in myocardial infarction. *Lancet* 2:693–700, 1968.

246. Menaker, W. Air pollution, smoking, and lung cancer (Letter to the Editor). *Brit. Med. J.* 2:416, 1956.

247. Merrington, M., and Spicer, C. C. Acute leukaemia in New England. *Brit. J. Prev. Soc. Med.* 23:124–127, 1969.

248. Metrakos, J. D. Congenital hypertrophic pyloric stenosis in twins. *Arch. Dis. Child.* 28:351–358, 1953.

249. Metropolitan Life Insurance Company. *Statistical Bulletin.* Metropolitan Life, New York, Monthly.

250. Miettinen, O. S. The matched pairs design in the case of all-or-none responses. *Biometrics* 24:339–352, 1968.

251. Miettinen, O. S. Individual matching with multiple controls in the case of all-or-none response. *Biometrics* 25:339–355, 1969.

252. Miettinen, O. S. Matching and design efficiency in retrospective studies. *Amer. J. Epidem.* 91:111–118, 1970.

253. Miettinen, O. S. Estimation of relative risk from individually matched series. *Biometrics* 26:75–86, 1970.

254. Miettinen, O. S., Reiner, M. L., and Nadas, A. S. Seasonal incidence of coarctation of the aorta. *Brit. Heart J.* 32:103–107, 1970.

255. Mill, J. S. *A System of Logic, Ratiocinative and Inductive* (5th ed.). Parker, Son and Bowin, London, 1862.

256. Miller, R. W. Delayed radiation effects in atomic-bomb survivors. *Science* 166:569–574, 1969.

257. Ministry of Health. *Mortality and Morbidity During the London Fog of December, 1952.* Report by a Committee of Departmental Officers and Expert Advisers appointed by the Minister of Health. Reports on Public Health and Medical Subjects No. 95. Her Majesty's Stationery Office, London, 1954.

258. Mirick, G. S., and Shank, R. E. An epidemic of serum hepatitis studied under controlled conditions. *Trans. Amer. Clin. Climat. Ass.* 71:176–190, 1959.

259. Monson, R. R., and MacMahon, B. Peptic ulcer in Massachusetts physicians. *New Eng. J. Med.* 281:11–15, 1969.

260. Moriyama, I. M. Uses of vital records for epidemiological research. *J. Chronic Dis.* 17:889–897, 1964.

261. Moriyama, I. M., Baum, W. S., Haenszel, W. M., and Mattison, B. F. Inquiry into diagnostic evidence supporting medical certifications of death. *Amer. J. Public Health* 48:1376–1387, 1958.

262. Moriyama, I. M., Dawber, T. R., and Kannel, W. B. Evaluation of diagnostic information supporting medical certification of deaths from cardiovascular disease. In Haenszel, W. (Ed.), *Epidemiological Approaches to the Study of Cancer and Other Chronic Diseases.* Nat. Cancer Inst. Monogr. 19. U.S. Govt. Printing Office, Washington, D.C., 1966.

263. Morris, J. N., Heady, J. A., Raffle, P. A. B., Roberts, C. G., and Parks, J. W. Coronary heart-disease and physical activity of work. *Lancet* 2:1053–1057, 1111–1120, 1953.

264. Munck, W. Autopsy findings and clinical diagnosis. *Acta Med. Scand.* (Suppl. 266) 142:775–781, 1952.

265. Mustacchi, P., David, F. N., and Fix, E. Three tests for space-time interaction: A comparative evaluation. *Proceedings of the Fifth Berkeley Symposium on Mathematical Statistics and Probability.* Vol. 4:229–235, University of California, Berkeley and Los Angeles, 1967.

266. Myers, R. J. Limitations in the use of OASDI records for health studies. *Amer. J. Public Health* 55:1787–1791, 1965.

267. Naeye, R. L., Benirschke, K., Hagstrom, J. W. C., and Marcus, C. C. Intrauterine growth of twins as estimated from liveborn birth weight data. *Pediatrics* 37:409–416, 1966.

268. National Academy of Sciences, Advisory Committee from the Division of Medical Sciences. *Radiation Exposure of Uranium Miners.* Federal Radiation Council, Washington, D.C., 1968.

269. National Center for Health Statistics. *Origin, Program and Operation of the U.S. National Health Survey.* Public Health Service Publ. No. 1000, Series 1, No. 1. U.S. Govt. Printing Office, Washington, D.C., 1963.

270. National Center for Health Statistics. Comparability of mortality statistics for the Fifth and Sixth Revisions: United States, 1950. *Vital Statistics Special Reports* 51, No. 2:131–178, 1963.

271. National Center for Health Statistics. *Plan and Initial Program of the Health Examination Survey.* Public Health Service Publ. No. 1000, Series 1, No. 4. U.S. Govt. Printing Office, Washington, D.C., 1965.

272. National Center for Health Statistics. *Plan, Operation, and Response Results of a Program of Children's Examinations.* Public Health Service Publ. No. 1000, Series 1, No. 5. U.S. Govt. Printing Office, Washington, D.C., 1967.

273. National Center for Health Statistics. Provisional estimates of selected comparability ratios based on dual coding of 1966 death certificates by the Seventh and Eighth Revisions of the International Classification of Diseases. *Monthly Vital Statistics Report* 17, No. 8. Suppl. Oct. 25, 1968.

274. National Center for Health Statistics. *Disability Days. United States—July 1965–June 1966.* Public Health Service Publ. No. 1000, Series 10, No. 47. U.S. Govt. Printing Office, Washington, D.C., 1968.

275. National Center for Health Statistics. *Plan and Operation of a Health Examination Survey of U.S. Youths 12–17 Years of Age.* Public Health Service Publ. No. 1000, Series 1, No. 8. U.S. Govt. Printing Office, Washington, D.C., 1969.

276. National Center for Health Statistics. *Eighth Revision International Classification of Diseases, Adapted for Use in the United States. Vols. 1 and 2.* Public Health Service Publ. No. 1693. U.S. Govt. Printing Office, Washington, D.C., 1967, 1969.

277. National Center for Health Statistics. *Report of the Twentieth Anniversary Conference of the U.S. National Committee on Vital and Health Statistics.* Public Health Service Publ. No. 1000, Series 4. U.S. Govt. Printing Office, Washington, D.C., 1970.

278. National Center for Health Statistics. *Vital Statistics of the United States. Vols. I and II.* U.S. Govt. Printing Office, Washington, D.C., Annual.

279. National Center for Health Statistics. *Monthly Vital Statistics Report.* U.S. Dept. of Health, Education and Welfare, Public Health Service, Washington, D.C., Monthly.

280. National Center for Health Statistics. Public Health Service Publ. No. 1000. U.S. Govt. Printing Office, Washington, D.C., Periodic.

281. National Committee on Vital and Health Statistics, Subcommittee on National Morbidity Survey. *Recommendations for the Collection of Data on the Distribution and Effects of Illness, Injuries, and Impairments in the United States.* Public Health Service Publ. No. 333. Reprinted in National Center for Health Statistics, *Origin, Program and Operation of the U.S. National Health Survey.* Public Health Service Publ. No. 1000, Series 1, No. 1. U.S. Govt. Printing Office, Washington, D.C., 1963.

282. National Committee on Vital and Health Statistics. *Use of Vital and Health Records in Epidemiologic Research.* Public Health Service Publ. No. 1000, Series 4, No. 7. U.S. Govt. Printing Office, Washington, D.C., 1968.

283. National Communicable Disease Center. *Morbidity and Mortality Weekly Report. Annual Supplement. Summary 1968.* National Communicable Disease Center, Public Health Service, Atlanta, 1969.

284. National Communicable Disease Center. *Morbidity and Mortality. Weekly Report.* National Communicable Disease Center, Public Health Service, Atlanta, Weekly.

285. National Heart Institute, Diet-Heart Review Panel. *Mass Field Trials of the Diet-Heart Question.* American Heart Association Monogr. No. 28. American Heart Association, New York, 1969.

286. National Office of Vital Statistics. Classification of joint causes of death. *Vital Statistics Special Reports* 5, No. 47:385–469, 1938.

287. National Office of Vital Statistics. Deaths from selected causes

by marital status, by age and sex: United States, 1940. *Vital Statistics Special Reports* 23, No. 7:117–165, 1945.

288. National Office of Vital Statistics. The effect of the Sixth Revision of the International List of Diseases and Causes of Death upon comparability of mortality trends. *Vital Statistics Special Reports* 36: No. 10, 1951 (Reprinted 1960).

289. National Office of Vital Statistics. Mortality from selected causes by marital status, United States, 1949–51. *Vital Statistics Special Reports* 39: No. 7, 301–429, 1956.

290. Neel, J. V., and Schull, W. J. *Human Heredity*. University of Chicago Press, Chicago, 1954.

291. Neel, J. V., Shaw, M. W., and Schull, W. J. (Eds.). *Genetics and the Epidemiology of Chronic Diseases*. Public Health Service Publ. No. 1163. U.S. Govt. Printing Office, Washington, D.C., 1965.

292. Newcombe, H. B. Multigeneration pedigrees from linked records. In Acheson, E. D. (Ed.), *Record Linkage in Medicine*. Williams & Wilkins, Baltimore, 1968.

293. Newcombe, H. B. Products from the early stages in the development of a system of linked records. In Acheson, E. D. (Ed.), *Record Linkage in Medicine*. Williams & Wilkins, Baltimore, 1968.

294. Newell, D. J. Errors in the interpretation of errors in epidemiology. *Amer. J. Public Health* 52:1925–1928, 1962.

295. Newell, G. R., Cole, S. R., Miettinen, O. S., and MacMahon, B. Age differences in the histology of Hodgkin's disease. *J. Nat. Cancer Inst.,* in press, 1970.

296. Newill, V. A. Distribution of cancer mortality among ethnic subgroups of the white population of New York City, 1953–58. *J. Nat. Cancer Inst.* 26:405–417, 1961.

297. Newman, H. H., Freeman, F. N., and Holzinger, K. J. *Twins: A Study of Heredity and Environment*. University of Chicago Press, Chicago, 1937.

298. Nielsen, H. The personal numbering system in Denmark. In Acheson, E. D. (Ed.), *Record Linkage in Medicine*. Williams & Wilkins, Baltimore, 1968.

299. Nitzberg, D. M. Results of research into the methodology of record linkage. In Acheson, E. D. (Ed.), *Record Linkage in Medicine*. Williams & Wilkins, Baltimore, 1968.

300. Norton, A. Incidence of neurosis related to maternal age and birth order. *Brit. J. Soc. Med.* 6:253–258, 1952.

301. Novitski, E., and Sandler, L. The relationship between parental age, birth order and the secondary sex ratio in humans. *Ann. Hum. Genet.* 21:123–131, 1956.

302. Ødegaard, Ø. Emigration and insanity. *Acta Psychiat. Neurol. Scand.* Suppl. 4, 1932.

303. Ødegaard, Ø. Emigration and mental health. *Ment. Hyg.* 20:546–553, 1936.

304. Osler, W. *The Principles and Practice of Medicine* (7th ed.). Appleton, New York and London, 1909. P. 364.

305. O'Sullivan, J. B. *Childbearing and Diabetes Mellitus.* National Center for Health Statistics, Series 11, No. 21. U.S. Govt. Printing Office, Washington, D.C., 1966.

306. Paffenbarger, R. S., Jr., and Williams, J. L. Chronic disease in former college students. V. Early precursors of fatal stroke. *Amer. J. Public Health* 57:1290–1299, 1967.

307. Paffenbarger, R. S., Jr., Wolf, P. A., Notkin, J., and Thorne, M. C. Chronic disease in former college students. 1. Early precursors of fatal coronary heart disease. *Amer. J. Epidem.* 83:314–328, 1966.

308. Pan American Sanitary Bureau. *Weekly Epidemiological Report.* Pan American Sanitary Bureau, Washington, D.C., Weekly.

309. Panum, P. L. Observations made during the epidemic of measles on the Faroe Islands in the year 1846. Reproduced in Delta Omega Society, *Panum on Measles.* American Public Health Association, New York, 1940.

310. Peñaloza, D., Arias-Stella, J., Sime, F., Recavarren, S., and Marticorena, E. The heart and pulmonary circulation in children at high altitudes: physiological, anatomical and clinical observations. *Pediatrics* 34:568–582, 1964.

311. Penrose, L. S. A method of separating the relative aetiological effects of birth order and maternal age, with special reference to mongolian imbecility. *Ann. Eugenics* 6:108–127, 1934.

312. Penrose, L. S. Parental age and mutation. *Lancet* 2:312–313, 1955.

313. Penrose, L. S. Parental age in achondroplasia and mongolism. *Amer. J. Hum. Genet.* 9:167–169, 1957.

314. Penrose, L. S., and Berg, J. M. Mongolism and duration of marriage (Letter to the Editor). *Nature* 218:300, 1968.

315. Perrott, G. St. J., Tibbitts, C., and Britten, R. H. The National Health Survey—scope and method of the nation-wide canvass of sickness in relation to its social and economic setting. *Public Health Rep.* 54:1663–1687, 1939.

316. Petras, J. W., and Curtis, J. E. The current literature on social class and mental disease in America: critique and bibliography. *Behav. Sci.* 13:382–398, 1968.

317. Pifer, J. W., Toyooka, E. T., Murray, R. W., Ames, W. R., and Hempelmann, L. H. Neoplasms in children treated with X-rays for thymic enlargement. I. Neoplasms and mortality. *J. Nat. Cancer Inst.* 31:1333–1356, 1963.

318. Pike, M. C., and Smith, P. G. Disease clustering: A generaliza-

tion of Knox's approach to the detection of space-time inter-actions. *Biometrics* 24:541–556, 1968.

319. Pike, M. C., Williams, E. H., and Wright, B. Burkitt's tumour in the West Nile District of Uganda 1961–5. *Brit. Med. J.* 2:395–399, 1967.

320. Pinkel, D., Dowd, J. E., and Bross, I. D. J. Some epidemiological features of malignant solid tumors of children in the Buffalo, N.Y. area. *Cancer* 16:28–33, 1963.

321. Pintner, R., and Forlano, G. Season of birth and mental differences. *Psychol. Bull.* 40:25–35, 1943.

322. Polk, R. L. & Co. *City Directories.* Polk, Detroit, Annual.

323. Pollack, E. S. Use of census matching for study of psychiatric admission rates. *Proc. Social Stat. Sect., Amer. Statist. Ass.:* 107–115, 1965.

324. Pollard, A. H. Methods of forecasting mortality using Australian data. *J. Inst. Actuaries* 75:151–182, 1949.

325. Pollin, W., Allen, M. G., Hoffer, A., Stabenau, J. R., and Hrubec, Z. Psychopathology in 15,909 pairs of veteran twins: evidence for a genetic factor in the pathogenesis of schizophrenia and its relative absence in psychoneurosis. *Amer. J. Psychiat.* 126:597–610, 1969.

326. Pollin, W., Stabenau, J. R., Mosher, L., and Tupin, J. Life history differences in identical twins discordant for schizophrenia. *Amer. J. Orthopsychiat.* 36:492–509, 1966.

327. Pollock, T. M. *Trials of Prophylactic Agents for the Control of Communicable Diseases.* World Health Organization, Geneva, 1966.

328. Poskanzer, D. C., Schapira, K., and Miller, H. Multiple sclerosis and poliomyelitis. *Lancet* 2:917–921, 1963.

329. Poskanzer, D. C., and Schwab, R. S. Cohort analysis of Parkinson's syndrome. *J. Chronic Dis.* 16:961–973, 1963.

330. Price, B. Primary biases in twin studies. *Amer. J. Hum. Genet.* 2:293–352, 1950.

331. Public Health Conference on Records and Statistics. *The 1970 Census and Vital and Health Statistics* (Appendix II). Public Health Service Publ. No. 1000, Series 4, No. 10. U.S. Govt. Printing Office, Washington, D.C., 1969.

332. Public Health Conference on Records and Statistics, Study Group on Record Linkage. *Progress Report.* National Center for Health Statistics, Document No. 603.5, mimeographed, Washington, D.C., 1966.

333. Public Health Service, Advisory Committee to the Surgeon General. *Smoking and Health.* Public Health Service Publ. No. 1103. U.S. Govt. Printing Office, Washington, D.C., 1964.

334. Pugh, T. F. The population explosion and the future num-

ber of mental-hospital inpatients. *New Eng. J. Med.* 271:672, 1964.

335. Pugh, T. F., and MacMahon, B. *Epidemiologic Findings in United States Mental Hospital Data.* Little, Brown, Boston, 1962.

336. Record, R. G., and McKeown, T.  Observations relating to the aetiology of patent ductus arteriosus. *Brit. Heart J.* 15:376–386, 1953.

337. Redmond, C. K., Smith, E. M., Lloyd, J. W., and Rush, H. W. Long-term mortality study of steelworkers. III. Follow-up. *J. Occup. Med.* 11:513–521, 1969.

338. Reed, W., Carroll, J., Agramonte, A., and Lazear, J. W.  The etiology of yellow fever. A preliminary note. *Phila. Med. J.* 6:790–796, 1900.

339. Registrar General for England and Wales. *The Registrar General's Decennial Supplement, England and Wales, 1931. Part IIa. Occupational Mortality.* His Majesty's Stationery Office, London, 1938.

340. Registrar General for England and Wales. *The Registrar General's Statistical Review of England and Wales for the Years 1938 and 1939.* Her Majesty's Stationery Office, London, 1947.

341. Registrar General for England and Wales. *The Registrar General's Statistical Review of England and Wales for the Two Years 1950–1951. Supplement on General Morbidity, Cancer and Mental Health.* Her Majesty's Stationery Office, London, 1955.

342. Registrar General for England and Wales. *The Registrar General's Decennial Supplement, England and Wales, 1951. Occupational Mortality, Part II. Vol. 1, Commentary. Vol. 2, Tables.* Her Majesty's Stationery Office, London, 1958 and 1957.

343. Registrar General for England and Wales. *The Registrar General's Statistical Review of England and Wales. Parts 1 and 2.* Her Majesty's Stationery Office, London, Annual.

344. Reid, D. D.  Studies of disease among migrants and native populations in Great Britain, Norway, and the United States. 1. Background and design. In Haenszel, W. (Ed.), *Epidemiological Approaches to the Study of Cancer and Other Chronic Diseases.* Nat. Cancer Inst. Monogr. 19. U.S. Govt. Printing Office, Washington, D.C., 1966.

345. Reid, D. D., Cornfield, J., Markush, R. E., Seigel, D., Pedersen, E., and Haenszel, W.  Studies of disease among migrants and native populations in Great Britain, Norway and the United States. III. Prevalence of cardiorespiratory symptoms among migrants and native-born in the United States. In Haenszel,

W. (Ed.), *Epidemiological Approaches to the Study of Cancer and Other Chronic Diseases.* Nat. Cancer Inst. Monogr. 19. U.S. Govt. Printing Office, Washington, D.C., 1966.

346. Rennie, T. A. C., Srole, L., Opler, M. K., and Langner, T. S. Urban life and mental health. Socio-economic status and mental disorder in the metropolis. *Amer. J. Psychiat.* 113:831–837, 1957.

347. Roberts, J., and Cohrssen, J. *Hearing Levels of Adults by Education, Income, and Occupation.* National Center for Health Statistics, Series 11, No. 31. U.S. Govt. Printing Office, Washington, D.C., 1968.

348. Rogot, E. A note on measurement errors and detecting real differences. *J. Amer. Statist. Ass.* 56:314–319, 1961.

349. Royal College of Physicians of London. *Smoking and Health.* Pitman, London, 1962. American Edition, Pitman, New York, 1962.

350. Salber, E. J., MacMahon, B., and Feldman, J. J. A test of apparent geographic clustering in breast cancer. *Amer. J. Epidem.* 87:110–111, 1968.

351. Salber, E. J., Trichopoulos, D., and MacMahon, B. Lactation and reproductive histories of breast cancer patients in Boston, 1965–66. *J. Nat. Cancer Inst.* 43:1013–1024, 1969.

352. Sartwell, P. E., Masi, A. T., Arthes, F. G., Greene, G. R., and Smith, H. E. Thromboembolism and oral contraceptives: an epidemiologic case-control study. *Amer. J. Epidem.* 90:365–380, 1969.

353. Sawyer, W. A., Meyer, K. F., Eaton, M. D., Bauer, J. H., Putnam, P., and Schwentker, F. F. Jaundice in army personnel in the Western Region of the United States and its relation to vaccination against yellow fever. *Amer. J. Hyg.* 39:337–430; 40:35–107, 1944.

354. Schapira, K., Poskanzer, D. C., and Miller, H. Familial and conjugal multiple sclerosis. *Brain* 86:315–332, 1963.

355. Schar, M., Lindenmann, J., Scholer, H., Goff, A. P., and Pollock, T. M. Beurteilung der Unschädlichkeit und Wirksamkeit der Sabinschen Viren bei Massenimpfungen im Kanton Basel-land. *Schweiz. Med. Wschr.* 93:421–427, 1963.

356. Schilling, R. F. S. (Chairman). Symposium on confidentiality of medical records and related problems. In Acheson, E. D. (Ed.), *Record Linkage in Medicine.* Livingstone, Edinburgh, 1968.

357. Scrimshaw, N. S., Trulson, M., Tejada, C., Hegsted, D. M., and Stare, F. J. Serum lipoprotein and cholesterol concentrations. Comparison of rural Costa Rican, Guatemalan, and United States populations. *Circulation* 15:805–813, 1957.

358. Segall, A. J. Personal communication, 1970.

359. Selikoff, I. J., Hammond, E. C., and Churg, J. Asbestos exposure, smoking, and neoplasia. *J.A.M.A.* 204:106–112, 1968.

360. Seltser, R., and Sartwell, P. E. The influence of occupational exposure to radiation on the mortality of American radiologists and other medical specialists. *Amer. J. Epidem.* 81:2–22, 1965.

361. Semmelweis, I. P. *The Etiology, the Concept and Prophylaxis of Childbed Fever* (1861). Translated and republished in *Medical Classics* 5:350–773, 1941.

362. Shapiro, S., Jacobziner, H., Densen, P. M., and Weiner, L. Further observations on prematurity and perinatal mortality in a general population and in the population of a prepaid group practice medical care plan. *Amer. J. Public Health* 50:1304–1317, 1960.

363. Shapiro, S., Strax, P., and Venet, L. Evaluation of periodic breast cancer screening with mammography. *J.A.M.A.* 195:731–738, 1966.

364. Shapiro, S., Strax, P., and Venet, L. Periodic breast cancer screening. The first two years of screening. *Arch. Environ. Health* 15:547–553, 1967.

365. Shapiro, S., Strax, P., Venet, L., and Fink, R. The search for risk factors in breast cancer. *Amer. J. Public Health* 58:820–835, 1968.

366. Shapiro, S., Weinblatt, E., Frank, C. W., and Sager, R. V. Incidence of coronary heart disease in a population insured for medical care (HIP). *Amer. J. Public Health* 59 (Suppl. June): 1–101, 1969.

367. Shepard, O. (Ed.). *The Heart of Thoreau's Journals.* Houghton Mifflin, Boston, 1927. P. 58 (Nov. 11, 1850).

368. Shields, J. *Monozygotic Twins Brought Up Apart and Brought Up Together.* Oxford University Press, London, 1962.

369. Sigler, A. T., Lilienfeld, A. M., Cohen, B. H., and Westlake, J. E. Radiation exposure in parents of children with mongolism (Down's syndrome). *Bull. Johns Hopkins Hosp.* 117:374–399, 1965.

370. Simpson, C. L., Hempelmann, L. H., and Fuller, L. M. Neoplasia in children treated with X-rays in infancy for thymic enlargement. *Radiology* 64:840–845, 1955.

371. Simpson, R. E. H. Infectiousness of communicable diseases in the household (measles, chickenpox, and mumps). *Lancet* 2:549–554, 1952.

372. Slater, P. *Survey of Sickness, October 1943 to December 1945.* The Social Survey. Her Majesty's Stationery Office, London, 1946.

373. Smith, A. Automatic linkage of medical and vital registration records. *Brit. J. Prev. Soc. Med.* 17:185–190, 1963.

374. Smith, R. L., Salsbury, C. G., and Gilliam, A. G.  Recorded and expected mortality among the Navajo, with special reference to cancer. *J. Nat. Cancer Inst.* 17:77–89, 1956.

375. Snedecor, G. W., and Cochran, W. G.  *Statistical Methods* (6th ed.). Iowa State University Press, Ames, Iowa, 1967.

376. Snow, J.  *On the Mode of Communication of Cholera* (2d ed.). Churchill, London, 1855. Reproduced in *Snow on Cholera*. Commonwealth Fund, New York, 1936. Reprinted by Hafner, New York, 1965.

377. Society of Actuaries.  *Build and Blood Pressure Study, 1959. Vols. 1 and 2.* Society of Actuaries, Chicago, 1959, 1960.

378. Spiegelman, M.  *Introduction to Demography* (rev. ed.). Harvard University Press, Cambridge, Mass., 1968.

379. Srole, L., Langner, T. S., Michael, S. T., Opler, M. K., and Rennie, T. A. C.  *Mental Health in the Metropolis. The Midtown Manhattan Study. Vol. 1.* McGraw-Hill, New York, 1961.

380. Stark, C. R., and Mantel, N.  Effects of maternal age and birth order on the risk of mongolism and leukemia. *J. Nat. Cancer Inst.* 37:687–698, 1966.

381. Stark, C. R., and Mantel, N.  Lack of seasonal—or temporal—spatial clustering of Down's syndrome births in Michigan. *Amer. J. Epidem.* 86:199–213, 1967.

382. Stern, C.  *Principles of Human Genetics* (2d ed.). Freeman, San Francisco, 1960.

383. Stevenson, A. C., Johnston, H. A., Stewart, M. I. P., and Golding, D. R.  Congenital malformations. A report of a study of series of consecutive birth in 24 centres. *Bull. WHO* 34 (Suppl.): 9–127, 1966.

384. Stewart, A., Webb, J., and Hewitt, D.  A survey of childhood malignancies. *Brit. Med. J.* 1:1495–1508, 1958.

385. Stocks, P.  *Sickness in the Population of England and Wales in 1944–1947.* Studies on Medical and Population Subjects No. 2. Her Majesty's Stationery Office, London, 1949.

386. Stoller, A., and Collmann, R. D.  Incidence of infective hepatitis followed by Down's syndrome nine months later. *Lancet* 2:1221–1223, 1965.

387. Susser, M. W., and Stein, Z.  Civilization and peptic ulcer. *Lancet* 1:115–119, 1962.

388. Susser, M. W., and Watson, W.  *Sociology in Medicine* (2d ed.). Oxford University Press, London, 1970.

389. Swaroop, S.  *Introduction to Health Statistics.* Livingstone, Edinburgh, 1960.

390. Sydenstricker, E.  A study of illness in a general population group. *Public Health Rep.* 41:2069–2088, 1926.

391. Sydenstricker, E., Wheeler, G. A., and Goldberger, J.  Disabling sickness among the population of seven cotton mill

villages of South Carolina in relation to family income. *Public Health Rep.* 33:2038–2051, 1918.

392. Taylor, F. H.   The relationship of mortality and duration of employment as reflected by a cohort of chromate workers. *Amer. J. Public Health* 56:218–229, 1966.

393. Taylor, I., and Knowelden, J.   *Principles of Epidemiology* (2d ed.). Little, Brown, Boston, 1964.

394. Terris, M. (Ed.).   *Goldberger on Pellagra.* Louisiana State University Press, Baton Rouge, 1964.

395. Tetlow, C.   Psychoses of childbearing. *J. Ment. Sci.* 101:629–639, 1955.

396. Thurnam, J.   *Observations and Essays on the Statistics of Insanity and on Establishments for the Insane.* Gilpin and Huntin, York, 1845.

397. Till, M. M., Hardisty, R. M., Pike, M. C., and Doll, R.   Childhood leukaemia in Greater London: a search for evidence of clustering. *Brit. Med. J.* 3:755–758, 1967.

398. Topley, W. W. C., and Wilson, G. S.   *The Principles of Bacteriology and Immunity* (2d ed.). Wood, Baltimore, 1936.

399. Trulson, M. F., Clancy, R. E., Jessop, W. J. E., Childers, R. W., and Stare, F. J.   Comparison of siblings in Boston and Ireland. *J. Amer. Diet. Ass.* 45:225–229, 1964.

400. Tseng, W. P., Chu, H. M., How, S. W., Fong, J. M., Lin, C. S., and Yeh, S.   Prevalence of skin cancer in an endemic area of chronic arsenicism in Taiwan. *J. Nat. Cancer Inst.* 40:453–463, 1968.

401. United Nations.   *Demographic Yearbook 1962, 1963, 1964.* United Nations, New York, 1962, 1964, 1965.

402. United Nations.   *Demographic Yearbook 1965.* United Nations, New York, 1966.

403. United Nations.   *Demographic Yearbook 1966, 1967.* United Nations, New York, 1967, 1968.

404. United Nations, Population Division and Statistical Office. *Population Census Methods.* United Nations Publication XIII, 4. United Nations, New York, 1949.

405. United Nations, Population Division.   *Foetal, Infant and Early Childhood Mortality. Vol. 1. The Statistics.* Population Studies No. 13. United Nations, New York, 1954.

406. Van Buren, G.   Some things you can't prove by mortality statistics. *Vital Statistics Special Reports* 12:191–210, 1940.

407. Vecchio, T. J.   Predictive value of a single diagnostic test in unselected populations. *New Eng. J. Med.* 274:1171–1173, 1966.

408. Wada, S., Miyanishi, M., Nishimoto, Y., Kambe, S., and Miller, R. W.   Mustard gas as a cause of respiratory neoplasia in man. *Lancet* 1:1161–1163, 1968.

409. Wagoner, J. K., Archer, V. E., Lundin, F. E., Jr., Holaday, D. A.,

and Lloyd, J. W.   Radiation as the cause of lung cancer among uranium miners. *New Eng. J. Med.* 273:181–188, 1965.

410. Walker, A. E., and Jablon, S.   *A Follow-up Study of Head Wounds in World War II.* Veterans Administration Medical Monograph. U.S. Govt. Printing Office, Washington, D.C., 1961.

411. Walker, J. B., and Kerridge, D.   *Diabetes in an English Community.* Leicester University Press, Leicester, 1961.

412. Weinberg, W.   Die Anlage zur Mehrlingsgeburt beim Menschen und ihre Vererbung. *Arch. Rass. GesBiol.* 6:322–339, 470–482, 609–630, 1909.

413. Wheelis, J. M., Jr.   A time-study of morbidity and mortality in the United States Navy. *Amer. J. Public Health* 28:1291–1297, 1938.

414. White, C.   Sampling in medical research. *Brit. Med. J.* 2:1284–1288, 1953.

415. White, C., and Bailar, J. C., III.   Retrospective and prospective methods of studying association in medicine. *Amer. J. Public Health* 46:35–44, 1956.

416. Wilder, C. S., and Rivers, C. W.   *Current Estimates from the Health Interview Survey.* Public Health Service Publ. No. 1000, Series 10, No. 52. U.S. Govt. Printing Office, Washington, D.C., 1969.

417. Wilkerson, H. L. C., and Krall, L. P.   Diabetes in a New England town. A study of 3,516 persons in Oxford, Mass. *J.A.M.A.* 135:209–216, 1947.

418. Willcox, W. F.   Introduction to Graunt, J., *Natural and Political Observations made upon the Bills of Mortality,* London, 1662, as republished by The Johns Hopkins Press, Baltimore, 1939.

419. Woodhall, B., and Beebe, G. W.   *Peripheral Nerve Regeneration: A Follow-up Study of 3,656 World War II Injuries.* Veterans Administration Medical Monograph. U.S. Govt. Printing Office, Washington, D.C., 1957.

420. Worcester, J.   Matched samples in epidemiologic studies. *Biometrics* 20:840–848, 1964.

421. World Health Organization.   *Manual of the International Statistical Classification of Diseases, Injuries and Causes of Death. Sixth Revision, 1948. Vols. 1 and 2. Bull. WHO* Suppl. 1, 1948, 1949.

422. World Health Organization.   Text of the Constitution of the World Health Organization. *Off. Rec. World Health Organ.* 2:100, 1948.

423. World Health Organization.   Comparability of statistics of causes of death according to the fifth and sixth revisions of the International List. *Bull. WHO* Suppl. 4, 1952.

424. World Health Organization.   Poisoning in accidents, suicides

and homicides; 1950–1956. *Epidem. Vital Statist. Rep.* 11:364–375, 1958.

425. World Health Organization. The use of twins in epidemiological studies. *Acta Genet. Med. (Roma)* 15:109–128, 1966.

426. World Health Organization. *International Classification of Diseases, Injuries and Causes of Death. Eighth Revision.* World Health Organization, Geneva, 1969.

427. World Health Organization. *World Health Statistics Report.* (Previously *Epidemiological and Vital Statistics Report.*) World Health Organization, Geneva, Monthly.

428. Wotiz, H. H., Shane, J. A., Vigersky, R., and Brecher, P. I. The regulatory role of oestriol in the proliferative action of oestradiol. In Forrest, A. P. M., and Kunkler, P. B. (Eds.), *Prognostic Factors in Breast Cancer.* Livingstone, London, 1968.

429. Yates, P. O. A change in the pattern of cerebrovascular disease. *Lancet* 1:65–69, 1964.

430. Yen, S., and MacMahon, B. Genetics of anencephaly and spina bifida? *Lancet* 2:623–626, 1968.

431. Yerushalmy, J., and Hilleboe, H. E. Fat in the diet and mortality from heart disease. A methodologic note. *New York J. Med.* 57:2343–2354, 1957.

432. Yuasa, S., and MacMahon, B. Lactation and reproductive histories of breast cancer patients in Tokyo. *Bull. WHO* 42:195–204, 1970.

433. Zalokar, J. B. Marital status and major causes of death in women. *J. Chronic Dis.* 11:50–60, 1960.

434. Zinsser, H. Varieties of typhus virus and the epidemiology of the American form of European typhus fever (Brill's disease). *Amer. J. Hyg.* 20:513–532, 1934.

435. Zukel, W. J., Cohen, B. M., Mattingly, T. W., and Hrubec, Z. Survival following first diagnosis of coronary heart disease. *Amer. Heart J.* 78:159–170, 1969.

# Index